WITHDRAWN

the
Courage
to Rise

4c 6m

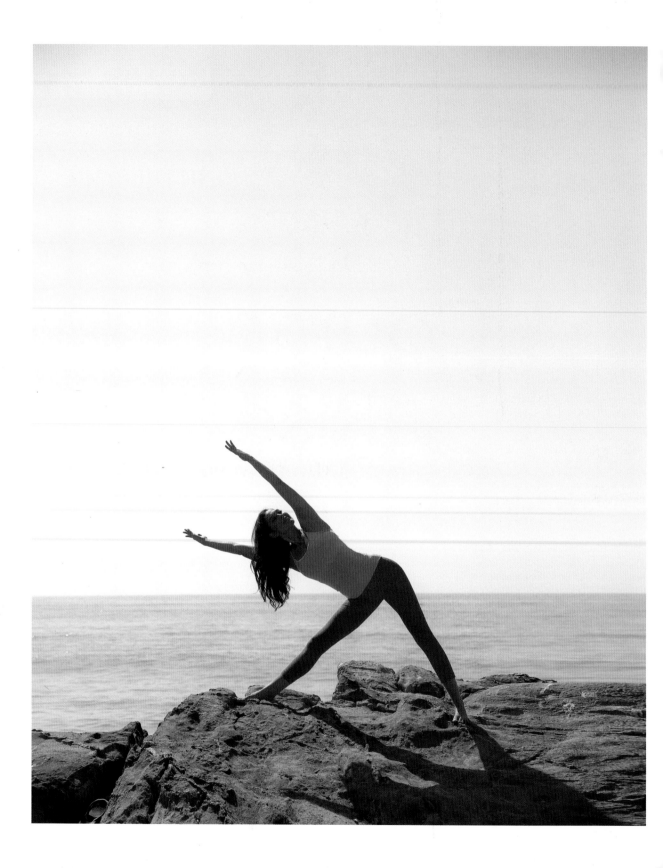

the Courage to Rise

Using Movement, Mindfulness, and Healing Foods to Triumph over Trauma

LIZ ARCH

WILLIAM MORROW
An Imprint of HarperCollinsPublishers

THE COURAGE TO RISE. Copyright © 2018 by Liz Arch. All rights reserved. Printed in China. No part of this book may be used or reproduced in any manner whatsoever without written permission except in the case of brief quotations embodied in critical articles and reviews. For information, address HarperCollins Publishers, 195 Broadway, New York, NY 10007.

HarperCollins books may be purchased for educational, business, or sales promotional use. For information, please email the Special Markets Department at SPsales@harpercollins.com.

FIRST EDITION

Designed by Diahann Sturge
Lifestyle and movement photography by Collin Stark
Food photography by Christina Peters
Recipes by Elise Museles
Food styling by Nicole Kruzick
Prop styling by Aneta Florczyk

Library of Congress Cataloging-in-Publication Data has been applied for.

ISBN 978-0-06-269423-2

18 19 20 21 22 SCP 10 9 8 7 6 5 4 3 2 1

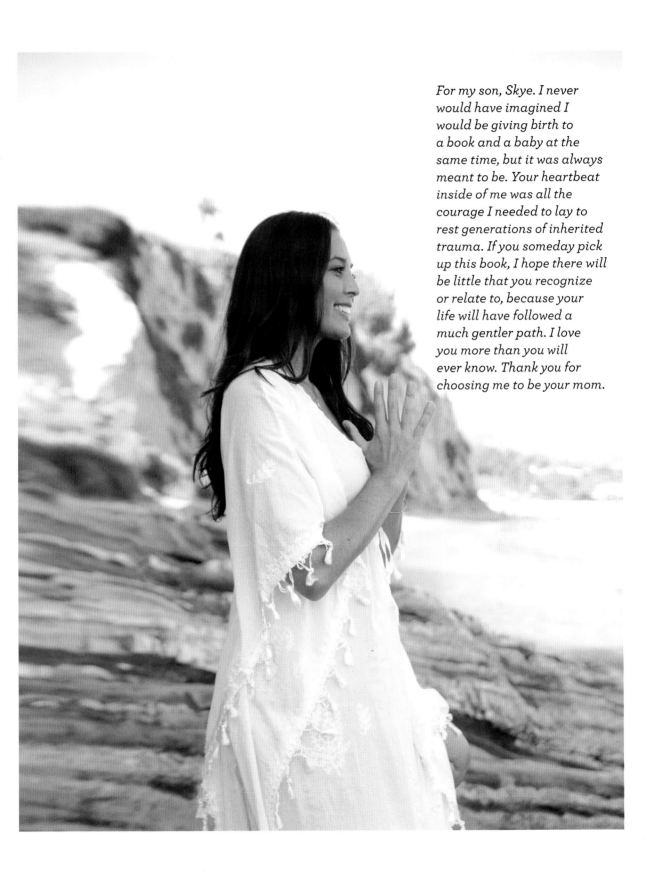

For my son, Skye. I never would have imagined I would be giving birth to a book and a baby at the same time, but it was always meant to be. Your heartbeat inside of me was all the courage I needed to lay to rest generations of inherited trauma. If you someday pick up this book, I hope there will be little that you recognize or relate to, because your life will have followed a much gentler path. I love you more than you will ever know. Thank you for choosing me to be your mom.

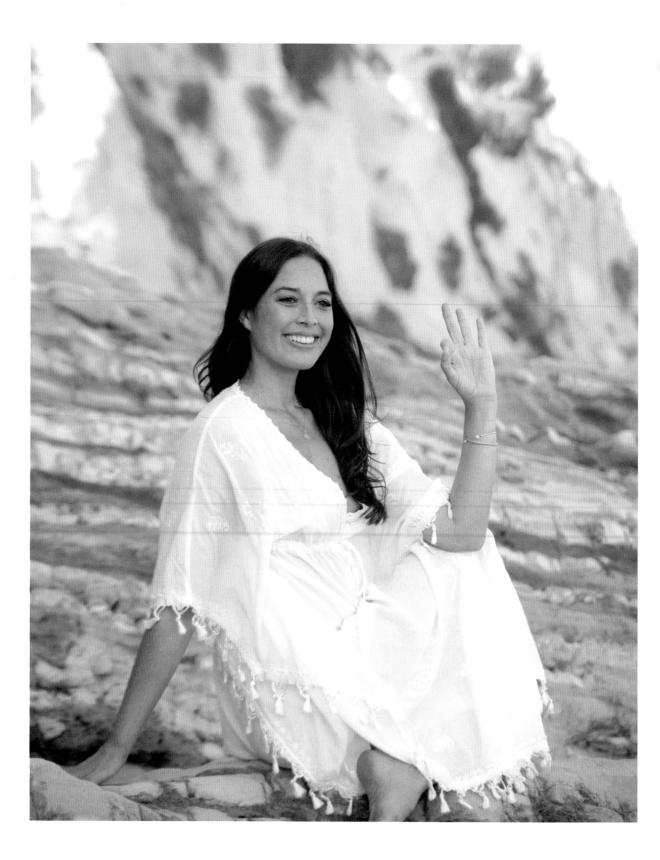

Contents

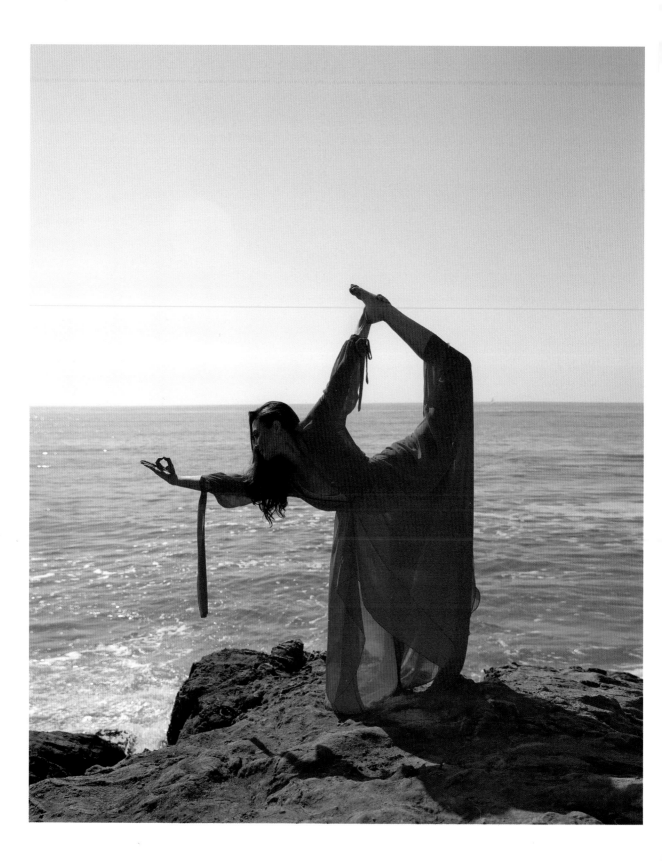

Introduction

The thing you are most afraid to write. Write that.
—Nayyirah Waheed, *salt.*

Here's the truth: I was scared shitless to write this book. Filling these pages with the wisdom of my wounds has been the most vulnerable and courageous act of my life. While I have led a charmed existence by many accounts—I was raised by loving parents, earned a college degree, and have always had a roof over my head—the deeper story of my life is not so shiny. It has been dark, messy, turbulent, confusing, terrifying, and filled with more shame and setbacks than I can count.

I was given an entire year to write this book—a long time in the world of publishing—and I missed every single editorial deadline along the way. Every time I sat down to write, I was plagued by self-doubt and feelings of deep unworthiness. I came up with a million ways to procrastinate, then blamed myself for being lazy. The truth is, I wasn't lazy at all. I was afraid. Terrified, in fact.

When I first told an acquaintance outside of my close circle of friends and family that I had a book deal, he said incredulously, "Wow, how did *you* get a book deal? You don't even have a PhD next to your name!" Immediately, I felt myself shrink. He was right. I'm not a doctor, psychiatrist, psychologist, or licensed therapist. Who the heck was I to think I was qualified enough to tackle the incredibly complex issue of trauma? What the fuck was I thinking? And then it hit me. I wasn't thinking. I was *feeling.*

My experience with trauma comes from feeling the grip of its dark claws closing around my throat. It comes from hitting rock bottom and climbing my way out, only to find I had so much further to fall. I know trauma because it burrowed into my body and lived in the marrow of my bones. For most of my life, it has fed my fear, fueled my anger, sabotaged my relationships, shut me down, and shut me up with shame.

A few years ago, I stepped onto a stage to speak publicly about my trauma. Although, to be honest, *trauma* wasn't a part of my vocabulary back then, so I called it by the only name I knew: *domestic violence.* My voice wavered and tears streaked down my face as I bared my soul to the one hundred people in the room and more than half a million more watching online. I had shared my story before in smaller, safer spaces—at advocacy meetings for domestic violence survivors and charity events where everyone championed the same cause. I always left those gatherings feeling empowered, uplifted, and more resilient.

This time felt different. Though my voice was reaching an audience bigger than I could have imagined, somehow I felt infinitely smaller. There was no wave of relief, only the familiar knot of fear. It was the most important stage I had ever stood on, and I felt a responsibility to distill the darkest chapter in my life into something neat and tidy that would inspire people rather than make them turn away. Looking back, I know why there was no solace to be found. I spoke only a part of my truth and kept hidden what hadn't yet healed. In all fairness, at that time I didn't fully comprehend all the wounds I still carried. We do the best we can with the tools we have. On that day, I stood onstage with a hammer but no nails.

Outwardly, I was a vision of health and success, but on the inside I felt damaged and lost. We like stories with happy endings. But trauma robs us of a clean narrative. I didn't know how to give voice to the fact that I still had nightmares all the time and slept with a hammer under my bed—and sometimes even a knife under my pillow. I didn't know how to find words to describe my crippling anxiety. I didn't know how to talk about my trust issues, jealousy, or explosive rage. I didn't know that so much of the "healing" work I thought I had done was actually spiritual bypassing. And I certainly didn't know that it was possible to wind up in another incredibly toxic relationship that would blow the lid off all the years of progress I thought I had made and leave me feeling like a failure and a fraud.

What I did not understand at the time was that the tracks of trauma had been laid long before domestic violence was ever part of my story. It started as early as age five. As I now know, childhood trauma can set us up for a lifetime of setbacks, making us more prone to posttraumatic stress disorder (PTSD), depression, dissociation, substance abuse, and a range of health problems as an adult.[1] Specifically, trauma that occurs during childhood (including emotional, physical, and sexual abuse; neglect, substance abuse, mental illness, loss of a parent, divorce, and violence or criminal behavior in the household) has been shown to have a lifelong impact on an individual's health and quality of life, including increased risk of obesity, diabetes, sexually transmitted diseases, heart disease, cancer, and stroke.[2]

Unresolved trauma can rob us of our physical and emotional health, our connection to self and others, and our connection to life. Yet many times we're not even consciously aware that we have been traumatized, which makes us blind to all the ways in which trauma has shaped our lives, relationships, and behavior. I, like many others, was stuck in an unconscious pattern of reenacting my trauma over and over again that would last until I eventually broke down—or broke through.

My breakdown moment came after I stood on that stage and made a sacred vow to myself and the world to never be in an abusive relationship again, only to find myself right back where I had started. The partner was different, but the pattern was the same, and all the years of work I had done to suture my soul were unraveled in an instant.

The floor of my rock bottom fell out from under me when I received a call from the founder of the online platform that hosted my speech, informing me that my speech had been removed from the site following a letter from my abuser, who claimed slander and threatened legal action, despite the fact that I never revealed his name or identity in my speech. Like many abusers, he set out on a mission to harass, intimidate, and publicly discredit me. He sent letters to companies I worked with, calling me mentally unstable, a liar, and an abuser in disguise. Fortunately, every company stood behind me in solidarity, with the exception of the one that pulled my speech. Despite the overwhelming support, the shame I felt threatened to swallow me whole.

The soil for my shame was the deeply buried belief that maybe he was right and I was an abuser in disguise. In my work with survivors of intimate partner violence, a common thread among most is the feeling they are somehow at fault. Abusers deny, minimize and blame, while survivors feel shame. Make no mistake, every bit of the abuse I experienced was very real, as it is for all the survivors I have worked with. I had been kicked, strangled, threatened with death on multiple occasions, verbally abused, financially controlled, and psychologically manipulated. But like so many survivors, I blamed myself, not only for winding up in an abusive situation but also for being a part of the cycle of violence. I couldn't reconcile what I knew to be my own personality with the rage and the sometimes explosive reactions that uncontrollably erupted when I was attacked or triggered, nor could I understand the hurtful words and shocking profanities that came out of my mouth when I felt harmed or threatened. It was like the invasion of the body snatchers; the kind, easygoing, nonconfrontational person that I knew myself to be in all other situations disappeared within the walls of those toxic relationships. As Bessel van der Kolk—a Dutch psychiatrist, renowned trauma expert, and author of *The Body Keeps the Score*—explains:

> Trauma robs you of the feeling that you are in charge of yourself. . . . The challenge of recovery is to reestablish ownership of your body and your mind—of your self. This means feeling free to know what you know and to feel what you feel without becoming overwhelmed, enraged, ashamed, or collapsed. For most people this involves (1) finding a way to become calm and focused, (2) learning to maintain that calm response to images, thoughts, sounds, or physical sensations that remind you of the past, (3) finding a way to be fully alive in the present and engaged with the people around you, (4) not having to keep secrets from yourself, including secrets about the ways that you have managed to survive.[3]

The first time I spoke my dark secret out loud to a trauma therapist, I wept uncontrollably and hid my face in shame. She didn't flinch as she handed me an article on the Karpman Drama Triangle, a model developed by psychiatrist Stephen Karpman in the early 1970s for understanding toxic relationships and the cycle of domestic violence. She also explained to me that many abusers are narcissists and victims are often either empaths or what psychologists refer to as highly sensitive people (HSP). The two attract each other like magnets and engage in a cycle that is hard to break free from, made all the more challenging by the fact that it's a common tactic of narcissists and abusers to blame and discredit the victim. The cycle of abuse is about exerting power and control to create dependency. Abusers isolate victims from vital support systems and use financial, physical, and psychological intimidation to keep their survivors quiet. And it works. I was threatened with violence and public humiliation if I ever spoke out and was repeatedly told, "No one will believe you," "I'll tell everyone you're crazy," and "It's all your fault."

It's said that our pain gives us our purpose. My breakthrough moment came when I realized I had a choice. I could let my unresolved shame and trauma destroy me or I could learn everything possible about my pain and transform it into my greatest power.

The path of courage is paved with fear. Healing from trauma is not linear. Often we take one step forward, followed by a giant leap back. Setbacks are *not* failures. They are a necessary part of the journey. Our setbacks reveal the blind spots where unresolved trauma still lurks and give us an opportunity to shine a light on our shadow. We can't see what's hidden in the dark or heal what we don't allow ourselves to feel. It takes strength to bounce back from something once. It takes *courage* to bounce back from something twice. It takes the *heart of a lion* to bounce back from something a third, fourth, or fifth time. If you are holding this book in your hands, you stand among the lion-hearted.

I may not have a medical degree hanging on my wall, but I am the expert on my own trauma. I wrote this book to help you become the expert on *your* own trauma, so you may also become the expert in your own healing. Don't let anyone tell you the power of healing is outside of yourself. Your greatest healer lives within. You are a keeper of light, and your job is simply to remember that.

A Proper Introduction

Now that I've shared some of the most intimate details of my life with you, let me step back and properly introduce myself. I am the founder of Primal Yoga, a yoga and martial arts fusion system designed to tap into our innate healing potential. I am also a mental health advocate, certified life coach, and the director of a nonprofit organization called Purple Dot Yoga Project, which uses yoga as a healing tool to support and empower individuals impacted by domestic violence and trauma. My passion and purpose is to give people the tools to overcome trauma and create physical health and emotional resilience through yoga, martial arts, mindfulness, and healing foods.

I work with people from all walks of life who are struggling with anxiety, depression, mood swings, fatigue, brain fog, chronic pain, gastrointestinal issues, and a general crisis of well-being. While a wide variety of environmental, genetic, and lifestyle factors can play a role in the symptoms of dis-ease listed above, what has astounded me is how much these crises of physical and mental health can be linked back to trauma of some nature. What I mean by *dis-ease* is quite literally a lack of ease in mind, body, or spirit, not to be confused with *disease*, which refers to illness. It may sound like new-age semantics, but viewing our health through the lens of "dis-ease" empowers the individual to reclaim their natural state of ease and well-being.

The Triad Approach to Healing

In the following chapters, I share a powerfully effective triad approach to *whole being healing*. Together, we will address the three key areas where dis-ease lives: the body, the brain, and the gut. I offer science-based, research-backed tools, specifically in the areas of yoga and martial arts (the body), mindfulness and meditation (the brain), and dietary interventions (the gut). You can implement some or all of these tools immediately to help you feel better in your body, more at ease in your mind, and more whole in spirit.

While each modality stands solidly on its own, these tools are most potent when used together. The main detour in my own healing was attempting to treat each symptom individually, rather than looking at the root cause of my own dis-ease. Treating symptoms rather than people is one of the major flaws in Western medicine today. Doctors are trained to diagnose and treat symptoms without a deeper understanding of how each part affects the whole. We see specialists for individual issues and search for a single solution to a complex question that often has more than one answer. This kind of approach leads to ineffective, one-dimensional results. Our health and vitality demands a better way.

Yoga was my first introduction to holistic healing. Yoga made me aware of my body and breath in the present moment. It grounded me and allowed me to finally *feel* what I had formerly kept numb. Yoga has long been touted as an effective way to help reduce stress and anxiety, boost mood, and create an overall sense of balance and well-being.

A seminal 2014 study in the *Journal of Clinical Psychiatry* found that yoga decreased PTSD symptoms to a degree comparable to that of pharmaceutical and psychotherapeutic counterparts. It concluded, "Yoga may improve the functioning of traumatized individuals by helping them to tolerate physical and sensory experiences associated with fear and helplessness and to increase emotional awareness and affect tolerance."[1]

I am a yoga teacher by trade, and there is no one who believes more wholeheartedly in yoga's benefits than me, but I can say with complete transparency that the physical practice of yoga is not enough—or at least it wasn't for me. It eased many of my symptoms, but it didn't cure everything. Fortunately, yoga led me to meditation, which is where even more life-changing shifts began to occur.

Like yoga, breathwork and meditation are being increasingly recognized for their ability to alleviate anxiety and depression. Twenty minutes of mindfulness meditation activates our prefrontal cortex, the part of our brain that staves off feelings of worry. When our anxiety *decreases* as a result of this, the activity in our anterior cingulate cortex *increases*. This is good news, because it is here in our anterior cingulate cortex that rational thought displaces worry.

Recently, there have been a ton of studies about how meditation positively impacts anxiety, but the most definitive study was published by *JAMA Internal Medicine* in 2014.[2] Researchers from Johns Hopkins University concluded that mindfulness meditation reduces symptoms of anxiety by counteracting our natural tendency to worry about things that might happen or fall into a rut of insomnia, both of which serve only to further heighten anxiety. Mindfulness does this by teaching us to stay in the moment, to recognize thoughts for what they are as they occur, and to prevent those thoughts from escalating. In this study, the researchers found that just twenty to thirty minutes of daily meditation could serve to significantly alleviate anxiety. This same study also showed that mindfulness meditation was also effective in treating depression and physical pain.

Mindfulness techniques and meditation played a monumental role in helping me ultimately eliminate my panic attacks for good, but I was still experiencing chronic fatigue, brain fog, mild depression, and digestive issues. I also began to notice that many of my meditation teachers, while completely at ease and content in mind, were unhealthy in body. It made me wonder, *What good is a healthy mind without a healthy body?* And vice versa. And that led me to the last piece in my healing puzzle—the gut—which, I discovered, is where both healthy minds and healthy bodies are made.

No amount of exercise or meditation can make up for a lousy, nutrient-poor diet. I would even go so far as to say that no single factor has a bigger impact on our physical and mental health than the food we put in our body. In his book *The Mind-Gut Connection*, Dr. Emeran Mayer writes that gut issues are more common than we think. In fact, nearly 15 percent of the United States population suffers from them. The problems include irritable bowel syndrome, chronic constipation, indigestion, and heartburn, all of which fall into the category of brain-gut disorders. Most important, Dr. Mayer writes that new studies point to the gut's influence on our emotions, pain sensitivity, relationships, and even our decisions. He writes, "As incredible as this may sound, your gut microbes are in a prime position to influence your emotions, by generating and modulating signals the gut sends back to the brain. Thus, what starts as an emotion in the brain influences your gut and the signals generated by your microbes, and these signals in turn communicate back to the brain, reinforcing and sometimes even prolonging the emotional state."[3]

When I was diagnosed with panic disorder, I was eating a primarily vegetarian diet, but I was what you might call a "junk food vegetarian." I consumed loads of inflammatory foods, such as processed sugar, bread, pasta, and dairy. I would soon learn that many of the foods I was eating were contributing to my anxiety and overall health issues. I began taking courses in nutrition and earned my plant-based nutrition certification from Cornell University. I also began working with a naturopath, a functional medicine doctor, and a nutrition coach. I read every book and took every course on gut health and nutrition I could find.

I had long heard that our gut effectively acts as a second brain, but was shocked to learn that more than 95 percent of our body's serotonin, a crucial brain neurotransmitter and mood balancer, is actually produced in the gut. By eliminating common foods that promote inflammation and have been connected with gastrointestinal distress, mood disorders, and a host of other health issues and adding gut-healing, mood-boosting foods to our diets, we can begin to take control of our mental health and physical well-being without having to reach for a bottle of pills.

How to Use This Book

I have divided this book into four parts. The first part, "Understanding Trauma," clearly defines trauma, identifies the causes and symptoms of trauma, and lays out the physical and emotional impact unresolved trauma can have on our lives. It also provides an overview of the latest neuroscience research coming out of the trauma field to help you understand how trauma works on a neurobiological level. You will see how trauma quite literally changes the brain, altering the balance of our autonomic nervous system and shaping our behavior, reactions, and relationships—often to devastating effect.

While it may be tempting to skip over this information and jump right into the movement, mindfulness, and nutrition practices in the following chapters, I strongly urge you to spend some time in this first section. Understanding the nature of trauma creates critical awareness that helps heal shame, dismantle self-blame, and lay the foundation for healing to unfold.

One of the biggest obstacles in healing trauma is shame. Shame disrupts our ability to connect with others and form healthy relationships and prevents us from leading healthy, meaningful, and fulfilling lives. According to Brené Brown—best-selling author, prominent shame researcher, and one of my personal heroes—"Shame corrodes the very part of us that believes we are capable of change."[4] Shame perpetuates the lie that we are alone in our darkness. It makes us feel dirty and unworthy of belonging and connection. Before we can truly begin to feel healthy and whole in mind, body, and spirit, we must tackle shame. The first part of this book will help you understand that some of your most shame-producing negative behaviors and emotional responses are not under your conscious control.

In part II of the book we delve into how important our physical body is to the healing process. This section details why traditional talk therapy might have failed you in the past and explains why a better approach to healing begins with the body. I share the latest scientific research about why yoga in particular (as compared to other movement modalities) is being used effectively in the treatment of PTSD and reveal powerful stories of healing and transformation from clients I have worked with firsthand.

We then begin the work of creating safety within your own body as I give the exact exercises I offer to my clients and in my therapeutic trainings, so you can begin befriending your body and taking back control of your life. You'll learn exercises to help shake off anxiety in under five minutes, promote restful sleep, bolster self-worth, release anger, increase energy to combat chronic fatigue, and more. These movements are most effectively used on a consistent basis, but you can also use them on an as-needed basis.

The movements I share blend together the soothing fluidity and mindfulness of yoga with empowering elements of martial arts techniques like tai chi and qigong. The martial arts influence is a unique and crucial component of this book that will provide you with an additional sense of agency, empowerment, and self-confidence.

In part III we examine how mindfulness literally rewires your brain. I show exactly why meditation is one of the most effective methods to reduce stress and create greater emotional well-being. I guide you through the science of mindfulness, sharing how meditation literally changes our brain for greater focus, self-control, and emotional regulation and giving simple yet deeply transformative techniques to start your own home meditation practice. These techniques include specific meditations for a variety of common challenges, including releasing anger, befriending fear, relieving anxiety and depression, and overcoming both physical and emotional pain. This section also helps you develop mindfulness skills to combat stress, ease anxiety, eliminate panic attacks, and create the ability to self-regulate. As with the movement portion of this book, these meditation and mindfulness practices are most effectively used on a consistent basis, but you may also reach for them as needed, in whatever amount of time you have available.

In part IV we learn why all health starts in the gut and how the food choices you've been making might be secretly sabotaging your physical health and mental well-being. I share a list of common food culprits that have been linked to inflammation, mood disorders, and a range of other issues, including bloating, brain fog, fatigue, acne, and more, and introduce you to feel-good foods and natural supplements that have been shown to boost energy, alleviate anxiety, regulate mood, and fuel the body. Finally, I offer more than twenty-five simple, delicious, and nutritious recipes, created in partnership with my dear friend Elise Museles, a nutrition expert, certified holistic health coach, and certified eating psychology coach, and the author of the book *Whole Food Energy*.

The tools in this book put the power of healing into your own hands and are meant to help you find *immediate* relief from symptoms of anxiety, depression, and trauma. However, it's also important to understand that the information and practices here are not intended to diagnose, treat, or assess any kind of physical, mental, emotional, or psychological condition, disorder, or disease. Professional therapy and/or psychiatric care is recommended in cases of severe trauma or if you have been diagnosed with any of the following mental health conditions: bipolar disorder, schizophrenia, multiple personality disorder, PTSD, or clinical depression. If you are currently on medication for depression, anxiety, bipolar disorder, or any kind of anxiety disorder, always consult your doctor, psychotherapist, or mental health counselor before making any changes to dosages or prescriptions. And understand that while the practices in this book may ultimately help you move toward a natural, drug-free life, they are not intended as a replacement nor should they be used as a substitution for any medication you are currently taking.

Over time, adopting these practices into a consistent lifestyle will create the most dramatic and lasting transformation. The tools in this book are not a magical overnight cure for PTSD, depression, or anxiety, and I certainly can't and won't promise you a time-stamped guarantee for your personal trauma resolution. Healing from trauma is unique to each individual, and there is no one-size-fits-all cure. But I do know from personal experience that when you're struggling to get out of bed under the weight of depression or are in the throes of a panic attack, simply surviving the next five minutes, let alone the next twenty-four hours, can feel like a lifetime.

So, while there are no timelines in this book, what you *will* find are quick tips for everything from calming breathing techniques to 5-minute stress-busting movement exercises to dietary interventions and even on-the-spot stress-reducing olfactory strategies (like sniffing a lemon!) that you can implement whenever anxiety strikes.

I remember forking over $200 to a top-rated cognitive behavioral therapist when I was at the height of my panic disorder, only to have him tell me that it would take a minimum of ten sessions over a period of a few months to find even the most minimal relief. I left his office in tears. Unnecessarily, I might add, because as you will see, there most definitely *are* some tricks that will offer temporary relief.

This book is designed to support you moment to moment when you need it the most while simultaneously helping you craft long-term strategies to achieve your greatest health and well-being. Take what you need from this book; use what works for you and discard what doesn't. No single modality is a complete cure. *The Courage to Rise* takes an integrated approach to empower you with the knowledge and tools from a variety of healing modalities to take control of your own healing and create dramatic shifts in your energy, mood, and resiliency.

Let's get started.

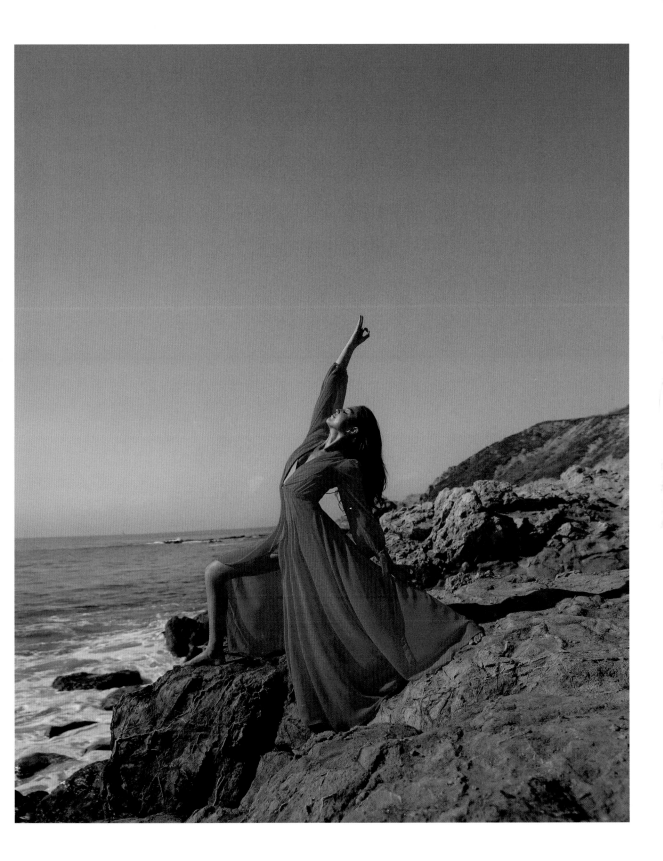

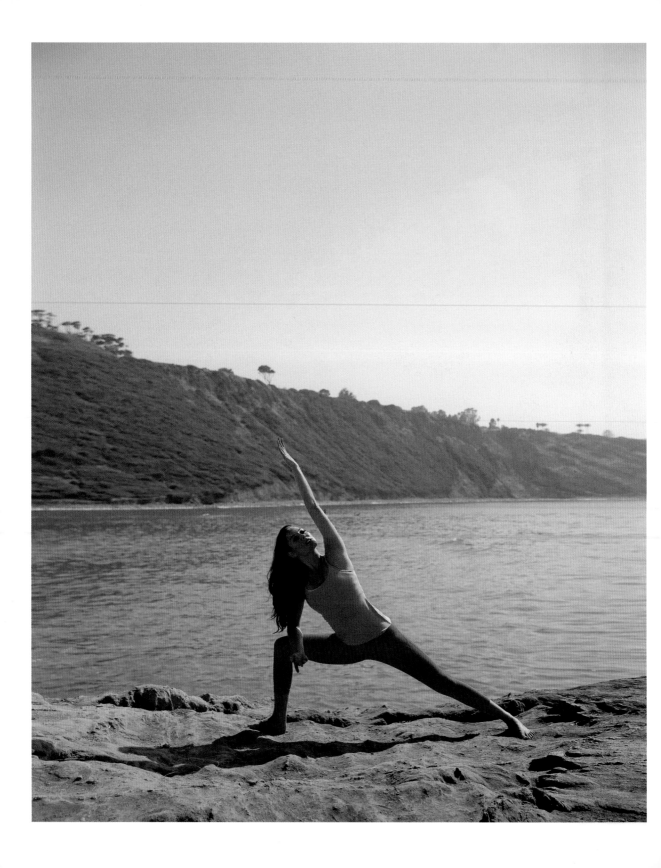

Part I

Understanding Trauma

Chapter 1

Trauma Is More Common
Than You Think

How can I be substantial if I do not cast a shadow?
I must have a dark side also if I am to be whole.
—C. G. Jung

As the rest of the world celebrated the impending new year, lighting fireworks and popping champagne corks to ring in 1988, I clutched my legs tightly against my chest. I was sitting on the roof of my family's car in my hometown of Kailua, Oahu, watching the floodwaters rise higher and higher. Just five years old at the time, I had done what little I could to secure those things I loved, which didn't include much more than putting my pet mice in their cage on top of our refrigerator so they wouldn't drown.

It felt like a race against time as my family's living room was submerged, our rattan furniture bobbing like rotten apples in the murky brown water. Huddled together with my family shivering in the dark, I plugged my ears in a futile attempt to block out a cacophony of car alarms wailing as their wires short-circuited. Scariest of all was the look of palpable panic that registered on my parents' faces as we anxiously awaited the arrival of the boat that would rescue us.

It wasn't until many years later, when I started working with a trauma therapist as an adult, that I understood the significance of the flood and the impact it had on my life, my patterns, and my relationships. When I was only five years old, the flood taught me that I wasn't safe in my own home. This sense of impending danger would be reinforced one night a few years later when I watched in horror as an intruder's shadowy hand reached through my window. It was drilled into me yet again a few years after that, when I awoke to a strange man standing over me, watching me as I slept.

My personal experience of danger was compounded by exposure to secondhand trauma everywhere I turned. Thankfully, violence was not a part of my direct experience with my mother and father as a child, but it existed on the periphery of my family tree. At a very young age, I became aware of the horrifying number of ways in which the world wasn't safe for the people I loved. I didn't have to look far to see the devastating effects of domestic violence, molestation, addiction, and mental health conditions.

"Scared animals return home, regardless of whether home is safe or frightening," writes leading trauma researcher Bessel van der Kolk.[1] One of the more perplexing hallmarks of trauma is that it leads people back into abusive households and dangerous situations, despite the inevitable harm that awaits. Feeling safe was foreign to me, so I, like so many other traumatized people, unconsciously reached for what was familiar. In my adult life, this manifested as choosing abusive men as my partners. Not surprisingly, my home was never safe. My life consisted of one volatile situation after another that often erupted into violence with little warning.

Unresolved trauma can manifest itself in a variety of physical, mental, and emotional ways, and often the symptoms show up years later. My symptoms as a child included hyperarousal—increased heart rate, sweaty palms, racing thoughts, nightmares, and hyper-vigilance. I was also excessively shy and had a difficult time expressing my emotions. In adulthood, after I accumulated even more notches on my trauma belt, these symptoms manifested as debilitating panic attacks, severe anxiety, agoraphobia, abrupt mood swings (crying uncontrollably, anger, and rage, followed by feelings of deep shame and low self-worth), fatigue, and mild depression.

I never connected my volatile mood swings, chronic fatigue, digestive issues, anxiety, or depressive thoughts with any of my past trauma. Like many people who have experienced trauma, I had little awareness of the insidious ways that trauma was impacting my health and well-being. Instead, I internalized everything and blamed myself for being a colossal train wreck of a human being.

The truth about trauma is that we've all experienced it. No one is spared. And while it may have only minor effects on some, it can have a devastating impact on others. The first step in reclaiming our lives is recognizing that we are wounded.

Healing Our Wounds

The wound is the place where the light enters you.

—Rumi

Trauma comes from the Greek word for "wound." Like all wounds, trauma inevitably leaves behind a scar. When the body experiences a physical wound, even something minor like a small cut or burn, scarring is part of the body's natural healing response. Some scars are jagged, discolored, indented, or raised. Others are faded, and some leave no visible trace at all. But regardless of the physical evidence left behind, a fundamental reorganization of tissue occurs at the site of the wound. In the smallest or deepest way, we are forever changed.

It is the same with trauma. We all experience trauma at some point in our lives. Some traumatic experiences leave behind physical scars, while others leave behind emotional scars. If we're lucky, these scars will fade into the background, serving as nothing more than a distant reminder of something that happened in the past, but that no longer holds any power over our present. But for others, the pain is like a fresh wound that never scabs over.

If your wounds are still open, know this: by nature, wounds are designed to heal. Healing is messy and not always linear, but it is also what our bodies do best. I once told a therapist that I wished I could go back in time to who I was before all of the bad decisions and traumatic memories. She told me there was no going back. There was only moving forward into who I was always meant to become.

Your trauma will change you, but it doesn't have to define you. If you allow it, your trauma can grant you your greatest courage and reveal to you your deepest strength. As one of my beautifully brave students said about her own journey of healing from abuse, "My memories do not need to hold me prisoner, and there are tools out there that can resolve our traumas and show others how to heal from theirs. Trauma is not merely an ocean to drown in, but a current that shepherds us to shore."

What Is Trauma?

Trauma is generally defined as an event that is life-threatening or psychologically devastating to the point where a person's ability to cope is overwhelmed. Many psychotherapists refer to trauma as "anything that is too much, too soon, or too fast for our nervous system to handle."[2]

Trauma has been around for as long as humans have walked the earth. Survival of the fittest had us fighting off saber-toothed tigers and warring with neighboring clans. But PTSD wasn't officially introduced into the *Diagnostic and Statistical Manual of Mental Disorders* (DSM) until 1980. In its original inclusion, the American Psychiatric Association described trauma as being "outside the range of usual human experience." However, human history and simple statistics reveal that, unfortunately, trauma is not rare at all. In fact, about 60 percent of men and 50 percent of women experience at least one trauma in their lives.[3] Women are more likely to experience sexual assault and child sexual abuse. A staggering one in three women in the United States experiences some form of physical violence by an intimate partner in her lifetime.[4] Twenty-four people per minute are victims of rape, physical violence, or stalking by an intimate partner in the United States, and more than 15 million children witness violence in their homes each year.

Men are more likely to experience accidents, physical assault, combat, or disaster, or to witness death or injury. The National Center for PTSD reports that, depending on the service era, roughly 11 to 30 percent of combat veterans will have PTSD in their lifetime.[5] In the general population, seven or eight out of every one hundred people will experience PTSD at some point in their lives.

We tend to think of trauma as occurring when we directly experience a frightening or life-threatening event, but trauma can also result from witnessing an event occurring to others, repeated exposure to dangerous or traumatic situations (as is the case with first responders), or learning that a traumatic event happened to a relative or friend. In addition to PTSD, secondary traumatic stress (STS) is a real phenomenon that affects individuals who are exposed to other people's trauma. It often impacts people in professions that deal with trauma on a daily basis, such as counselors, nurses, and first responders, but it can also affect those whose friends or family members are victims of trauma.

The effects of secondhand trauma can mimic the symptoms of PTSD, including hypervigilance, intense fear, avoidance of public places, angry outbursts, nightmares, and more. Whether we are exposed to trauma directly or indirectly, powerful feelings such as fear, helplessness, despair, disconnection, isolation, rage, and shame can flood our system, altering our perception of our own worth, value, and purpose in the world.

Causes of Trauma

When most people think of trauma, obvious causes come to mind, such as war; severe emotional, physical, or sexual abuse; neglect, betrayal, or abandonment during childhood; experiencing or witnessing violence; rape or sexual assault; and major injuries or illness. But trauma can also occur as a result of seemingly ordinary events, leading to symptoms that can greatly alter our sense of being in the world, creating frustration, loss of connection, self-blame, and shame.

One of my yoga clients described moving a lot with her family as a child. As an adult, she dealt with attachment and codependency issues. A therapist later helped her realize that every time she moved, she experienced it as a deep loss. She was constantly leaving behind meaningful friendships, relationships, possessions, places, and people.

When the root cause is not readily apparent, many people blame themselves for their anxiety, depression, anger, fear, or addiction issues and determine that they're either "crazy" or that "something is wrong" with them. Connecting the dots and normalizing symptoms that make us feel less than human as a natural effect of traumatic stress can be a powerful breakthrough moment for people. Trauma affects us on a neurobiological level and quite literally changes our brain. It hijacks our nervous system, increases stress hormones such as adrenaline and cortisol, and bypasses our neocortex (our "higher thinking" brain), affecting our ability to make clear decisions, create healthy connections, and form safe relationships in the world. Vital structures in the brain are altered by trauma, impairing memory function and creating an inability to distinguish between past and present. As Bessel van der Kolk says, "Trauma results in the fundamental reorganization of the way mind and brain manage perceptions. It changes not only how we think and what we think about, but also our very capacity to think."[6]

This is important information to understand, because knowing that traumatic stress symptoms are not a character defect or a sign of weakness is what creates the fertile soil for healing to begin.

Chapter 2

How Trauma Works

One of the greatest roadblocks to healing trauma is that the source
often remains out of sight. Without a context for understanding
our symptoms, it can be difficult to know what steps to take.
However, when we can bring an inherited or early life trauma into
view, we can begin to disentangle from patterns of reliving.
—Mark Wolynn

Trauma of any nature can interfere with an individual's ability to live their best life. Trauma affects everyone differently. The same event can have a subtle effect on one person and a catastrophic effect on another. Yet some therapists differentiate between Trauma "with a big *T*" versus trauma "with a little *t*."

Trauma with a Big T

According to the DSM, Trauma with a big *T* is a major traumatic event that classifies as a "stressor" in making a clinical diagnosis for PTSD. These major stressors include exposure to death, threatened death, actual or threatened serious injury, or actual or threatened sexual violence. This can include:

- Physical or sexual assault
- Experiencing war or combat stress
- Experiencing or witnessing an act of terrorism
- Experiencing or witnessing rape, sexual assault, physical assault, violence, mugging, or violent robbery

- Natural disasters like fires, tornadoes, hurricanes, tsunamis, floods, or earthquakes
- Serious accidents like a car or plane crash
- Life-threatening illnesses or injuries

Trauma with a Little t

Less obvious causes of trauma can have an equally devastating impact on the lives and well-being of the people who experience them. Nonetheless, they are often overlooked as a valid source of distress by both the individual who has experienced the event and professional therapists, precisely because these occurrences don't seem out of the ordinary. Some of these causes of little-*t* trauma include:

- Childhood neglect or abandonment
- Bullying
- Betrayal and infidelity
- Experiencing repeated moves and relocations (as is the case with many military families)
- Experiencing the death or loss of a family member or friend
- Experiencing the death or loss of a pet
- Unemployment or prolonged financial stress
- Divorce
- Chronic illness
- Hospitalization
- Surgical or invasive medical or dental procedures, including the use of general anesthesia
- Exposure to extreme temperatures (for example, a child being locked in a hot car or left outside in freezing temperatures)
- Having or adopting a child
- Prenatal or birth stress
- Conflict with siblings, parents, children, significant others, friends, employers, or coworkers
- Legal issues

Little-t trauma often has a cumulative effect. Whether multiple little t's are experienced successively over a short period of time or accumulated over a lifetime, they can overwhelm an individual's ability to emotionally process, self-regulate, and cope. These types of trauma are often accompanied by shame or denial of their importance and reluctance to seek help or receive support.

Unfortunately, trauma of any kind has a stigma attached to it. Even when we've been exposed to notable trauma, many people have resistance to labeling an event as "traumatic." It's as if we think experiencing trauma somehow soils or weakens us. Curiously, others distance themselves from trauma because they don't feel their experience was catastrophic enough compared to someone else's trauma.

RECONNECTING WITH OUR FELT SENSE

Jenny is a regular yoga student of mine who works as a licensed clinical social worker. She completed a Purple Dot Yoga Project trauma-informed Yoga Teacher Training program I co-led to help supplement her work with her clients. Throughout the course of this training, Jenny unconcealed her own trauma.

I considered yoga as something deeply personal, but trauma as something outside of me. I didn't know what it would feel like to blend the two. In my work, I bear witness daily to the painful experiences of my clients but never considered my own trauma history. I have a relatively healthy relationship with both of my parents and felt adored and safe through my childhood. I've never experienced interpersonal violence or PTSD symptoms. For me, that meant that I had it pretty good and had no right to claim trauma as mine. When I started this training, I thought of myself as an outsider looking in on the traumas of others.

During the training, we had opportunities to consider our individual histories through various prompts and exercises. I didn't think I had much to share. However, on the third day of the training, I found myself returning to September 11. At the time, I was a junior at a high school just blocks away from the World Trade Center. After school, my friends and I frequented the shopping mall at the Towers. Even as I shared this with the group, I found myself listing the ways that 9/11 wasn't as bad for me as it was for some of my friends.

My first-period classroom was on a lower floor, which meant that we didn't see the first building fall from our windows. Because my homeroom was on the ground floor, I was enlisted to set up folding tables for a triage center while other classmates were evacuated to the West Side Highway. They saw the second tower fall, and I was spared.

Because of these details, I've always been resistant to consider 9/11 a personal trauma. And yet, as I shared this story out loud in the group, I felt—and still feel—a tightness in my throat and tears in my eyes. Through the course of the training, I realized my body reacted when I heard someone speak about that day; I grew tense and my fingers started to tingle. This was a trauma that I was carrying deep within, and because I was comparing it to the experiences of others, I was resistant to naming it.

The power of identifying this in myself has impacted me both personally and professionally. The training truly helped to heal some of the wounds of my personal trauma. I stopped comparing and felt part of a shared experience. This training has shifted the way I think about and define trauma, increasing my empathy and understanding of the different appearances of trauma. I know this will change the way I approach and relate to my clients.

Jenny was able to tune into her "felt sense," tracking her emotions and sensations back to her experience on September 11. Deepening our connection to our felt sense allows us to understand where trauma lives in our bodies and how it manifests in symptoms like chronic tension, shortness of breath, or numbness. Trauma can disconnect us from our capacity to feel. Reestablishing our connection to what we are feeling is one of our most potent tools for healing.

Identifying Our Own Traumas

As you read through the lists of potential big-*T* and little-*t* traumas, did anything hit home? Did anything on the lists create a visceral reaction in your body or trigger a memory from the past? Read through the lists again and pay close attention to any physiological reactions in your body, including elevated heart rate or respiration, sweaty palms, or muscle tension. Notice any mental reactions, such as wanting to dismiss any of the things on the lists above as common or unworthy of a traumatic stress response.

A therapist I once worked with asked me to write out a list of all my traumas from birth to present day. Initially, all I could come up with was my experience of intimate partner violence. She asked me to dig deeper. I never once considered how so many other seemingly innocuous events in my life had slowly chipped away at my physical and emotional well-being. My list ended up being pages long, providing me a with a startlingly clear blueprint of all the ways trauma had shaped my life, my relationships, my patterns, my thoughts, and my actions.

If you've experienced one or more of the items mentioned in this chapter, it does not mean you have PTSD. In fact, most people who experience a traumatic event will *not* develop the disorder.

Before we go any further, this seems like a good place to mention that I'm not particularly fond of the word *disorder*, nor am I a fan of the widespread use of psychiatric diagnoses as defined by the DSM. While diagnostic labels can be helpful if they create a framework for deeper empathy for what an individual is experiencing and provide a map for how to more effectively guide care, they can also be very stigmatizing and disempowering because they pathologize symptoms as sickness for which only a doctor has the cure.

The truth of trauma is that our suffering can be transformed into wisdom and strength. In many traditional cultures around the world, suffering is a path that leads to spiritual enlightenment. This is not to say we should seek out suffering as a necessary means for awakening. Cult leaders and narcissists hiding under the guise of "guru" have long taken advantage of that narrative. It's instead to say that suffering is part of the human condition. If we can make meaning of our suffering, we can access a deeper purpose and power. As psychiatrist and Holocaust survivor Viktor Frankl writes in his book *Man's Search for Meaning,* "For what then matters is to bear witness to the uniquely human potential at its best, which is to transform a personal tragedy into a triumph, to turn one's predicament into a human achievement."[1] What profound shifts might occur if we reframed trauma not as something that breaks people, but as something that can truly make people? But I digress.

After a traumatic event, there is a normal window of time and a normal set of stress-related responses that most people experience and ultimately move through. However, in the case of unresolved trauma, these stress responses can become programmed as our default mode, rather than onetime defense strategies to help protect us from harm. The smallest of stressors can make us feel like our world is collapsing. When our stress hormones are running the show, it becomes dangerously easy to shape a belief of ourselves as unstable and unfit to be a loving partner, a responsible parent, or a productive part of society. Unresolved trauma of this nature can lead to a diverse range of symptoms that may show up immediately or years down the road.

Symptoms of PTSD

There are four main categories of symptoms present in individuals with PTSD: intrusion, avoidance, hyperarousal, and negative changes in beliefs and feelings.

Intrusion

Intrusion symptoms refer to a visceral experience of reliving the event. Memories no longer become locked in a vault labeled "the past." Instead, they can come flooding back at any moment, creating the same feelings of terror and hopelessness that were present during the original trauma.

Common intrusion symptoms include nightmares or flashbacks. Intrusion symptoms can often be triggered by a sound, sight, or smell that causes you to relive an event in the past. For example, the sound of fireworks going off on the Fourth of July might trigger a traumatic memory of being back in an active war zone. Even though there's no danger in sight, a combat veteran's nervous system may still react with the same cascade of stress hormones as it would if he or she were under attack.

Avoidance

Avoidance refers to the act of avoiding certain situations, places, or people that remind you of a traumatic experience. After I got out of my abusive relationship, I avoided parks that my partner and I had frequented, restaurants where we'd celebrated birthdays or anniversaries, and even movie theaters, because they triggered traumatic memories. Familiar sights and sounds would flood my body with intense fear, hopelessness, and shame.

Avoidance can seem like a good strategy to keep traumatic memories at bay in the short term, but over time your world begins to shrink as the list of places, people, and activities you once enjoyed drastically diminishes. Avoidance can also manifest as an unwillingness to speak about, think about, or seek help for a traumatic experience.

Hyperarousal

Hyperarousal symptoms may show up as feeling jittery, easily startled, or always on edge. You might feel irritable, agitated, angry, or aggressive without warning or major provocation. Hyperarousal can also affect your sleep and impair your ability to concentrate and focus on tasks throughout the day.

Hyperarousal was one of my primary and most disruptive symptoms of trauma. I would experience uncontrollable outbursts of rage that would leave me feeling shameful and "bad." At times, my anger felt like an out-of-body experience. I would wonder, *Who is this crazy person screaming at the top of her lungs?* I also experienced major bouts of insomnia and would jolt awake at any small noise in the middle of the night, my entire body tense and ready to fight off an imaginary attacker. My heart constantly felt like it was about to beat out of my chest, and it would sometimes take hours for my nervous system to settle back down.

Negative Changes in Beliefs and Feelings

The final hallmark category of symptoms in PTSD is negative changes in beliefs and feelings. Trauma affects how we view the world and ourselves. It distorts our ability to see our own goodness and worth. Individuals with PTSD often believe they are "bad" at their core and are distrustful of themselves and others. The world is viewed as a dangerous place, and relationships do not feel safe. Negative self-talk is the overriding narrative, and positive emotions like joy and love may feel completely foreign. One woman who suffered from multiple abuses and inherited family trauma expressed it to me in this way: "I have no spark to get up in the morning. I have no desires, I have no goals, no sensations of love. I'm a shell. And the more I try to fix it, the emptier I feel."

Other Symptoms of Trauma

In my personal work, most, if not all, of the clients who reach out to me seeking a holistic antidote to their anxiety, panic attacks, or depression have a history of trauma that is revealed along the way. Unresolved trauma can manifest in a variety of physical, mental, emotional, and behavioral ways. Often, the symptoms show up years later and have a devastating impact on the lives of those affected. As Peter A. Levine, trauma researcher, psychologist, and creator of the Somatic Experiencing method, notes:

> Trauma is about a loss of connection—to ourselves, to our bodies, to our families, to others, and to the world around us. This loss of connection is often hard to recognize, because it doesn't happen all at once. It can happen slowly, over time, and we adapt to these subtle changes sometimes without even noticing them. These are the hidden effects of trauma, the ones most of us keep to ourselves. We may simply sense that we do not feel quite right, without ever becoming fully aware of what is taking place; that is, the gradual undermining of our self-esteem, self-confidence, feelings of well-being, and connecting to life.[2]

Physical Symptoms of Trauma

Trauma can announce itself through the presence of a variety of physical symptoms. Following is a list of some of the main culprits that show up in our physical bodies to warn us of trauma:

- Chronic pain
- Chronic fatigue
- Muscle tension, joint pain
- Headaches, migraines, neck and back pain with no known cause
- Autoimmune disorders
- Thyroid conditions
- Skin disorders
- Digestive issues, such as bloating, irritable bowel syndrome, spastic colon, celiac disease, and GERD
- Loss of appetite
- Eating disorders
- Insomnia

- Nightmares, night terrors
- Flashbacks, intrusive memories
- Panic attacks
- Hyperarousal, racing heart, trouble breathing, nervous sweating
- Hypervigilance, always being "on edge" or "on guard," jumpy, easily startled
- Hyperactivity
- Hyperventilation
- Hypersensitivity to noise and light
- Lacking physical sensation, feeling numb
- Loss of sex drive

Emotional and Mental Symptoms of Trauma

Trauma may also present itself through a variety of mental or emotional manifestations. The following may be warning signs of traumatization:

- Easily overwhelmed
- Irritable, outbursts of anger
- Abrupt mood swings (crying, rage, frequent anger, despair)
- Anxiety
- Phobias
- Fear of dying
- Emotionally numb
- Hopelessness, despair
- Depression
- Feelings of detachment
- Loneliness, isolation
- Shame, guilt, low feelings of self-worth
- Self-blame or blame of others
- Terror, intense fear
- Grief
- Inability to concentrate and focus, feeling "spaced out," short attention span
- Difficulty learning new things
- Impaired memory
- Difficulty planning for the future
- Confusion
- Paranoia; frightening, racing, or obsessive thoughts
- Reduced ability to cope with stress
- Suicidal thoughts
- Distrust
- Loss of faith in family, community, relationships, or higher power

Behavioral Symptoms of Trauma

Finally, trauma can sneak through the cracks of our behavior. The following behaviors may actually be symptomatic of traumatization:

- Self-destructive behaviors
- Substance abuse and addictive behaviors (overeating, drinking, smoking)
- Sexual promiscuity
- Self-mutilation
- Antisocial behaviors, social withdrawal
- Violent behavior
- Co-dependency issues
- Avoidance of people, places, conversations, activities, objects, or situations
- Attraction to dangerous situations, people, or activities
- Loss of interest in activities previously enjoyed
- Dissociation, immobility, freeze response
- Obsessive-compulsive behaviors, controlling

Detecting Trauma

While some of these symptoms may present themselves immediately in the aftermath of a traumatic event, others can take years to show up. This gap can create a disconnect between the original cause and the long-term effects, leading to misdiagnosis and mistreatment of symptoms. Sadly, misdiagnosis often occurs in cases of children diagnosed with "behavioral issues."

Trauma is typically classified into two main types: shock trauma and complex trauma. Shock trauma refers to a single unexpected event that overwhelms the nervous system and normal coping mechanisms of the body, triggering feelings of intense fear, a sense of helplessness, and loss of control. Examples of shock trauma include some of the big-*T* traumas, such as sexual assault, violent crimes, natural disasters, and automobile accidents.

Complex trauma, on the other hand, is characterized by the experience of and exposure to multiple, chronic, and prolonged traumatic events, often of an interpersonal nature, such as abuse or severe neglect. Complex trauma often begins early in life within a child's primary caregiving system and interferes with the child's ability to form secure attachments, impairing healthy cognitive, emotional, physical, and social development.

Childhood Trauma and the ACE Study

From 1995 through 1997, Kaiser Permanente and the Centers for Disease Control and Prevention surveyed more than seventeen thousand adults in one of the largest scientific research studies of its kind to understand the relationship between childhood trauma and the risk for physical disease and mental health issues in adulthood. The study, known as the Adverse Childhood Experiences (ACE) Study, identified ten "ACEs" or areas of childhood trauma:

1. Psychological abuse
2. Physical abuse
3. Sexual abuse
4. Emotional neglect
5. Physical neglect
6. Loss of a parent (for any reason)
7. Mother treated violently
8. Substance abuse
9. Mental illness
10. Criminal behavior in the household

The study determined that ACEs are strongly related to the development of risk factors for disease, addiction issues, mental health issues, and risky behavior. They are even a predictor for early death. As the number of ACEs a child is exposed to increases, so does the risk for the following behaviors and physical and mental health crises:

- Severe obesity
- Diabetes
- Depression
- Suicide attempts
- Sexually transmitted diseases
- Heart disease
- Liver disease
- Cancer
- Stroke
- Broken bones
- Smoking

- Alcoholism and alcohol abuse
- Poor work performance and missed work
- Financial stress
- Risk for intimate partner violence
- Multiple sexual partners
- Unintended pregnancies
- Early initiation of sexual activity
- Adolescent pregnancy
- Risk for sexual violence
- Poor academic achievement

The study showed that almost two-thirds of participants reported at least one ACE, and more than one in five reported three or more ACEs, demonstrating that childhood trauma is far more pervasive than ever imagined. People with six or more ACEs died nearly twenty years earlier on average than those without any childhood trauma.[3]

The ACE study serves as a cautionary tale about the devastating impact unresolved childhood trauma can have on an individual's life trajectory. It can also serve as the impetus to create a greater societal understanding of and support network for trauma survivors so that they can find healing and reclaim their lives.

Chapter 3

The Trauma Cycle

The truth is that our finest moments are most likely to occur when we are feeling deeply uncomfortable, unhappy, or unfulfilled. For it is only in such moments, propelled by our discomfort, that we are likely to step out of our ruts and start searching for different ways or truer answers.
—M. Scott Peck

There is a stigma around trauma that keeps it shrouded in secrecy and spoken of in whispered tones. Those who experience trauma are often too ashamed or fearful to bring it into the light. For the casual bystander, sadly, trauma is a topic that is better left untouched; once it is spoken of aloud, it requires the bystander to make a choice. Judith Herman addresses this in her seminal book *Trauma and Recovery: The Aftermath of Violence—From Domestic Abuse to Political Terror*:

> To study psychological trauma is to come face to face both with human vulnerability in the natural world and with the capacity for evil in human nature. . . . When the events are natural disasters or "acts of God," those who bear witness sympathize readily with the victim. But when the traumatic events are of human design, those who bear witness are caught in the conflict between victim and perpetrator. It is morally impossible to remain neutral in this conflict. The bystander is forced to take sides.
>
> It is very tempting to take the side of the perpetrator. All the perpetrator asks is that the bystander do nothing. He appeals to the universal desire to see, hear, and speak no evil. The victim, on the contrary, asks the bystander to share the burden of pain. The victim demands action, engagement, and remembering.[1]

As humans, we prefer to forget things that make us squirm. Or worse, we glorify the perpetrator and blame and discredit the victim, so we don't have to share in the victim's suffering.

Tragically, in many cases of childhood sexual abuse or incest, one parent will side with the other and blame the child for lying and making up stories. If the relationship dissolves, the parent may even blame the child for "making" their partner leave. Assigning accountability to the victim removes the responsibility for action. Psychologically, victim blaming also helps people feel safer in the world. If we can make ourselves believe that someone was sexually assaulted because they "asked for it," then we can continue on in blissful ignorance, believing such things will never happen to us.

Turning a blind eye to trauma, especially when it's of an interpersonal nature, has tragic consequences, not just for the victim but also for society at large. Childhood trauma, abuse, and neglect are associated with a higher risk of criminality, including incarceration for violent crimes.[2] According to data, a staggering 75 percent of perpetrators of child sexual abuse reported being victims of sexual abuse themselves during childhood.[3] A study conducted by the Bureau of Justice Statistics found that among state prison inmates 61 percent of male inmates and 34 percent of female inmates with reported histories of childhood and/or adulthood abuse were serving a sentence for a violent offense.[4] Other studies have shown that between 77 and 90 percent of incarcerated women have reported extensive histories of emotional, physical, and sexual abuse.[5] The data are clear: childhood trauma is a predictor of criminality across the board. Multiple studies have also revealed that childhood trauma is associated with a higher risk for mental health issues like depression and anxiety, alcoholism, drug abuse, and antisocial behaviors in adulthood.

FROM SURVIVOR TO THRIVER

In 2017 I met Sheri Poe, an entrepreneur, speaker, advocate, and all-around powerhouse of a woman. Sheri founded Ryka, the first and only athletic footwear designed exclusively for women; holds several honorary doctorate degrees; has appeared on *Today* and *The Oprah Winfrey Show*; and has been featured in *Newsweek*, the *Wall Street Journal*, the *New York Times*, and more. We instantly connected over our shared passion for helping people heal from trauma and transition from survivor to thriver.

Sheri is the epitome of a "thriver," but she's had to overcome enormous trauma to get where she is today. She shares her story in her own words:

Forty-five years ago I was a thriving college freshman when I was held at gunpoint for a number of hours by a stranger. The incident culminated with him sexually assaulting me. I was not only traumatized by the rape but terrified for my life. I was in a state of shock when the campus police showed up at my dorm. Nonetheless, they questioned me in a manner that conveyed they doubted my experience, and laughed with one another as I recounted my ordeal. They threw my underwear around the interrogation room at the police station and told me I must have done something for the perpetrator to choose me to attack. In short, the incident was my fault.

At the hospital, the nurse and the doctor were disgusted by me and told me I must have "asked for it." The doctor refused to examine or even touch me.

The one person I was sure would support and understand me was my therapist. Unfortunately, when I recounted my ordeal to him, he also insinuated that I must have done something to bring on this attack.

I was further traumatized as a result of this victim blaming. I felt embarrassed, ashamed, dirty, and disgusting. I made a decision not to tell people what had happened to me, including my parents, family, and friends. For many years, the only people in my life who knew were my college roommate and my brother. I decided to live in denial of the experience, stuffed it down emotionally, and did not seek help for many, many years. As a result of my denial and secrecy, I suffered from severe bulimia, PTSD, and chronic trauma and adopted impulsive sexual behaviors. I became extremely physically depleted and, as a result, was hospitalized for two months in my twenties.

After dropping out of college, I decided to immerse myself in my spirituality and lived in meditation centers for six years. I found these centers to be a very nurturing and grounding environment. I discovered how healing yoga and exercise were in terms of connecting me with my body. These daily practices helped me find some peace in the midst of my complex emotional state. Meditation, mindfulness practices, and daily exercise have been powerful healing tools for me. These practices connect us to our bodies, our emotions, and our spirituality.

I started speaking publicly about my sexual assault experience and the aftermath in 1991. It has been life changing, deeply powerful, and healing. The process of sharing with others and encouraging them to have hope and get the help they need has become my life's work.

In my trauma recovery, I discovered the power of our words and thoughts. Each thought is accompanied by a feeling. I noticed that the word *survivor* felt dark, scary, and heavy, and I didn't want to feel that way over and over again. On the other hand, the word *thriver* feels very happy, light, and healthy. We have a choice to take our power back and to live as thrivers. Today, I identify as a thriver rather than a survivor.

Healing Shame

As Sheri's story illustrates, shame is one of the biggest obstacles in healing trauma. Trauma is so destructive because it makes us feel like an outcast from society.

Healing happens when we are able to speak the unspeakable. Speaking out requires a safe space to house our shame. As speaker, author, and renowned shame researcher Brené Brown says, "Our stories are not meant for everyone. Hearing them is a privilege, and we should always ask ourselves this before we share: 'Who has earned the right to hear my story?' If we have one or two people in our lives who can sit with us and hold space for our shame stories, and love us for our strengths and struggles, we are incredibly lucky."[6]

Finding someone safe to share our shame with is often no easy task, and sharing with the wrong person can inflict pain worse than the original trauma. I will never forget the day when my older sister, whom I love more than anything but haven't always had the smoothest relationship with, bluntly said, "I will never understand why people just don't leave." She was, of course, referring to the abuse I had experienced in my past relationships. Then she twisted the knife with five simple words that, to this day, remain seared into my soul: "I will always judge you."

As if finding a safe place to house our shame weren't hard enough, there's also the issue of rampant misguided self-help advice that, when misinterpreted, can dangerously perpetuate self-blame. My abuser called himself my "teacher," and whenever he would physically or emotionally inflict harm he would tell me he was simply my "mirror" reflecting back to me all my own worst qualities. It was always *my* responsibility to look in the mirror.

During one of the darkest moments of my life, I spent the night in jail on a domestic violence charge. My partner and I had had an altercation the night before that ended with him strangling and threatening to kill me. I had finally had enough and called the police. When they came, I got scared. In my mind it suddenly didn't matter that I could barely swallow as a result of the force of his hands around my throat or that he had brutally ripped off my clothes as I had tried to run to safety. What mattered was that I had participated in the violence, and the only person I saw fit to blame was myself. The police separated and handcuffed us both to take us in for questioning. My partner admitted to nothing, while I naively told the police it must have been my fault because he was simply my mirror. "Spiritual" words have never tasted so toxic.

Recognizing the people and situations in our life that are "mirrors" is a fundamental concept in many self-help programs. And at times it's incredibly useful. It can help reveal unhealthy patterns and offer us a tool of awareness to break free. But when people who have been through trauma are told that every situation is a mirror and that we "attract" our own reality, it can reinforce shame and the belief that we are deserving of every pain inflicted upon us. Let yourself call bullshit on that right now. No one asks to be assaulted in a dark alley or abused by a parent at home. Use your mirror to see your blind spots, but please do not use it as a weapon of self-blame.

Understand also that if mirrors reflect our darkness, then it only stands to reason that they must also reflect our light. How powerful would it be if we started seeing our light everywhere we looked? Drown out the voices that whisper you are bad, broken, unlovable, and unworthy. And listen instead to the voice that says you are capable, loved, worthy, and whole. In yogic philosophy, our soul or true self (known as "Ātman") is eternally whole. Recovering from trauma means reconnecting to our transcendent nature. We don't have to "fix" ourselves, because we were never broken.

Trauma Reenactment

One of trauma's most fascinating symptoms, which also often contributes to shame, is what Peter A. Levine calls the "compulsion to repeat." Victims of trauma commonly end up reenacting their original trauma throughout their life in a variety of ways that are both obvious and not so obvious. For example, perhaps not surprisingly, many women and men who have been sexually assaulted end up engaging in risky and impulsive sexual behaviors. An even more obvious and tragically common reenactment scenario is a young girl who is raped and grows up to become a prostitute. Bessel van der Kolk explains, "Compulsive repetition of the trauma usually is an unconscious process that, although it may provide a temporary sense of mastery or even pleasure, ultimately perpetuates chronic feelings of helplessness and a subjective sense of being bad and out of control."[7]

There has been much debate in the trauma research field about why victims repeat trauma. Freud took particular interest in the subject, postulating that reenactment was ultimately a way for people to gain mastery over their original wound. More modern thinkers disagree, arguing that reenactment often ends up not in mastery, but in retraumatization. Research into the neurobiology of trauma also points to very real changes in a traumatized person's brain, which alters the individual's perception of safety and danger.

There's a structure in our brain called the hippocampus, which is primarily responsible for forming, storing, and retrieving memory, along with spatial navigation. The hippocampus encodes memory and plays a role in consolidating short-term memory to long-term memory. You can think of the hippocampus as a time-date stamp for your memories and experiences.

Let's say, for example, that you were attacked by a large dog as a child. The hippocampus stores the information that large dogs are dangerous for later use. As an adult, you are out for an evening walk when a large dog suddenly comes running toward you. Your hippocampus retrieves the archived memory from childhood, and in a coordinated effort with your autonomic nervous system, creates your reaction to the approaching canine, which most likely involves running away or getting in a defensive position to ward off a potential attack.

If, on the other hand, you had overwhelmingly positive experiences with dogs in your past, your reaction would be very different. Perhaps you might kneel down to pet the dog rather than tensing all your muscles in preparation to fight. Essentially, the hippocampus allows us to recognize situations, events, objects, or people that we have previously encountered so that we can scan our environment for signs of safety or danger.

Trauma has been shown to affect the hippocampus. Brain imaging technology (MRI and PET scans) performed on people with PTSD demonstrates that the volume of the hippocampus can actually shrink in size in traumatized individuals. When our hippocampus shrinks, our ability to recognize danger can too. This may be one of the reasons traumatized individuals often repeatedly find themselves in unsafe situations.

Reenactments are not limited to replicating the original trauma. As Peter A. Levine notes, trauma reenactments can appear in a variety of forms, such as recurring accidents like repeated bodily injuries or falls, and even psychosomatic diseases. Reenactments can also take place on notable dates or anniversaries of a traumatic experience.

When I was asked by my therapist to make a list of all my past traumas from childhood to present, I was shocked not only by the number of traumatic events I had experienced in my life, but also by the fact that many of these events happened on or around the same date, years apart. Turns out it was by no coincidence that many of my traumas big and small played out on the anniversary of the flood I described in the opening chapter.

A client I worked with relayed her experience of domestic violence within the timeline of her three pregnancies. Emotional abuse was a constant within the relationship, but physical abuse was rare. She now has three beautiful and healthy children; however, exactly four months into each pregnancy her (now ex-) husband was physically violent toward her. The more work I do with people who have experienced trauma, the more patterns of reenactment come to light.

How About You?

Are there any seemingly random events or mishaps that keep showing up in your life? Do you have a strong emotional reaction to any special occasions or specific dates, like your birthday or certain holidays? Do you feel more depressed, anxious, angry, or fall ill at a certain time every year? While there is certainly room for coincidences in life, when it comes to trauma, very little is coincidental.

If you suspect you have unresolved trauma in your past, you are not alone. The tools and practices in the pages to come will provide you with a road map to healing. Trauma can be resolved and harmful patterns dissolved. Once I became aware that the anniversary of the flood was a trauma trap for me, it helped me understand why I would get flooded with feelings of fear and sadness, seemingly out of nowhere almost every New Year's Eve. I had filed the flood away as unimportant, but my body remembered its significance. Awareness allows us to change the pattern. It doesn't mean that I don't still get triggered, anxious, or sad as one year gives way to the next. Sometimes I do. But now I have the tools to meet my emotions so they don't run the show. I connect with my felt sense. I actively check in and ask myself what I'm feeling and where I'm feeling it in my body. I remind myself that while my body and mind have been patterned to react a certain way, I can make a different choice. Viktor E. Frankl, a psychiatrist and Holocaust survivor, is commonly quoted as having said, "Between stimulus and response there is a space. In that space is our power to choose our response. In our response lies our growth and our freedom."

FINDING YOUR INNER RESOURCE

An inner resource is anything that mentally creates a sense of comfort and support for you. To find your inner resource, think about anything real or imagined that makes you feel at ease. It can be a special location in nature like a tranquil lake, a favorite room, a person or pet you love, a treasured memento, an activity you enjoy, a color, or any image that makes you feel happy, calm, or centered. Mentally paint the scene of your inner resource with as much detail as possible—what does it look like, sound like, smell like, taste like, and feel like? Use your inner resource as an anchor before you practice the movement sequences or mindfulness techniques in this book. Come back to your inner resource any time you feel overwhelmed or ungrounded.

Chapter 4

Trauma and Your Brain

When a person continually faces danger he is powerless to overcome,
his final line of defense is at last to avoid even feeling the danger.
—Rollo May

There's a reason we can't just "get over" trauma. Trauma fundamentally changes our brain, maladaptively affecting memory, emotional regulation, and our stress and fear responses.

Our Three Brains

To understand trauma, we must first get acquainted with the wondrously complex organ responsible for thought, emotion, movement, sensation, and communication: the human brain. In 1990, Paul D. MacLean, a physician and neuroscientist, suggested that we have three brains in one: the reptilian brain, the mammalian brain, and the neocortex. His theory is now known as the triune brain model and serves as a simplified way to view the very complex functioning of the human brain.

This is important information for our purposes because the task of resolving trauma must address all three brains, as well as our physical body, which ultimately becomes the battlefield where trauma plays out.

The Reptilian Brain

The brain develops from the bottom up, starting with the reptilian or "lizard" brain. This part of the brain ensures our survival. The reptilian brain is the oldest and most primitive part of our brain.

It consists of the brain stem and cerebellum and is responsible for our survival instincts, including our fight-or-flight response. It controls automatic, involuntary processes that we don't have to think about, like sleep, digestion, circulation, respiration, heartbeat, and sexual arousal. It governs instincts and reflexes and makes automatic, instinctual survival decisions.

The Mammalian Brain

The mammalian brain—appropriately named because all mammals have one—sits right above the reptilian brain and serves as our emotional center. It houses attachment, motivation, behavior, memory, sense of smell, and how we see and perceive the world.

Also known as the limbic system, our mammalian brain acts as our memory vault, remembering and encoding both pleasant and unpleasant experiences. It plays a critical role in the detection and perception of outside threats by comparing our past and present experiences. It makes decisions designed for our survival based on stored history, rather than logical analysis.

The Rational Brain

Finally, we have the neocortex, also known as our "rational" or "cognitive" brain. The neocortex is the youngest part of the brain and is responsible for higher cognitive functions, such as language, reasoning, planning, abstract thought, and voluntary movement. The neocortex develops last because it is the least essential part of our brain from a purely primitive survival standpoint. The capacity for abstract thought holds little value if our basic involuntary survival functions like respiration, heartbeat, and digestion are offline.

Under ordinary, everyday conditions, the neocortex helps manage the more instinctual reptilian brain and emotional limbic system, applying rational thought and reasoning to decision-making. However, when we're in distress or faced with a threat, our neocortex gives up the reins to the limbic system, which works in tandem with the reptilian brain to activate what's known as our fight-or-flight response.

How Our Brain Responds to Threats

Fight-or-flight response is an evolutionary mechanism designed for primitive survival. In times of real or perceived threat, our nervous system is flooded with stress hormones, which spring us into action to flee from or fight off an attack. In fight-or-flight mode, the neocortex goes offline, allowing us to act first and think later. Consider the example of Emily suddenly coming upon a snake while walking around her backyard. She jumps back instinctively, only to realize moments later that it is just a garden hose.

This lightning-fast chain of reactions prompted by the limbic system and reptilian brain goes something like this: upon seeing the snake, the sensory thalamus—a structure located in the limbic system that acts as a central information hub for our all of our senses except for smell—alerts the amygdala of the snake-like shape. The amygdala, an almond-shaped structure in the limbic system that plays a central role in processing fear, acts as an "alarm bell" when danger is detected. In this case, the amygdala processes the incoming sensory information as a threat and sends an instant message to the hypothalamus and the brain stem, recruiting the stress hormone system and the autonomic nervous system (ANS) to mobilize the body to leap away from danger.

Neuroscientist Joseph LeDoux calls this almost instantaneous pathway to the amygdala the "low road." The low road bypasses the neocortex completely and sends information directly from the thalamus to the amygdala, prompting us to act. We also have another pathway called the "high road." The high road directs the same sensory information to the medial prefrontal cortex (MPFC); once the higher thinking brain has assessed the information, it relays the appropriate message back down to the amygdala.

The difference between the low road and the high road is that the high road takes about eight times longer than the low road. Although this time difference can be measured in milliseconds, in a dangerous situation it can mean the difference between life and death. By the time the neocortex kicks in, our body has already responded to the threat by jumping away.

Trauma primarily plays out along the "low road" in the limbic system. PTSD has been shown to affect critical structures in the limbic system, including the amygdala, hippocampus, and hypothalamus. Trauma also affects a part of the neocortex called the medial prefrontal cortex.

The Thalamus

The thalamus is like an international phone operator, directing calls where they are supposed to go. The thalamus provides the amygdala with sensory input, which the amygdala then interprets to determine whether the incoming information poses a threat to our lives.

The Amygdala

If the thalamus is a phone operator, the amygdala is like the translator, interpreting the content of each call. The amygdala plays a starring role in our danger detection.

Our brain is wired with a negativity bias, which means it is constantly scanning for threats and detects negative information faster than positive information to help ensure our survival. If danger is sensed, the amygdala instantly alerts the sympathetic nervous system to mobilize us for fight or flight.

The Hippocampus

As you may recall, the hippocampus is responsible for memory. When the amygdala sounds the alarm bell, the hippocampus scans our memory to relate any past experiences to what is currently happening.

Remember, too, that the hippocampus can shrink in those suffering from depression and PTSD, thus affecting how they process and perceive safety and danger.

The Hypothalamus

The main role of the hypothalamus is to regulate hormones. When the amygdala and hippocampus agree that danger is present, the hypothalamus kicks into gear, signaling the pituitary, thyroid, and adrenal glands to release stress hormones like cortisol and adrenaline.

The hypothalamus receives information not just from the brain, but also from the heart, vagus nerve, digestive system, and skin. While the hypothalamus controls the release of hormones, it does not possess the ability to determine whether a stressor poses an actual threat to our survival or not. The hypothalamus can release the same flood of stress hormones in response to someone honking at us in traffic and a car actually hitting us and causing an accident. One event is life-threatening, the other is not; it's not the hypothalamus's job to tell the difference between the two.

The Medial Prefrontal Cortex

While trauma plays out largely in the limbic system, the malfunctioning of certain regions of the neocortex also contributes to the development of PTSD. In the traumatized brain, a region of the neocortex, the MPFC, is affected. Neuroimaging techniques performed on patients with PTSD showed diminished activation within the MPFC when patients were exposed to trauma-related stimuli, while activation was elevated in the amygdala.[1]

In a nontraumatized brain, the MPFC has the ability to help regulate amygdala activity and dampen distressing emotions like fear and anxiety. However, in the traumatized brain, the MPFC is unable to keep the amygdala in check, which results in significant emotional and psychological distress. Essentially, the brain under the influence of trauma loses its ability to think rationally, leaving us operating purely from our animal instincts.

Quick Tip:
Tame Your Amygdala by Tapping

If someone can be traumatized in thirty seconds, why can't they be healed in a day, an hour, a minute?

—Rick Wilkes, Emotional Freedom Technique (EFT) expert

Emotional Freedom Technique (EFT), also known as tapping, combines the ancient wisdom of Chinese acupressure with modern psychology to rewire the brain; calm the nervous system; and help with PTSD, anxiety disorders, phobias, and negative thought patterns.

While we cover a variety of tapping techniques based on principles from Chinese medicine in the movement section of this book, EFT employs a very specific tapping sequence based on nine different acupressure points, located on our hands, head, and upper torso. Proponents of EFT claim that tapping works by "turning off" the amygdala, which dampens our response to stress.

To start tapping immediately, check out thetappingsolution.com/tapping-101 and click on "Introduction to the Tapping Points" for a free four-minute video that guides you through the nine basic points of the tapping sequence. If you're interested in learning more about tapping, I highly recommend reading *The Tapping Solution,* by Nick Ortner.

Scanning for Danger

We receive an incredible amount of sensory information from the outside world every second of every day. As you're reading this book, your thalamus is processing the temperature of the air on your skin, the brightness of the lights in the room, the weight and texture of this book in your hands, and so on.

If the temperature of the room you are in right now is relatively mild, your thalamus will likely file that information away as unimportant. If, however, the temperature suddenly becomes burning hot, your thalamus will send a signal to your amygdala to alert it of potential danger. Without any conscious thought, the amygdala will help mobilize you into action almost instantaneously.

In people with PTSD, the amygdala appears to be hyperactive, constantly scanning for danger where none exists. With this in mind, it's important to note that the amygdala can't discern between past and present; that job is reserved for the hippocampus. Because the amygdala doesn't process time, danger can feel ever-present, locking traumatized individuals into a chronically overstimulated and hyperaroused state. The trap of trauma is that it feels like it has no beginning or end.

In panic disorder, which affects many people who have experienced trauma, the hypothalamus triggers the release of stress hormones constantly, so danger feels like it's lurking around every corner. This constant stream of stress hormones can lead to adrenal fatigue because these glands are working overtime without a break. Our internal alarm system never goes quiet, and the result is complete physical and mental exhaustion.

At the height of my panic disorder, I was so fatigued that I could barely function, yet my nervous system refused to call off the alarm. My body desperately craved sleep, but I was completely wired and could sleep only an hour or two per night—if I was lucky. During those sleepless nights, I was plagued by deep fears of dying. I thought if I closed my eyes I would never wake up again. During a particularly intense episode, I stayed up for a full forty-eight hours, thinking that I would rather end my life than continue to live in fear and panic for the rest of my life. In the coming chapters, we'll learn movement techniques that retrain our body and mind to recognize the fact that scary sensations and uncomfortable experiences have a concrete beginning, middle, and end. This frees us from the fear that our suffering will last forever.

The Autonomic Nervous System

A key player in our fight-or-flight response is the autonomic nervous system, which is like the on/off switch for the body's response to danger. It is divided into two branches: the sympathetic nervous system and the parasympathetic nervous system.

The sympathetic nervous system prepares our body to spring into action. It activates our fight-or-flight response and produces chemicals like adrenaline and cortisol to mobilize us to fight off an attacker or flee from danger.

The parasympathetic system is our rest, digest, and freeze response, which regulates basic body functions like digestion, wound healing, sleep, and dream cycles. When we're in sympathetic arousal or fight-or-flight mode, our body puts the brakes on normal bodily functions deemed nonessential by the autonomic nervous system in order to concentrate on the present task of saving our life. Our heart rate increases, our respiration quickens, our pupils dilate to let in more light for improved vision, our perception of pain diminishes, our muscles tense, and our digestion slows in an attempt to preserve energy and divert blood to the limbs and muscles that need it the most to successfully fight or flee.

People who are chronically stressed often complain of digestive issues because their digestive system essentially shuts off in sympathetic arousal. We'll discuss the importance of the gut and its role in depression, anxiety, fatigue, and overall dis-ease in the body and present a protocol for healing the gut in part IV. For now, it's important to know that the fight-or-flight response was biologically designed with our survival in mind, and that it happens automatically without our conscious thought.

When we're in parasympathetic dominance, our heartbeat slows, our pupils constrict, and activity in the stomach is stimulated and saliva production increased to help facilitate digestion.

The two branches of the nervous system are also involved in sexual arousal and orgasm. It may sound counterintuitive, but it is actually the parasympathetic nervous system that promotes sexual arousal and erection, which explains why when we're stressed out or anxious we may have a difficult time getting "in the mood." During actual orgasm, however, the sympathetic nervous system momentarily kicks in to help facilitate ejaculation and vaginal contraction. After that, our bodies settle back into parasympathetic dominance, which is why we're often sleepy after sex. This natural rhythm between arousal and calming creates a balanced state for our bodies and minds to thrive. Being in a chronic state of stress and sympathetic activation can lead to sexual dysfunction like premature ejaculation and impotence, which creates feelings of embarrassment, shame, and inadequacy. If you're dealing with sexual dysfunction related to stress or trauma, the tools in this book can help alleviate these symptoms as the underlying trauma stored in the body is addressed and released.

In a healthy individual, there is a functioning balance between the sympathetic and parasympathetic nervous systems. Even during times of stress, a balanced nervous system will follow up sympathetic arousal with parasympathetic calming, creating a natural cycle of charge (sympathetic activation), followed by discharge (parasympathetic release). This rhythm of charge and discharge creates homeostasis in the body and mind. A balanced autonomic nervous system gives us the ability to process and assess certain experiences, situations, and emotions, and to respond appropriately while maintaining our health and well-being. In people with PTSD, however, the sympathetic and parasympathetic nervous systems can swing wildly out of balance, leaving people stuck in either the "on" or "off" position.

And it's not only people with PTSD whose nervous systems suffer. People who work or live in high-stress environments (hello, most of us!) are also affected. While our fight-or-flight response was helpful when we had to summon all our strength to fight off wild animal attacks as cave people, in the modern world it has become counterproductive and, frankly, destructive. We're flooded by the same stress hormones when we get called into the boss's office at work as we were when our lives were threatened in more primitive times. This is problematic because elevated cortisol levels over the long term can weaken the immune system; create gastrointestinal issues, including poor nutrient absorption and inflammation; increase the risk for heart disease; and lead to weight gain and other disruptive issues like insomnia, chronic fatigue, depression, and more.

Fight, Flight, or Freeze

Much of what we know about how the body stores and releases trauma today comes from observing animals in the wild. All animals, including humans, respond to threats with the same set of evolutionarily programmed defense strategies: fighting, fleeing, or freezing. Fleeing is usually the first line of defense. If we can't outrun a predator, we will turn to our second line of defense and put up a fight. If we lack the physical capacity to fight or know we will be overpowered, we may instinctively invoke the freeze response as a last resort.

The freeze response occurs in extremely dire circumstances, when our brain determines that we can neither outrun nor outfight a threat. From an evolutionary perspective, the freeze state is a merciful one because it temporarily physically and mentally numbs the body to pain in the event of imminent death.

Many sexual assault survivors and survivors of incest describe going into a freeze or dissociative state while their bodies are under attack. This dissociative state helps numb out the physical and emotional pain of the violation. A childhood sexual assault survivor I spoke with recalled how she was sexually abused by multiple men within her own home from age four to sixteen. She describes her experience of dissociation: "I learned how to leave my body. I would check out and simply go away." She went on to explain that "going away" was what enabled her to survive and endure.

Dissociation or going into the freeze response during a traumatic event is thought to be one of the biggest predictors for developing PTSD in the future because the trauma never had the chance to be fully discharged from your system. A primary goal of trauma healing is to release or discharge the energy that can get trapped in the body at the moment of freezing.

Trauma researchers and somatic therapists believe that traumatic responses occur when an individual's attempts to fight or flee are unsuccessful, which is often the case in car accidents, combat, rape, abuse, and other violent crimes in which an individual is overwhelmed or overpowered, or simply doesn't have enough time to run or fight because everything happens so fast.

The fight-or-flight response generates a massive amount of energy, and our bodies naturally want to see this response through to successful completion. That's part of the reason the physical exercises and breathwork practices in this book are so important. They can help you complete interrupted fight-or-flight responses by discharging stuck energy that has been frozen in your nervous system. Successful discharge lays the groundwork for deeper healing to unfold.

Animal Instincts

Researchers have noted that animals living in their natural habitat are exposed to trauma on a daily basis. Despite this, we don't see lions walking around the savannah displaying signs of PTSD. This is because animals naturally discharge their traumatic stress by involuntarily shaking from head to toe. Video footage often used to demonstrate this discharge shows an impala completely frozen and immobilized under the jaws of a cheetah. Before the cheetah can bite down, a feisty baboon wanders into the frame, distracting the cheetah. The cheetah gets up and leaves the frozen impala unharmed. Once the cheetah has left the scene, the impala comes out of its freeze state and launches into a full-body shake. Researchers have cited this full-body trembling as something animals instinctively do to effectively release traumatic stress from their nervous system after escaping an attack. After a few moments of trembling, the impala bounds back to life and goes on its merry way, having successfully discharged the trauma.

Another classic video example is a 1997 *National Geographic* clip that shows a polar bear running from wildlife researchers who are armed with tranquilizer guns. The polar bear gets hit with a tranquilizer and is completely immobilized. When the polar bear comes out of his immobilized state, he breaks out into full-body tremble. Slowing down the footage reveals that the trembling isn't completely at random. The polar bear gnashes his teeth (fight response), and his legs move as if he were running (flight response), thereby completing the interrupted autonomic nervous system response. After the trembling subsides, the polar bear begins to involuntarily take deep belly breaths, thereby releasing the remaining stress so his nervous system can return back to homeostasis.

Unfortunately, we humans often disrupt our own natural instincts of discharge of trauma, leading to PTSD, anxiety disorders, hypervigilance, flashbacks, depression, and more. Peter A. Levine's book *In an Unspoken Voice: How the Body Releases Trauma and Re-*

stores Goodness recounts the author's own traumatic experience of being hit by a car while crossing the street. In the ambulance, Levine was able to track his body sensations and allowed his body to naturally shake and tremble, which effectively "reset" his nervous system, giving him a better likelihood of avoiding PTSD in the aftermath of the accident.

Levine goes on to note that the general public often isn't so lucky to have this experience. Most paramedics are trained to stop people from shaking by strapping them down or sedating them with drugs. This kind of intervention can interfere with the body's natural fight-or-flight response, thus keeping patients frozen or trapped in their own trauma. Levine summarizes: "It is my observation that a precondition for the development of posttraumatic stress disorder is that a person is both frightened and perceives that he or she is trapped. The interaction of intense fear and immobility is fundamental in the formation of trauma, in its maintenance and in its deconstruction, resolution, and transformation."[2]

The good news is that our body is incredibly resilient and our brain possesses the ability to rewire itself. What was once trapped can be released.

RELEASING TRAPPED TRAUMA

One of the most deeply touching and profound experiences of physical trauma release I've had the privilege to witness and help facilitate was with Tori, a radiant young woman who took a Purple Dot Yoga Project Trauma Informed Teacher Training I co-taught. Tori, who had experienced abuse in her past, describes her experience of going through one of our trauma-release breathwork techniques:

I was truly fascinated by the breathwork exercise. I anticipated an emotional reaction, perhaps accompanied by memories resurfacing and tears, but the results have profoundly transformed my reactions to my past traumas. As the breathing began, I almost immediately felt strong emotions rising to my chest, similar to the precursor of a panic attack. Powerful memories began to surge through my body. I am not sure how much time passed before I became consciously aware of my corporeal surroundings and cognizant of my body sliding upward on my mat.

My legs, independent of my conscious control, were actively jerking up and down at my hip flexors, my back arching away from the mat. My arms were bent at right angles at the elbows, fists clenched and waving wildly, whether in an innate reaction to fight or aid my flight, I am unsure, but the physical reaction was astounding. I was running. In the course of this flashback, I was moving through the actions that were denied to me at the time of my trauma. I had read about this phenomenon, but was astonished to experience it myself. I gradually felt my legs slow as my pent-up emotions began to dissipate.

We were then instructed to begin taking calming breaths, and my instincts took over once more. This time, as we cooled, I completed the action I had not been able to take at the time of my trauma. In my mind's eye, I walked toward my past self and lifted her into an embrace. I guided her gently out of the house where she had lived with her abuser and we left. I left. After years of futile anguish about a past I couldn't change, my body completed the motion it wasn't able to take previously.

The freedom and lightness I felt in my body was indescribable. This experience—this beautiful, wondrous, miraculous experience gifted to me by my body—has completely rewired my reactions to both my abuser and to myself. The memories remain, but they are no longer coupled with panic attacks and swells of suffocation. My trauma had been resolved, and I was given new hope that the hurt can be healed.

Chapter 5

Creating a Healing Path

*The human soul doesn't want to be advised or fixed or saved. It
simply wants to be witnessed—to be seen, heard and companioned
exactly as it is. When we make that kind of deep bow to the soul of a
suffering person, our respect reinforces the soul's healing resources,
the only resources that can help the sufferer make it through.*
—Parker J. Palmer, *The Gifts of Presence, the Perils of Advice*

There are two main approaches to treating trauma: top down or bottom up. Top down refers to addressing trauma from the neocortex down. It is referred to as such because the
neocortex is the youngest part of our brain and the last to develop. Bottom up refers to addressing trauma from the oldest part of our brain, the reptilian brain, and moving up from there.

Healing from the Top Down and the Bottom Up

Traditional talk therapy is a top-down approach. It requires the client to access language,
which is housed in the neocortex, to talk about traumatic events and experiences. It should be
noted, though, that some critics of talk therapy argue that talking about traumatic events over
and over again is akin to reliving them and can actually be retraumatizing.

Strong research is now emerging that a bottom-up approach may be a more effective
means of healing trauma, because traumatized individuals need to feel safe in their bodies and
regulated in their autonomic nervous system before they can begin to access and make sense
of their experiences in a top-down way. A bottom-up approach uses body-oriented techniques
and can include various forms of movement therapy (yoga, dance, martial arts), body sensing,
tapping, breathwork, and other specialized body-based interventions, such as Somatic Experiencing (created by Dr. Peter A. Levine) and Tension, Stress, and Trauma Release, or TRE
(created by Dr. David Berceli).

Remember that when our body is in fight-or-flight mode, our higher thinking brain lets go of the wheel and allows the lower two brains to do the driving. Many traumatized individuals simply don't yet have the language to describe what they're feeling because the higher brain has, in effect, been disconnected.

I believe that talk therapy can be a profoundly healing tool that offers awareness about how our patterns play out and provides the space to process feelings of shame in a safe container. Giving voice to the terrifying thoughts and sensations that hold us captive allows us to begin reintegrating the body and mind back into its original state of wholeness. However, getting to that point requires us to *feel* into our bodies first. This is why talk therapy may be best used either in tandem with a body-based, bottom-up approach or introduced further down the road once an individual has worked through resolving any trauma stored in the body first. Although it should be noted that if an individual has been diagnosed with schizophrenia, multiple personality disorder, bipolar disorder, borderline personality disorder, or clinical depression or is experiencing suicidal thoughts or behaviors, the first course of action should always be to seek professional psychiatric help. And in any case, of course, you should always consult with a qualified mental health care practitioner, psychotherapist, or medical doctor before starting this or any other type of program.

This book employs both a top-down and a bottom-up approach by integrating movement, breathwork, mindfulness, and nutrition to help resolve trauma and restore vitality and well-being to the body, mind, and spirit.

In part II we walk through the science of physical exercise (a bottom-up approach) and specific Primal Yoga movement practices that draw from the ancient wisdom of yoga and martial arts. The physical exercises and poses outlined emphasize a connection to the felt sense in present-time awareness. When trauma gets trapped in the body, it can feel like it exists in the ever-present now, rather than being something that happened in the past. Various yoga postures and movements will help you become gradually aware of your body and the fluctuating sensations that live there, which will allow you to shift your perception of time and learn to separate the past from the present.

Yoga also requires a deep awareness of and connection to the breath. Breathwork is another bottom-up approach that works with the most primitive parts of our instinctual brain. When introduced mindfully and practiced with care, breathwork can be one of the most powerful and profoundly healing tools of traumatic stress release available. Breathing practices allow us to both activate and soothe the autonomic nervous system, and through specific breathing exercises, traumatized individuals can discharge traumatic stress and learn to self-regulate.

Part III of this book utilizes some top-down tools of healing by introducing a variety of simple and effective mindfulness and meditation techniques. Mindfulness strengthens the capacity of our medial prefrontal cortex to monitor our body's sensations. When practiced consistently over time, meditation can actually change our brain, increasing the gray matter and cortical thickness in several key structures of the brain. The bulking up of the brain in specific areas has been linked to greater emotional regulation, improved learning, memory, focus, and even greater compassion and empathy. Mindfulness has also been shown to decrease the size of the amygdala, which you'll remember is responsible for sounding the alarm that kicks off our fight-or-flight response.

Last, in part IV we come back to the body, discussing why the food we eat has such a radical and often overlooked impact on our physical, emotional, and mental health and well-being. In some ways, I'm most excited about this portion of the book because the nutritional component of healing is a game-changer. No one told me that the trauma symptoms I was suffering from—like anxiety, depression, and fatigue—were being magnified and perpetuated by the state of my gut. It is my mission to tell you what no one told me, and to offer you medicine not from the pharmacy but from the refrigerator that will help you put all the pieces of trauma recovery together.

The Problem with the Current Medical Model

The topic of mental health and the very personal decision about whether or not to take psychiatric drugs as a way to manage symptoms carries a stigma and is often accompanied by judgment or shame. Psychiatric drugs have helped many of my friends and loved ones manage very real symptoms of depression and anxiety. It's unhelpful and, frankly, harmful to pass judgment on anyone who has used or benefited from prescription medications.

If you are currently on medication for any psychiatric diagnosis, including schizophrenia, multiple personality disorder, bipolar disorder, borderline personality disorder, severe depression, anxiety disorders, or PTSD, *never* discontinue medical treatment or change your dosage without the guidance of a qualified mental health professional. The physical exercises, mindfulness techniques, and nutritional guidelines in this book can be helpful as supplemental treatments, but they should never be used as substitutes for medication.

If you have been courageous enough to seek out professional help and were handed a prescription, I commend you for being proactive about your health. I will, however, point out some of the flaws in the pharmaceutical industry today and provide research-backed evidence about the risks and long-term side effects that antidepressants and antianxiety medications carry.

The Problem with Big Pharma

Big Pharma is a multibillion-dollar industry. In 2015, the amount of money spent on prescription drugs in the United States reached an all-time high of $424.8 billion. With these skyrocketing treatment costs, it would stand to reason that depression and suicide rates would simultaneously decrease. But the reality is that depression and suicide rates are on the *rise*.

The Centers for Disease Control and Prevention (CDC) published a report in January 2017 that showed the suicide rate had increased from 11.3 suicides per 100,000 people in 2007 to 12.6 suicides per 100,000 people in 2013. The report also found that the depression rate in teenagers has increased from 8.3 percent in 2008 to 10.7 percent in 2013.[1] Ironically, one possible reason for this increase may be the overprescription and misuse of medications. While prescription drugs may help treat and manage symptoms of depression and anxiety, they are far from a cure. Antidepressants and antianxiety medications come with a lengthy list of side effects, which can include depression, anxiety, and suicidal thoughts—the very things they are meant to treat.

Psychiatric drugs work by artificially adjusting brain chemistry. The commonly accepted view of depression in the biomedical field is that it is a result of insufficient levels of serotonin in the brain. Drugs like Prozac and other selective serotonin reuptake inhibitors (SSRIs) work by increasing levels of serotonin in the brain by blocking its reabsorption.

The problem is that the evidence supporting the serotonin hypothesis is circumstantial at best. To date, there have been no human studies that definitively show that low serotonin causes depression. In fact, new research reveals that we may have it all backward. According to a 2015 paper published in *Neuroscience & Behavioral Reviews*, researchers found that depression may actually be linked to *elevated* rather than decreased levels of serotonin. Lead author Paul Andrews, an assistant professor of psychology, neuroscience, and behavior at McMaster University in Canada, points to the fact that, although antidepressants increase serotonin within minutes to hours of ingestion, the effectiveness of these drugs takes much longer to kick in. "You'd think that if the low serotonin hypothesis was true, the anti-depressant drugs would work rapidly too," he says. "But they don't—it takes three to four weeks for their symptom-reducing effects to kick in. So there's always been this disconnect between the onset of the pharmacological effects of the anti-depressants and their therapeutic effects."[2]

To cast further doubt on the low serotonin hypothesis, there is an antidepressant on the market today called tianeptine, which goes by the trade names Coaxil and Stablon. Tianeptine actually works by lowering serotonin. This drug has been shown to be just as effective as Prozac, which raises the question: how much do we really know about the way serotonin reacts chemically in our brain? As Irving Kirsch, associate director of the Program in Placebo Studies at Harvard Medical School and author of the book *The Emperor's New Drugs: Exploding the Antidepressant Myth*, says, "If depression can be equally affected by drugs that increase serotonin and by drugs that decrease it, it's hard to imagine how the benefits can be due to their chemical activity."[3]

All signs point to the truth that depression cannot be so easily attributed to one isolated chemical. Humans are incredibly complex beings, and the current biomedical model does not take into account the myriad lifestyle, environmental, social, and developmental factors that can play a role in depression. Nutrient-deficient diets that are high in processed foods, sedentary lifestyles, environmental and chemical toxins, history of trauma, chronic stress, and the lack of a strong social support system can all significantly contribute to the onset of depression.

As functional medicine doctor and *New York Times* best-selling author Mark Hyman says, "Depression is not a deficiency of Prozac, any more than cholesterol issues are a deficiency of statin drugs. There is a root cause, and while a medication might be lifesaving as short-term triage, it's not about addressing the root cause."[4]

So how did we become such a pill-happy nation? Partly because we've been sold the idea that Prozac, Paxil, Zoloft, and the like are the singular cure to a complex problem. An analysis of budget spending of ten of the world's biggest pharmaceutical companies revealed that a whopping nine out of ten spend more on marketing than on research.[5]

The bottom line is that drug companies want to sell as many drugs as possible. As a result, there is a major lack of transparency in terms of how the pharmaceutical industry reports drug study findings, not to mention huge and often undisclosed conflicts of interest.

Drug companies are not required by law to publish findings from every study they conduct. The result is a selectively high reporting of studies with positive results that support the agenda of the pharmaceutical companies and a grossly underreported number of studies revealing negative results. In a 2008 study published in the *New England Journal of Medicine*, researchers took a critical look at the drug industry's reporting to uncover possible bias. They analyzed seventy-four FDA-registered studies of twelve different antidepressants involving more than twelve thousand participants and found that thirty-seven out of thirty-eight studies viewed by the FDA as having positive results were published, while only fourteen out of thirty-six studies viewed by the FDA as having negative or questionable results were published. Researchers also found that, according to published literature, it appeared that 94 percent of the trials conducted were positive, yet the full FDA analysis showed that only 51 percent were positive.[6]

One reason drug companies are selective about publishing all findings is that multiple studies show that in cases of mild or moderate depression, SSRIs are no more effective than placebos, and, in some cases, the placebos are actually more effective than the drug itself! In 2010, a meta-analysis of six large studies published in the *Journal of the American Medical Association* (*JAMA*) issued a major blow to the antidepressant industry. The paper concluded: "The magnitude of benefit of antidepressant medication compared with placebo . . . may be minimal or nonexistent, on average, in patients with mild or moderate symptoms."[7]

While the *JAMA* paper did show that antidepressants had a slight advantage in effectiveness over placebos in cases of severe depression (about 13 percent of cases), the major takeaway, says Steven Hollon, psychology researcher at Vanderbilt University and coauthor of the *JAMA* paper, was: "Most people don't need an active drug. For a lot of folks, you're going to do as well on a sugar pill or on conversations with your physicians as you will on medication."[8]

Irving Kirsch goes a step further, saying that not only are most, if not all, of the benefits of antidepressants due to the placebo effect, but "instead of curing depression, popular antidepressants may induce a biological vulnerability, making people more likely to become depressed in the future."[9] Kelly Brogan, a holistic women's health psychiatrist and *New York Times* best-selling author, agrees. In her book *A Mind of Your Own: The Truth About Depression and How Women Can Heal Their Bodies to Reclaim Their Lives*, she writes, "Despite what you've been led to believe, antidepressants have repeatedly been shown in long-term scientific studies to worsen the course of mental illness—to say nothing of the risks of liver damage, abnormal bleeding, weight gain, sexual dysfunction, and reduced cognitive function that they entail. The dirtiest little secret of all is the fact that antidepressants are amongst the most difficult drugs to taper from, more so than alcohol and opiates."[10]

If you're considering antidepressants as a short-term treatment plan to help you get through a difficult patch, consider the risk that you might be signing up for a much longer-term prescription. Many people on antidepressants cite the return of negative symptoms they experience when trying to wean off their prescriptions as evidence for the drugs' effectiveness. However, current research is debunking this. In her book, Brogan points to the work of Dr. Paul Andrews of the Virginia Institute for Psychiatric and Behavioral Genetics. Dr. Andrews suggests that the symptoms people feel upon stopping an antidepressant are not a return of the original mental health condition, but withdrawal symptoms from the drug itself. Not only that, but patients who opt for medication may actually prolong the duration of their symptoms. Brogan quotes Andrews's explanation from a 2011 article published in *Frontiers in Psychology*: "Unmedicated patients have much shorter episodes, and better long-term prospects, than medicated patients. . . . The average duration of an untreated episode of major depression is twelve to thirteen weeks."[11]

I want to circle back to say that none of the information presented here is intended to demonize antidepressants or diminish their very real role in saving numerous lives. It's simply to help you weigh the risks and be better informed about what is right for you.

Sometimes the right thing to do is to take the meds. A friend of mine described her decision to take medication to me like this: "When I'm drowning in depression, antidepressants help me swim back up to the surface. I might still be a ways off from land, but at least I'm no longer at the bottom of the ocean." Swimming is always better than sinking. There is no shame in doing whatever you can to keep yourself afloat.

But if medications don't feel right for you or you have a goal to eventually taper off, know this: our bodies are incredibly resilient and made for self-healing. When we have a cut, our skin naturally repairs itself. Likewise, low moods and even bouts of anxiety and depression can also resolve themselves naturally over time. While some cases may certainly require medical intervention, a growing body of research confirms that lifestyle changes such as exercise, stress reduction through mindfulness practices, and dietary changes, including natural supplementation, can be equally powerful and have the benefit of far fewer side effects. When we start treating our body as a whole, rather than treating parts and individual symptoms, we create a vibrant path toward long-term health and well-being.

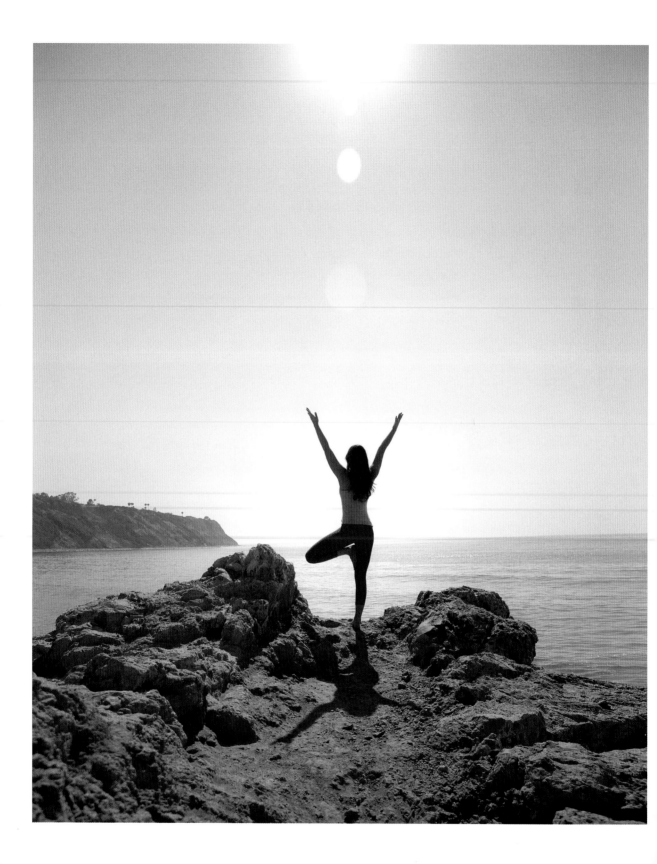

Part II

Releasing Trauma from Our Body

Chapter 6

Movement Is Medicine

There is more wisdom in your body than in your deepest philosophy.
—Friedrich Nietzsche

What if a natural prescription for anxiety and depression already exists within each one of us and is, moreover, encoded into our very own biology? What if all we had to do to begin to tap into it was get off the couch and get moving? Maybe it sounds too good to be true—but it's not!

Decades of scientific research have confirmed that exercise is one of the most powerful and accessible tools we have at our disposal to combat physical and mental dis-ease. Beyond the physical benefits of increased strength, stamina, flexibility, balance, and coordination, exercise is also a potent antidote for stress. It promotes more restful sleep, and it increases feelings of self-worth and emotional well-being. Exercise also improves memory and learning, lowers the risk of dementia and age-related diseases, supports brain health, boosts mood, and, yes, can even help ward off depression and anxiety.

Western culture tends to look at the body and the brain as two separate entities. This critical disconnect between mind and body fails us time and time again because it places a narrow lens on alleviating singular symptoms, rather than holistic healing. The mind is inextricably linked to the body. What happens in one affects the other. We cannot optimize our brain without equally optimizing our body.

The Body–Brain Connection

Rodolfo Llinás, neurophysiologist and author of *I of the Vortex: From Neurons to Self*, writes, "That which we call thinking is the evolutionary internalization of movement." To illustrate this point, he describes a primitive sea creature called the sea squirt. In its larval life, the sea squirt has the ability to move around through the water until it eventually attaches itself to a stationary object, where it spends its adult life immobile, like a plant perched on a piece of coral. Once situated, the sea squirt passes its days by eating its own brain. Yum! Without the need for movement, the sea squirt's brain is no longer necessary.[1]

Our bodies were designed to move. Without physical activity, not only does our body begin to break down, but our mind deteriorates as well. In the absence of movement, our brain quite literally shrivels. Brain scans of people with sedentary lifestyles reveal a physical shrinking of key parts of the brain, including the hippocampus and the cingulate gyrus. Remember that the hippocampus is also one of the key structures known to shrink in the brains of people with depression and PTSD.

Animal studies have shown that exercise can increase the size of the hippocampus by stimulating the growth of new neurons while encouraging cell survival, which enhances learning and memory. Many of the diagnosed mental "disorders" we classically attribute to the brain are actually intimately tied to our physical body. People suffering from depression, anxiety, chronic fatigue, brain fog, digestive issues, and a host of other maladies might be better served with exercise, rather than pills, as a first line of defense.

Exercise regulates critical mood-balancing neurotransmitters—namely serotonin, dopamine, and norepinephrine—all three of which belong to a group known as monoamines. As we've already discussed, serotonin has taken center stage in the debate about the cause and treatment of depression. While there is conflicting information and still much more to be learned about the way serotonin functions in the body, one thing that researchers agree on is that serotonin is a key player in mood regulation. It also plays a role in sleep, libido, social behavior, memory, appetite, and digestion.

Dopamine, another important mood-regulating neurotransmitter, is linked to our "pleasure system," and plays a role in motivation, attention, addiction, reward, and desire. Unlike dopamine and serotonin, which are hailed as the "happiness heroes," norepinephrine is often pegged as a stress hormone and is overlooked for its role in brain health. Along with epinephrine (more commonly known as adrenaline), norepinephrine is released by the adrenal glands in the sympathetic nervous system as part of the fight-or-flight response. In a balanced nervous system, it kicks in when an emergency situation demands it, then eases off. Its job is to make us more aware, awake, focused, and alert when responding to stress.

When stress becomes chronic, our adrenals work overtime to produce these stress hormones, but they can't sustain this over the long term. Eventually they burn out. This is commonly known as adrenal fatigue. When we're in the initial "alarm" phases of adrenal fatigue, our bodies overproduce hormones like norepinephrine and cortisol, which get our heart racing, our palms sweating, and our body and brain alert and primed to fight or flee. However, when these hormones linger in our system longer than necessary, they can contribute to anxiety, insomnia, irritability, and unstable moods. Once we reach the burnout stage, we are operating at a deficit. Low levels of norepinephrine can contribute to fatigue, brain fog, depression, and disinterest in life and activities that once brought joy and excitement.

An imbalance of norepinephrine has also been linked to attention deficit hyperactivity disorder (ADHD). The common prescription for ADHD is drugs like Ritalin or Adderall, but Dr. John Ratey, clinical professor of psychiatry at Harvard Medical School and best-selling author of the book *Spark: The Revolutionary New Science of Exercise and the Brain*, has found that regular exercise can temper ADHD by instantaneously boosting baseline levels of both dopamine and norepinephrine. While Dr. Ratey does not recommend that those with ADHD toss out their Ritalin and replace it entirely with exercise, he has found that, for a number of his patients, daily exercise offers another powerful tool to manage their symptoms and even lower their dosage of medication.

No one, doctors and researchers included, fully understands the complexity of how these three neurotransmitters actually function and interact in the body. *But the one thing all experts agree on is that exercise benefits everyone.*

The impact of exercise on our mental health cannot be overemphasized. It's no coincidence that antidepressants target the exact same chemicals that exercise naturally boosts. In a landmark study, researchers at Duke University found that exercise was just as effective as antidepressants in relieving symptoms of patients with major depressive disorder. In what is now known as the SMILE (Standard Medical Intervention versus Long-term Exercise) study, James Blumenthal and his colleagues randomly divided a group of 156 older adults into three groups: an exercise-only group, a medication-only group (which used the antidepressant Zoloft), and a group that combined both exercise and medication.

The exercise group did thirty minutes of aerobic exercise (either walking or jogging) three times a week. After sixteen weeks, all three groups reported a significant decrease in depressive symptoms, with no major differences between them. This indicates that exercise is as effective as antidepressants.

However, one significant difference *was* noted in participants at a ten-month follow-up to the study. Participants in the exercise-only group showed notably lower rates of depression relapse compared to both the medication and combination groups. The participants who continued to engage in regular exercise during the follow-up period were also more than 50 percent less likely to be depressed at their ten-month assessment compared to those who did not exercise.

Let that sink in for a moment. While it's certainly heartening to confirm that exercise, indeed, has a powerful therapeutic benefit, it's equally alarming to discover that the natural antidepressant effect of exercise can be weakened over time when combined with long-term antidepressant use. *In other words, antidepressants can actually block some of exercise's most powerful mood-boosting benefits.*

Exercise as Prevention

We've all heard it before: the best medicine is preventative medicine. While exercise offers powerful benefits as an intervention when health issues arise, it is most effectively used as a preventative measure. It's far easier to step out of a small ditch than to climb your way out of deep, dark hole. Don't wait until you need a ladder! Exercise can help stop symptoms before they start.

But if you're already in the hole, focus on taking one small step at a time. Start wherever you're at, even if that just means sitting up on the couch instead of lying down. Take the stairs instead of the elevator. Walk your dog a half a block farther than usual. And most important, be kind to yourself and practice patience along the way.

What Kind of Exercise Is Best?

Certain types of exercise are better than others when it comes to increasing muscle strength and bone density; others are great for increasing cardiovascular health or reducing chronic pain; while still others excel at improving balance, coordination, and flexibility. However, when it comes to brain health, the latest research suggests that aerobic activity may be superior to other forms of exercise, such as weight training and high-intensity interval training (HIIT).

A study published in the February 2017 *Journal of Physiology* looked at new brain cell growth in rats based on three different types of workouts: running, weight training, and HIIT. Researchers from the University of Jyväskylä in Finland separated rats into groups, giving each group a different exercise regime for a period of seven weeks, then measured the creation of new brain cells (a process known as neurogenesis) in their hippocampal region (key for learning and memory). From there, the researchers determined which workout yielded the brawniest brain. They found that rats that aerobically exercised by running on wheels showed the highest number of new neurons in their hippocampus. The longer the distance they ran over the course of the seven weeks, the more new cells were measured.

The HIIT group had higher levels than the sedentary control group, but far fewer new neurons than the running group. The weight-training group, while physically stronger, wasn't brawnier in brainpower by the end of the experiment. In fact, their hippocampal tissue was comparable to that of the sedentary rats.[2]

Despite these results, study leader Dr. Miriam Nokia noted that the benefits of weight training and high-intensity training should not be discounted. These types of workouts likely benefit the brain in other ways, but they simply aren't as effective in creating changes in the hippocampus. This lack of positive impact on the hippocampus likely has to do with the fact that more intense workouts like HIIT are stressful on the body, and "stress tends to decrease adult hippocampal neurogenesis."[3]

For optimal brain function, most experts recommend some form of daily aerobic activity for forty-five minutes to an hour. Whether it's dancing, running, power walking, bike riding, or anything else, getting your heart rate up for longer durations has brain-boosting benefits.

That being said, when it comes to trauma and its accompanying symptoms, such as depression and chronic fatigue, telling someone to go run for an hour every day is not always realistic. Simply getting out of bed can be a big challenge, so the chances of making it to that high-energy dance class are unlikely at best.

It should also be acknowledged that not everyone has the ability to physically exercise, let alone run. If you use a wheelchair or live with a disability, it can feel incredibly insensitive and infuriating to hear someone blabber on about healing yourself through aerobic exercise. One of the many reasons I was drawn to yoga and internal martial arts like tai chi and qigong is that they are among the oldest and most inclusive forms of exercise available. *Internal* refers to a focus on more subtle energy flow and qi cultivation versus physical strength and outward power, which are classified as *external* styles (like kung fu). Not only that, but a growing body of research is now confirming the effectiveness of some of these internal styles in treating anxiety, depression, chronic pain, and PTSD.

If you have limited mobility, know that you can still benefit from many of the tools presented in this section. Each movement sequence in this book is paired with a breathing technique. If nothing else, start with your breath. Our breath lays the foundation for our physical and mental health. Yogis and martial artists are trained to develop deep awareness of their breathing patterns. It doesn't matter how strong or flexible you are; if you're not breathing with conscious intention, you're not doing yoga.

Our breath is truly one of the most effective ways to heal from the inside out. If all you do is learn how to breathe properly, you have already done enough. There are also a number of different restorative poses illustrated here that can be done seated or lying down, as well as a chair sequence that may be done in a wheelchair. Use what works from each sequence and leave what doesn't. And know that there are many other wonderful resources available that are tailored to support individuals with physical disabilities in creating a deeper connection to their bodies. One of my favorites is Warriors at Ease, a nonprofit organization that uses yoga and meditation to support the health and healing of service members, veterans, and their families. They have helped thousands of warriors in wheelchairs and with amputations use yoga as a part of their recovery. You can find out more about their programs at warriorsatease.org.

All that said, what type of exercise is best? My simplest and most honest answer is: the best kind of exercise is the one that you'll do, and stick to. What has personally stuck for me is yoga and martial arts. These two ancient practices have been my lifeline during some of the darkest moments in my life. In the words of one of my private clients who used yoga as a recovery tool to overcome addiction, "Yoga saved my life."

If you are new to either practice, I encourage you to keep an open mind. It may not be love at first tree pose (that's the name of a yoga pose, by the way), but once you tangibly experience the benefits in your own body and mind, what once felt challenging and uncomfortable may soon feel like home. I still remember the first yoga class I ever walked into. It was *not* my scene. All around me, people were contorting themselves into strange shapes, calling out the names of poses in a language I didn't understand, and breathing a little too heavily for my comfort. I awkwardly giggled my way through the entire thing and wrote it off as something I would never do again. I certainly never would have imagined that more than fifteen years later, yoga would have evolved into my greatest teacher and best friend.

Yoga

The headline for a recent article in *Time* magazine proclaims: "It's Official: Yoga Helps Depression." The article cites a study published in the *Journal of Alternative and Complementary Medicine*, which took a group of thirty people with clinical depression between the ages eighteen and sixty-four and split them into two groups. One group was prescribed a ninety-minute yoga class three times per week, as well as four thirty-minute sessions per week at home. The second group completed two ninety-minute yoga classes and three thirty-minute at-home sessions per week.

The participants selected were either not using any antidepressant medication at all or had been on a consistent dose for at least three months, meaning any relief of depressive symptoms could be attributed to the yoga classes rather than the antidepressants kicking in. After three months, the participants were given a depression-screening questionnaire. The majority of participants in both groups lowered their scores by at least 50 percent, with the group that did more yoga lowering their depression scores even more than those who did less yoga.[4]

A growing body of evidence is confirming what the ancient yogis intuitively knew: yoga heals. And it heals without any of the harmful side effects that come with pharmaceuticals. Here is just a taste of the physical, mental, and emotional benefits that yoga has now been scientifically proven to offer:

- It is increasingly being recognized as an effective treatment modality for reducing symptoms of PTSD.[5]
- Hatha yoga significantly increases heart rate variability (HRV), which is an important measure of our heart health and our body's ability to adapt to stress.[6] Low HRV is linked to sympathetic nervous system dominance (fight or flight), which can be associated with stress and inflammation. A high HRV, on the other hand, indicates increased parasympathetic tone, which can positively affect our sleep, recovery, digestion, and ability to manage stress.
- Thanks to yoga, in a 2013 study, a group of participants with PTSD showed a significant reduction in their symptoms as measured by the Clinician-Administered PTSD Scale, a clinical PTSD assessment tool.[7]
- A pilot study at Walter Reed Medical Center found that yoga nidra—a form of deep relaxation—resulted in a reduction in the severity of PTSD symptoms, including insomnia, depression, anxiety, and fear.[8]

Yoga Is for Everybody

Despite what some may tell you, yoga has nothing to do with religious beliefs, divine intervention, or mystical properties. If you've been hesitant to try it because you think you'll have to worship Hindu gods, dress in all white, or contort yourself into a pretzel, I have good news for you: none of the above is true. Yoga is an evidence-backed practice that harnesses its healing power from a combination of movement and breathing techniques that have been shown to support our autonomic nervous system in reestablishing balance. Where other traditional methods of mental health care have failed, the latest research is showing that the body may very well provide the best route to sustainable, holistic success.

Martial Arts

Over the years, many of my Primal Yoga students have commented that my combination of yoga and martial arts has empowered them in ways no other physical modality has. I started martial arts when I was a little girl and have trained in many different styles over the years.

I can personally attest that there's nothing more cathartic than being able to kick, punch, grunt, and scream in a safe and controlled environment.

If trauma is frozen energy left over in our body from an unsuccessful attempt to fight or flee, I can think of no better way to help complete our most primal survival instincts than martial arts. It is a powerful way to release anger and frustration, and to reestablish a sense of strength, autonomy, control, and self-discipline.

If your trauma, however, involved any kind of physical attack or assault on your body, you may understandably be hesitant to jump into a martial arts class. For a long time after my physical abuse, I had to stop martial arts because it felt too triggering to have kicks and punches flying at me. I would get emotionally flooded if someone got anywhere near my neck or throat. A friend once playfully tapped me on the head and I was instantly overcome by blind rage followed by profound grief. My first instinct was to strike him back, but instead I burst into tears. My poor friend sat there completely bewildered; of course, he had no idea that he had triggered the deepest wound inside me.

Fortunately, my love of martial arts eventually outgrew my fear and I started training again at an academy I trusted and respected. Within this safe container, I was able to breathe again and began releasing my fear and shame.

A few years after I had resumed my training, I had a profound realization during one of my jiu-jitsu classes. I had just finished three five-minute rounds of sparring with three different physically imposing men. In each of these rounds, I was placed in a chokehold. And each time, I calmly found my way out without panicking or becoming emotional. I was able to stay cool under pressure, and more important, I was having fun! It was during this experience that an incredible realization hit me like a lightning bolt: I was no longer afraid! Instead, I felt empowered. My fight-or-flight response was no longer running the show.

Internal Martial Arts (Qigong and Tai Chi)

The beauty of martial arts is that they can be both hard and soft. If kicking, punching, or ground grappling is triggering for you, you might want to consider looking into gentler internal forms of martial arts, such as tai chi and qigong. Both of these modalities have their roots in fighting arts but have been adapted over centuries for the purpose of profound self-healing.

Qigong is an ancient Eastern practice that was developed as a way of consciously exercising one's *qi* (also known as chi, or one's vital life force energy). Qigong is an important pillar of traditional Chinese medicine. It's based on the premise that nature is our most powerful medicine, and our bodies carry an innate wisdom and capacity for self-healing. By consciously cultivating our *qi*, it is believed that we can prevent disease and enhance our health and well-being. Research backs up these claims. The practice of qigong has been shown to lower blood pressure; increase vitality and stamina; reduce stress levels; enhance immune system function; improve cardiovascular, respiratory, circulatory, lymphatic, and digestive function; and improve balance.

Qigong typically involves a slow and easy-to-follow routine (also known as a "form"), a series of postures or gentle movements performed in connection with controlled breath. There are thousands of different styles of qigong, from medical to meditative.

Tai chi (or *taiji*, which translates to "supreme ultimate" or "universal harmony") is a form of moving meditation. Many today know it best as a calming, almost slow-motion exercise that is practiced by groups in parks. However, you might not know that it was originally coined as an explanation for the formation of the universe and the foundation of human life. Tai chi represents all that is yin (female) combining with all that is yang (male), to create two balanced aspects of "the One." You've probably seen this expressed in symbolic form through the circular black-and-white tai chi symbol (more commonly known as the yin and yang symbol).

The practices of tai chi and qigong aim to create harmony in the body, which is achieved when we have a balance of yin and yang. Everything in the universe, including ourselves, has both a yin and a yang aspect. Yin is the more feminine water energy. It is static, calming, and intuitive, and it corresponds to the earth. Yang is the more masculine fire energy. It is dynamic, stimulating, and logical, and it corresponds to the heavens. Our body's various organs are also considered to be either yin or yang. When yin and yang are in balance, health prevails.

Yin and yang provide a framework for the universe that is made up of opposing yet complementary forces. The Five Elements or Five Phases Theory expands upon this view of the universe by describing five stages of transformation as represented by five distinct elements: wood, fire, earth, metal, and water. In Chinese philosophy, these five elements correspond with various aspects of nature, the seasons, foods, senses, planets, and life itself. Each element is also paired with an organ system in the body, as well as mental qualities and emotions. Many acupuncturists use the five elements to diagnose and treat physical, emotional, and mental health conditions. Several styles of qigong also draw from the five elements to harmonize the body.

One of the most healing aspects of qigong is that it can be practiced by anyone, anywhere. No equipment is needed, no athletic prerequisites are required, and many forms are gentle enough to be done seated or lying down, using breathing and visualization techniques rather than physical movement to move the qi.

Chapter 7

The Healing Power of Breath

Instead of acting out, act in. When you're triggered, locate where you
feel uncomfortable in your body. Place your hand there. Bring your
breath there. Tell that young fragmented part of you: "I've got you.
I won't leave you. I'll breathe with you until you're at peace."
—Mark Wolynn

For those of you who live with chronic fatigue, an autoimmune disorder, or serious illness; are physically restricted from an injury; live with a disability; or are simply too exhausted from the emotional weight of depression or anxiety to even think about starting an exercise program, know that you can start small. You can start with your breath. Breath is movement. And it is one of the most the most powerful ways we as humans have to move our bodies and influence our own self-healing.

Conscious Breathing

Breathing is an involuntary function we're innately born to do without conscious thought. So what's the difference between breathing to sustain life and conscious breathing? Conscious breathing allows us to develop the ability to mindfully control and regulate our breath to achieve a desired effect, such as calming our anxiety when we're stressed out or energizing our body and mind when we're feeling lethargic. The ancient yogis developed a sophisticated and powerful system of breathing practices known as *pranayama* to control and harness the healing power of the breath. *Prana* means "life force," and *ayama* means "to extend or draw out." The yogis intuitively knew that by controlling our breath, we could not only train our mind, but also transform the state of our health and strengthen our vital life force energy.

There are two main categories of breathing practices: calming and energizing. Calming practices activate our parasympathetic nervous system to soothe, cool, and calm our body and mind. Energizing practices activate our sympathetic nervous system to wake us up and create more vital energy in the body. Calming breathing techniques are like taking a Valium, while energizing techniques are like a shot of espresso, but without any of the nasty side effects. Calming breathing practices are generally safe to be practiced for longer periods of time (anywhere from twenty minutes up to an hour), multiple times throughout the day.

Energizing practices should generally be practiced for much shorter durations (one to five minutes max). Energizing practices should also not be done by anyone with hypertension, epilepsy, or a history of seizures, hernia, aneurysm, recent surgery, glaucoma, retinal detachment, asthma, diabetes, or psychiatric conditions like bipolar disorder, psychosis, or paranoia. Stimulating breathing practices can cause manic symptoms, agitation, or irritability in people with these psychiatric conditions.

Discharging Traumatic Stress Through Breath

While many trauma-informed yoga classes are cautious about introducing energizing breath practices or avoid them altogether, I have personally experienced the powerful effect these stimulating breathing techniques can have on releasing the deepest traumatic wounds. Bearing witness to the transformations people go through during a breathwork session has been one of my greatest and most sacred honors as a teacher. Stimulating breathwork has also personally helped me release my own deep grief and toxic anger. I have trembled, I have wept, I have laughed, and I have screamed. Each time, I emerge humbled and awestruck by the level of catharsis breathwork has gifted me.

While it is always best advised to practice any kind of stimulating breathwork with a trained teacher who can support and guide you, I feel I would be doing more harm than good by withholding a few of the easier-to-learn techniques from those who can most benefit.

Stimulating breathing techniques are so effective at releasing trauma because they activate our sympathetic nervous system, where our fight-or-flight response gets trapped in cases of unresolved trauma. You might be thinking, *Wait a minute. Why the heck would I want to intentionally activate my fight-or-flight system? Won't that create more anxiety?* The answer is: it depends. If you just got rear-ended in your car and you're already in a state of fight or flight, creating additional stimulating breath can indeed create more anxiety. You would benefit more from a few deep belly breaths or some other sort of calming practice, like alternate nostril breathing.

However, if you are depressed, shut down, or frequently dissociate, when practiced in a safe environment, stimulating breathing techniques can help you discharge any frozen fight-or-flight energy locked in your nervous system. When we're in a state of freeze or collapse, our dorsal vagal complex is running the show. In order to climb out of this depressed, numb, and frozen state, we need to temporarily shift into our sympathetic nervous system, where our energy naturally operates at a higher frequency. The key is to not overstimulate the body to the point where we collapse into freeze again, but to keep it at a safe level where our nervous system is activated just enough to discharge any traumatic stress. Once our body has discharged that energy—which can manifest as tingling, trembling, shaking, flailing, punching, or kicking—deeply calming breath is introduced to bring balance back to the autonomic nervous system.

The concept of discharging traumatic stress from the body in a manageable way without overwhelming the nervous system is called *titration*. Titration creates a feeling of safety in the body, letting your body know it's okay to begin discharging and releasing stuck energy while staying within a safe window of tolerance. A feeling of safety within our own bodies is key to shifting into our social engagement system, where health and well-being thrive.

IT ALL BEGINS WITH BREATH

I first met Kristin when she signed up for one of my Yoga Teacher Trainings in 2014. She is a single mother with a rare blood disorder called ITP (immune thrombocytopenia). Because of this, her immune system destroys her own platelets and attacks her bone marrow. On the first day of the training, she was physically depleted and visibly fatigued. She warned the group that she might need to take things a little slower than everyone else.

Whenever I encounter someone with an autoimmune disorder, more often than not there's a link to past personal trauma. Kristin possessed an inner strength and quiet courage that only the bravest among us have. It's an astonishingly beautiful quality that I see time and again with people who have experienced trauma. There is a huge misconception that trauma creates broken people. Nothing could be further from the truth. Trauma creates warriors among those of us who have met life's battles with unwavering resilience. As it turns out, Kristin had endured a long history of trauma and abuse. It was her warrior spirit that led her to this particular teacher training.

The first day of teacher training, I was in so much pain. I was bleeding a lot, to the point where my blood soaked through my clothes and stained my mat. I was so vulnerable. I knew I had made it out of hell and that being at that training was the first light I could see at the end of the tunnel. I knew my life was going to move up from there. Just the thought of freeing myself induced anxiety and panic attacks. But my soul said, "Go on. You've already died—there is nothing left to lose. Reinvent yourself."

This reinvention started by taking five minutes to breathe before my day began. I knew I only had that. My body was broken and my hopes were too, but my survival instinct said, "Start with the breath."

From there, yoga soon turned into a love affair. I wanted to be with myself again. Through yoga, I had found home again. In movement and breath, I became aware of all the little parts of me—my toes, my hands, the creases of my hips in a certain pose. There I was. I started listening to my body, feeling everything instead of constricting in the face of pain and hardship. Yoga led me to gentleness, and that gentleness spilled over into strength.

Today, Kristin is a certified yoga teacher who shares her light and gifts with others by teaching trauma-informed yoga classes as an ambassador for Purple Dot Yoga Project. Her story is a powerful illustration of how something as small and seemingly insignificant as taking a few moments a day to consciously breathe can ultimately change your life.

Breathing with Purpose

Pause for a moment and take a full, deep breath. Inhale through your nose and sigh your breath out through your mouth. Did you notice how your body subtly shifted? Perhaps you felt your belly inflate or your chest expand? Our breath moves our body from the inside out. It has the power to stop anxiety in its tracks, reduce chronic pain, help lift depression, relieve insomnia, release anger, improve digestion, improve athletic performance, and enhance pleasure, and that's just the tip of the iceberg.

If you take only one thing away from this book and ignore everything else, begin to shift your focus to your breath. Think about it. Humans can survive for weeks without food, days without water, but only minutes (approximately three, to be exact) without air. Oxygen provides vital nourishment for every cell in our body, without which we literally could not survive. Think about how much money you spend on groceries each week to fuel your body and how much you spend on gas to fuel your car. Now ask yourself how much time and attention you spend fueling your cells with their most important energy source—oxygen. Of course we all breathe naturally to sustain life, but there's a difference between breathing for survival and breathing intentionally and with purpose.

Have you ever noticed that when you're anxious, stressed, nervous, or panicky, your breathing changes? Your heart rate increases and your breath becomes shallow and rapid as it shifts into your upper chest. This is our fight-or-flight response in action. When we are in danger, our body needs quick access to more oxygen so that we can rapidly respond to a threat. Unfortunately for many of us, upper chest breathing becomes the norm rather than just an emergency response.

Functional breathing starts with our diaphragm and should originate from our belly, rather than our chest. The diaphragm is a thin dome-shaped muscle that sits just below our lungs and is our primary muscle of respiration. This powerful muscle contracts and flattens downward when we inhale, allowing air to be pulled into our lungs as they expand. As the dome pulls downward, it compresses our abdominal organs, which move down and out, expanding our belly like a balloon. The diaphragm then relaxes back into its dome shape as we exhale and our belly softly draws back in. Slow, deep diaphragmatic breathing (also known as belly breathing or abdominal breathing) can slow our heart rate, lower blood pressure, ease anxiety, and calm our mind.

Breath Check

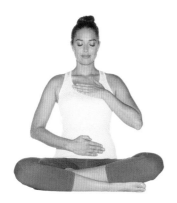

Breathing is one of those things we do on autopilot, so let's take a couple of minutes to become aware of how we're breathing.

Find a comfortable seated position or lie down on your back. Place one hand on your belly and the other on your chest. Take a full, deep inhalation through your nose and notice which hand moves more. Is it the one on your belly or the one on your chest?

Keep your hands on your body and observe the movement of your chest and abdomen as you exhale. If you're properly breathing from your diaphragm, your belly should inflate as you inhale and draw back in as you exhale.

If the opposite happens, and your belly inflates with your exhale, then you are stuck in a pattern called "reverse breathing." It will take some time and patience to retrain your body to breathe more functionally. It can be frustrating at first, like learning how to pat your head and rub your belly at the same time. But you'll get the hang of it soon!

Finally, if your belly didn't move at all, but your chest heaved up, then you are thoracic breathing, or "chest breathing." The breathing exercises in this book will be of huge benefit to you and you will be astonished to see how quickly your mood and energy transform once you start to shift your breath from your upper chest down into your belly.

Breath and Our Emotional State

Our emotional state can change our physiological state in an instant. The phone rings and you see it's an ex that you haven't spoken to in years. Before you even hear the sound of their voice or what they have to say, your sympathetic nervous system has already been activated and your breath is one of the first things affected.

We've already discussed the lightning-fast chain reaction of physiological responses that occur in the body when we feel an intense emotion like fear. But did you know it's not a one-way street? Just as your emotional state can change your breath, your breathing can change your emotional state. When we're stressed, we breathe more shallowly; when our breath is shallow, we feel more stress.

Breath and stress are like the chicken and the egg. Anxiety and chest breathing are a vicious cycle, and the more you get pulled into the loop, the more challenging it is to distinguish which came first. Dysfunctional, shallow chest-breathing patterns can create and worsen a host of issues, including panic attacks, anxiety, depression, concentration issues, memory problems, digestive issues, muscular pain, and high blood pressure. In his book *Anatomy of Hatha Yoga*, David Coulter writes, "Habitual chest breathing not only reflects physical and mental problems, it creates them. It mildly but chronically overstimulates the sympathetic nervous system, keeping the heart rate and blood pressure too high, precipitating difficulties with digestion and elimination, and causing cold and clammy hands and feet."[1]

The diaphragm separates the abdominal cavity from the chest cavity. The heart sits on top of the diaphragm, while our abdominal organs like the liver, stomach, and spleen reside below. The rhythmic movement of the diaphragm massages our internal organs and helps stimulate the wavelike movement of the intestines (known as peristalsis), which is vital for healthy digestion and waste elimination. Take a moment to do a quick gut check. When was the last time you had a great bowel movement? Yes, I'm asking about your poop. If your internal pipes are feeling clogged up, your breathing may be partly to blame. Deep diaphragmatic breathing can help get things flowing again, helping to relieve constipation, bloating, gas, and irritable bowel syndrome.

Our respiratory muscles, like any other muscle in our body, can become weakened and chronically tight. The diaphragm attaches to our ribs and lumbar vertebrae and also has fascial connections to our psoas muscle (our main hip flexor and our primary muscle of fight or flight) and our quadratus lumborum (QL), a muscle that has the important job of both stabilizing and mobilizing our spine and pelvis.

Because of these crucial connections, dysfunctional breathing is often a hidden culprit of lower back pain. Dysfunctional breathing also manifests as muscle tension and pain in our head, neck, shoulders, chest, and upper back. When our diaphragm isn't functioning properly, other muscles in our upper chest and neck—namely our scalenes, sternocleido-mastoid, trapezius, and pectoralis minor—jump in to help out. Despite their valiant efforts, these secondary muscles weren't designed to do the heavy lifting of the diaphragm. Over time, these overtaxed muscles wear out, which leads to pain and chronic tension. If you are a chest breather, chances are you are also carrying some unnecessary pain and tension in your neck and shoulders. While popping an aspirin might help in the short term, the long-term solution is to change the way you breathe.

Quick Tip:
Hum for Your Health and Happiness

Feeling down? Humming a happy tune may help! In a 2011 study, researchers discovered that chanting *om,* a sacred Sanskrit syllable commonly used in yoga and meditation that ends with a humming vibration, stimulates the vagus nerve and deactivates the amygdala and other key areas of the brain associated with depression.[2]

Find a comfortable seat. Close your eyes if that feels comfortable to you. Take a full, deep inhalation. On your exhalation, chant, "Om." Drag out the "mmmmm" sound for as long as you can, keeping your lips closed as you do so. Repeat three times.

Sit quietly and notice any sensations in your body, observing how you feel. Not into *om*? Try humming your favorite tune instead.

Chapter 8

Breathing Techniques

Whoever can swallow the breath like the tortoise or pull the breath in and circulate it like the tiger or guide and refine the breath like the dragon shall live a long and healthy life.
—Master Ge Heng, alchemist, second-century China

Before we begin delving into specific breathing techniques, take a few moments to set up your space. Find a quiet place and turn off any distractions, like the television or your phone.

Traditionally, many of these breathing practices are performed seated, with eyes closed. If you do not feel comfortable being seated, you may lie down or prop yourself up with pillows. If you don't feel safe or comfortable closing your eyes, it's absolutely fine to keep them open.

Some of these breathing practices employ what's known as resistance breathing. Resistance breathing intentionally creates airway resistance in the throat to induce a deeply soothing parasympathetic response. Think of a cat purring as it cuddles up on your chest. The vibration produced by your feline's purr has a calming effect on both you and your pet. Studies have shown that cats actually help their owners relieve stress and lower blood pressure more than any other pet, and purring may be a large part of that.

We will cover resistance breathing techniques like ocean breathing and pursed lip breathing. These breathing techniques create an audible sound that may be triggering to someone who has experienced sexual trauma. If any of the sounds in the breathing practices are triggering, stop the breath technique.

We will begin by learning belly breathing. Don't move on to any of the other techniques until you feel comfortable and confident breathing diaphragmatically into your abdomen. Next, get acquainted with the rest of the calming techniques before moving on to the energizing ones. If you feel light-headed or dizzy during any of the exercises, stop immediately. And remember not to practice the energizing breathing techniques if you have any of the conditions listed in the previous chapter (see page 54).

Belly Breath

Belly breath, also known as abdominal or diaphragmatic breath, is a deeply relaxing breath that activates the parasympathetic nervous system. In belly breathing, the diaphragm contracts and moves downward, drawing air into the lower portion of the lungs, which increases beneficial oxygenation of the cells throughout the body. When air moves down into the lower portion of the lungs, our belly softly inflates. On the exhalation, the diaphragm releases upward and our belly moves back in toward the spine. Deep, slow belly breathing also stimulates the vagus nerve, which has a calming effect on body and mind.

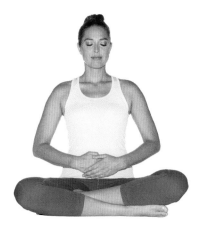

HOW TO DO IT:

- If this is your first time practicing belly breathing, it can be helpful to lie down in order to find full expansion of the abdomen. Once you are able to feel the rise and fall of your abdomen on your back, practice this calming breathing technique sitting up. It is safe to use in any position and situation throughout your day (sitting at your desk, standing in line at the grocery store, or lying down before bed). Wherever you are, create a comfortable surface for yourself where you feel supported. If it feels comfortable to you, close your eyes.

- Close your mouth and begin to breathe in and out slowly through your nose.

- Place one hand gently on your belly and feel your abdomen softly rising as you inhale and falling as you exhale. Relax the muscles of your abdomen and imagine your abdomen inflating like a balloon on the inhalation and naturally deflating on the exhalation. Be gentle with yourself. There is no need to actively push your abdomen out with force. Instead, just allow your breath to rise and fall within you. If you are having trouble feeling the expansion of your belly, place a small object like a light book, a deck of cards, or a small pillow on your abdomen.

- Take a few deep cycles of belly breath and encourage your body to release any muscular tension as you slowly breathe in and out through your nose.

- As you get more comfortable with belly breathing, see if you can stretch out your breathing to only 5 full cycles of breath per minute.

- Close your practice by sitting quietly for a few moments. Observe how you feel. Notice if any thoughts or sensations have shifted. Offer yourself gratitude for taking a few moments out of your day to practice self-care.

USE BELLY BREATH TO:

- calm anxiety and ease stress
- ground yourself during episodes of dissociation
- anchor into the present moment
- help ease chronic pain and release muscular tension
- promote deep and restful sleep

Pursed-Lip Breath

Pursed-lip breath is a variation of diaphragmatic breathing in which you inhale through the nose and exhale through the mouth with pursed lips. This pursing of the lips creates a little resistance, which helps slow down the breath. It's kind of like slowly letting air out of a tire through a tiny hole. As with belly breathing, pursed-lip breath activates your parasympathetic nervous system, stimulates your vagus nerve, and is deeply calming for body and mind.

HOW TO DO IT:

- Find a comfortable seated position. Sit with your spine erect and your shoulders gently dropping away from your ears.
- Inhale slowly through your nose and feel your abdomen softly rising as breath fills your lungs. Relax the muscles of your abdomen and imagine your belly inflating like a balloon. Remember, there is no need to actively push your abdomen out with force.
- Exhale the breath out through your mouth, pursing your lips together to create a smaller opening so the air can release at a slower rate, as if you were slowly deflating a balloon. Your exhalation should never be so forceful that you experience any strain. Feel your abdomen gently drawing in as you exhale out through your mouth.
- Take 5 to 10 cycles of pursed-lip breath, encouraging your body to release any muscular tension as you breathe.
- As you become more comfortable with pursed-lip breathing, see if you can stretch it out to only 5 full cycles of breath per minute.
- Close your practice by sitting quietly for a few moments. Observe how you feel. Notice if any thoughts or sensations have shifted.

USE PURSED-LIP BREATH TO:

- calm anxiety and ease stress
- prevent panic attacks
- ground yourself and anchor into the present moment during episodes of dissociation
- help ease chronic pain and release muscular tension
- promote deep and restful sleep
- ease nausea during pregnancy or chemotherapy

Open Palm/Closed Palm Belly Breath

This breathing exercise pairs belly breathing with the simple motion of opening and closing your hands. If you haven't paid much attention to the way you breathe for most of your life, learning to breathe properly can feel a little awkward at first. It's natural to get confused about when your abdomen should be expanding and when it should be deflating. This grounding practice uses the simple motion of opening your palm, then forming a tight fist to help you physically connect with the sensation of expansion as you inhale and contraction as you exhale.

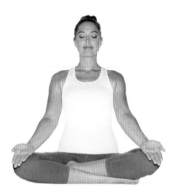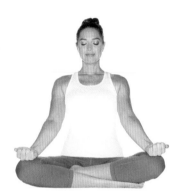

HOW TO DO IT:

- Find a comfortable seated position, with your spine erect and shoulders gently dropping down away from your ears.
- Place your hands on your knees with both palms facing up.
- As you inhale through your nose, open your palms and spread your fingers wide. Feel your belly softly expanding as your fingers open.
- Exhale through your nose and tightly curl your hands into fists. Feel the muscles in your forearms contract and your abdomen softly drawing in.
- Repeat for 5 to 10 cycles of breath.
- Sit quietly and observe how you feel. Were you able to more easily connect with the idea of expansion and contraction in your body?

USE OPEN PALM/CLOSED PALM BELLY BREATH TO:

- physically ground yourself in times of stress, anxiety, or dissociation
- warm up your wrists before beginning your yoga practice

Balloon Breath

Similar to open palm/closed palm belly breath, balloon breath pairs gentle movement of the arms with inhalation and exhalation to help you more deeply connect with the physical sensation of expansion and contraction. It is also a technique often used in meditation and qigong practices. The word *qi* doesn't have a direct English translation, so it often just gets described as "energy." If you're a *Star Wars* fan, you can think of *qi* as "the Force." The word *gong* translates as "skill" or "work." So *qigong* means "the skill of cultivating energy," or simply "energy work."

According to traditional Chinese medicine, the twelve main meridians (or energy pathways) in our body either start or end in our hands and feet. Our hands are thus powerful conduits of energy where we can receive and emit chi. Many acupuncturists and massage therapists will practice some form of qigong to get the energy flowing in their hands before they touch and treat their patients. When you practice balloon breath consistently, you may start to feel a palpable sensation of your own vital life force energy flowing through your hands. It can feel warm, tingly, or magnetic.

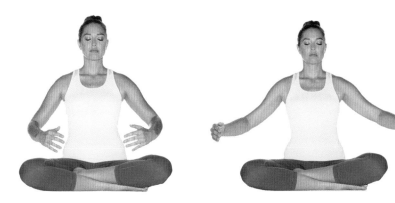

HOW TO DO IT:

- Start in a comfortable seated position with your spine erect and shoulders gently dropping down away from your ears.
- Hold your arms out in front you and gently cup your palms as if you were holding a small balloon or ball between your hands. Keep your shoulders relaxed and elbows slightly bent.
- As you inhale through your nose, expand your hands outward, as if the balloon were inflating between your palms. Feel your abdomen softly expanding as your hands drift apart.

- As you exhale through your nose, bring your hands back toward each other, as if the balloon were deflating. Feel your abdomen softly drawing in as your imaginary balloon shrinks down. The movement of your hands should be slow and smooth, as if they are moving through molasses or pulling apart taffy.

- Repeat for 5 to 10 cycles of breath. You can gradually increase your practice up to 20 minutes to allow yourself to drop into a deep meditative state and really begin to feel the cultivation of energy between your palms.

- Close your practice by resting your palms down on your lap, sitting quietly, and observing how you feel. Do you notice any sensations in your palms? Perhaps a sense of warmth or gentle tingling?

USE BALLOON BREATH TO:

- induce a meditative state that will calm you when you're feeling anxious, stressed, or overwhelmed

- cultivate vital life force energy in the body that can be used in times of fatigue and burnout

Ocean Breath

Ocean breath is a technique used by yogis while practicing the physical postures (known as *asana*) in yoga. In Sanskrit, this breathing technique is called *ujjayi*, which is commonly translated to "victorious breath." Because of its oceanic quality and sound, it is also commonly referred to as ocean breath. When used in synchronization with yoga postures, ocean breath creates a rhythmic flow that grounds you in the present moment and cultivates self-awareness during your practice. It also has a balancing meditative quality that helps soothe the nervous system.

It is a good idea to get comfortable with ocean breath before practicing the movement sequences described in the next chapters. Note that the deep sound of ocean breath can be triggering for some. Instead, you can practice belly breathing (page 61) or pursed-lip breathing (page 63).

HOW TO DO IT:

- Find a comfortable seated position and hold your spine erect.
- Ocean breath is practiced by breathing in and out through your nose with your mouth closed. However, to produce the oceanic sound, open your mouth and make a soft, slow, drawn-out *haaahhhhh* sound as you exhale, as if you were trying to fog up a mirror. The sound should have a whisper-soft quality.
- Once you feel comfortable producing this sound, close your mouth and explore making a similar sound with your lips closed while exhaling out through your nose. Imagine the sound of the ocean when you hold a seashell up to your ear.
- Now let's put it all together. Close your mouth and begin breathing in and out through your nose. Allow your inhalation to be long, slow, and full.
- As you exhale through your nose, gently constrict the back of your throat and release the breath slowly with a gentle oceanic sound. Note that the breath should never be practiced forcefully, as this may strain the back of your throat and vocal cords.
- As you continue breathing, visualize a continuous wave of breath that rises and falls from your abdomen to your upper chest. However, unlike belly breath, ocean breath doesn't actively inflate your belly like a balloon. While your belly may softly move, the focus is not exclusively on your abdomen.
- Repeat for 3 to 5 minutes.

USE OCEAN BREATH TO:

- accompany physical yoga postures
- steady your mind when stressed or agitated
- soothe your nervous system
- create mental focus and presence

Sun Breath

Sun breath is a great practice to introduce once you have learned ocean breath. It integrates ocean breath with gentle arm movements that create greater focus, presence, and body awareness.

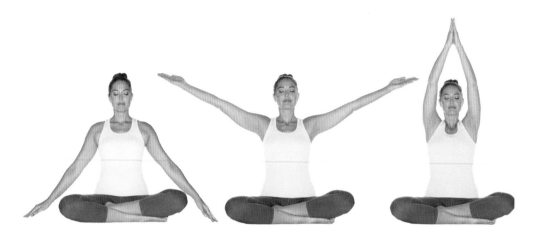

HOW TO DO IT:

- Start from a seated position, with your spine erect and your arms down by your side.
- Close your mouth and take a few slow, deep ocean breaths through your nose.
- On the inhalation, turn your palms outward and sweep your arms out and up toward the sky. Bring your palms to touch overhead with your arms held straight as you reach the peak of your inhalation.
- On the exhalation, sweep your arms back down by your side.
- Repeat for 5 to 8 cycles of breath.

USE SUN BREATH TO:

- prepare for a yoga practice
- balance and harmonize your nervous system
- ease agitated thoughts and worry
- oxygenate your body
- focus your mind

Three-Part Breath

This ancient yogic breathing technique known as the three-part breath, or *dirga pranayama* in Sanskrit, is particularly helpful during times of stress. *Dirga* means "complete." You can think of it as a complete breath that rises and falls in a continuous wave from your abdomen to your upper chest. Practicing the three-part breath for 5 to 15 minutes can help decrease stress and promote a sense of well-being and calm.

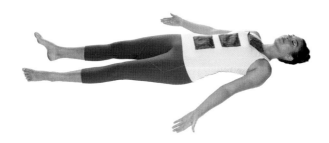

HOW TO DO IT:

- When first learning the three-part breath, lie down on your back. Find a comfortable position and support yourself with pillows as needed. To more easily feel the physical sensation of breath filling your body, try placing a small object on each of the three positions you will be breathing into: your belly, your rib cage, and your chest.

- Part 1 (breathing into your belly): Close your eyes and mouth and begin to breathe in and out slowly through your nose. Place one hand on your belly and feel your abdomen softly inflating like a balloon as you inhale and slowly deflating as you exhale. Practice 3 cycles of breath in this manner, noticing how your belly rises and falls with your breath.

- Part 2 (breathing into your rib cage): Inhale through your nose, filling your belly up with breath like a balloon. Continue inhaling the same breath up into your rib cage, feeling your middle lungs expand and your ribs widen. As you exhale through your nose, release the air first from your middle lungs and rib cage, then from your belly. Repeat this slow and steady breath, drawing up from your abdomen and into your rib cage, for 3 cycles of breath.

- Part 3 (breathing into your upper chest): Inhale through your nose, first feeling your belly expand, then your rib cage. Continue inhaling the same breath up into your upper lungs, expanding your upper chest all the way to your collarbones at the base of your throat. On your exhalation, first release the air from your upper chest, then your rib cage, then your belly. Practice this full three-part rhythm for 5 to 8 cycles of breath.
- Close your breathing practice by sitting quietly and observing how both your body and mind feel.

USE THREE-PART BREATH TO:

- temper anxiety or nervous energy
- help alleviate insomnia and induce sleep

Alternate Nostril Breath

Alternate nostril breath is an ancient yogic breathing practice known as *nadi sodhana*. It activates the parasympathetic nervous system and is particularly helpful in calming anxiety and aiding in restful sleep.

Nadis are energetic pathways in the body, through which our *prana*, or vital life force energy, flows. *Sodhana* means "to purify" in Sanskrit. *Nadi sodhana* is a practice that clears out or purifies the energy and circulation channels in the body. It is performed by alternating the breath from one nostril to the other. By balancing the airflow of the left and right nostril, you balance the left and right hemispheres of your brain, making this the perfect preparation for meditation practice.

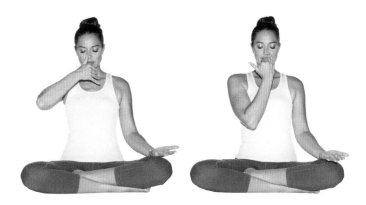

HOW TO DO IT:

- Find a comfortable seated position with your spine erect.
- Open your right palm wide with fingers spread. Curl your index and middle fingers in toward your palm, keeping your thumb, ring finger, and pinkie finger extended.
- Place your thumb against your right nostril and inhale slowly through your left nostril.
- Next, close your left nostril with your right ring finger, release your thumb from your right nostril, and slowly exhale through your right nostril.
- Inhale through your right nostril, then close your right nostril with your thumb, release your ring finger from your left nostril, and exhale through your left nostril. You have now completed one round of alternate nostril breathing.
- Repeat for 5 to 10 cycles.

USE ALTERNATE NOSTRIL BREATH TO:

- calm your nervous system in times of stress or anxiety
- stop a panic attack before it starts
- alleviate insomnia

Cautions and Contraindications

Do not perform alternate nostril breath if you have a cold, stuffy nose, or sinus congestion.

4–7–8 Breath

The 4–7–8 breath is a breathing technique used often in yoga classes and body-based therapy settings to quell anxiety and quickly induce a soothing effect on the nervous system. Dr. Andrew Weil, a world-renowned pioneer in the field of integrative medicine, is a huge proponent of the 4–7–8 breath and popularly prescribes it as an antidote to stress and as a powerful tool against insomnia. You can watch a video of him performing this breathing technique on his website at www.drweil.com.

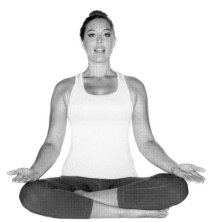

Note: If it feels uncomfortable or triggering to hold your breath, skip the breath retention step and just practice the inhalation and exhalation.

HOW TO DO IT:

- Find a comfortable seated position or practice lying down if you are using 4–7–8 breath to help you fall asleep.
- Place the tip of your tongue just behind your front teeth near the roof of your mouth. Your tongue will rest here throughout the duration of the practice.
- With your tongue in position, part your lips, and make a *whoosh* sound as you exhale completely through your mouth.
- Close your lips and inhale deeply through your nose, mentally counting to 4.
- Hold your breath as you silently count to 7.
- Exhale through your mouth, repeating the whoosh sound for a count of 8. This completes one cycle of breath. Complete 4 cycles of breath total.

USE 4–7–8 BREATH TO:

- calm anxiety and agitation
- help you fall asleep

Cooling Breath

This cooling yogic breathing technique is known as *sitali pranayama*. It works by drawing cool air into the mouth to diminish excess heat in the body, regulate body temperature, and soothe the nervous system during times of stress or agitation. An alternate option (described on the next page), for those who are unable to curl their tongue, is known as *sitkari pranayama*, or "teeth hissing breath." It works similarly to *sitali* by cooling the body and calming the nervous system.

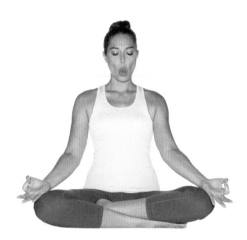

HOW TO DO IT:

- Find a comfortable seated position and sit with your spine elongated and shoulders relaxed.

- Curl the sides of your tongue in toward each other like a taco shell and stick your tongue out of your mouth like a straw.

- Lower your chin slightly and inhale through your mouth, sipping the air in through your curled tongue as if you were sipping cool water from a straw. As you inhale, slowly lift your chin up toward the sky, taking care not to lift so high that you strain the back of your neck.

- At the end of your inhalation, draw your tongue back into your mouth, close your lips, and exhale slowly through both nostrils as you slowly lower your chin back to your starting position.

- Repeat for 5 to 10 breaths.

ALTERNATE OPTION:

Note: The ability to curl your tongue is genetic. If you can't curl your tongue, try this alternate cooling breath practice; it is equally effective.

- With your mouth closed, curl the tip of your tongue upward so it touches the roof of your mouth right behind your front teeth.
- With upper and lower teeth gently touching, part your lips and inhale through your mouth, making a soft hissing sound as cool air fills your mouth.
- Close your lips and exhale slowly through your nostrils.
- Repeat for 5 to 10 breaths.

USE COOLING BREATH TO:

- reduce anger, frustration, agitation, and anxiety
- cool your body and release excess heat
- calm your nervous system in times of stress

Energizing Breathing Techniques

The following energizing breathing practices are safe for most when practiced as described. However, in cases of severe trauma or stress, activating breathing techniques can cause emotional flooding, agitation, increased anxiety, or overwhelm and are not advised. Do not practice these energizing breathing techniques if you are pregnant, have high blood pressure, a history of seizures, glaucoma, retinal detachment, asthma, or psychiatric conditions like bipolar disorder, psychosis, or paranoia, as they could trigger a manic episode.

Joyful Breath

You can think of joyful breath like a natural jolt of caffeine without the jittery side effects. It is a stimulating and uplifting breathing technique that energizes the body and wakes up the mind. It is often known as "ha" breath because of the sound made while practicing it. In Hawaiian, *ha* means "breath" or "spirit," and it is often translated to mean "breath of life." In Eastern self-healing traditions like qigong, the *ha* or *he* sound is a healing sound associated with the heart and the element of fire. The movement of the arms in this breathing technique also encourages blood flow to the heart.

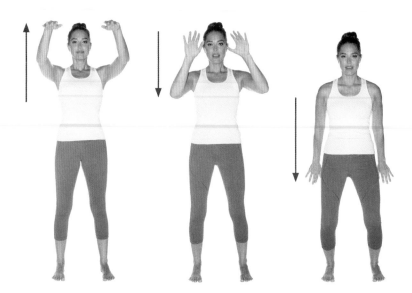

HOW TO DO IT:

- Start standing with your feet hip-width distance apart, spine erect, and a slight bend in your knees. Rest your arms gently down by your sides.

- Inhale through your nose as you raise your arms straight out in front of you at eye-level height. Keep your elbows slightly bent and shoulders, wrists, and fingers relaxed as you float your arms up.

- Exhale through your mouth, making a loud *ha* sound as you powerfully bring your arms straight back down, pushing your palms down toward the floor. Visualize yourself releasing any negative thoughts, feelings, energy, or emotions as you swing your arms down to the floor. Allow the earth to absorb and neutralize any negative energy so it is no longer stored in your body, mind, and spirit. This completes one cycle.

- Repeat for 5 to 10 cycles.

USE JOYFUL BREATH TO:

- provide a mental or physical pick-me-up
- ease lethargy, sluggishness, and depression
- enliven your body and brain

Breath of Fire

Breath of fire is a powerful breathing technique that quickly oxygenates the blood, creating an immediate effect of mental and physical alertness. In the Kundalini yoga tradition, this breath is also believed to help clear mental and creative blockages.

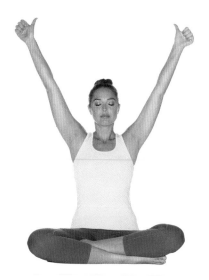

Tip: You may want to keep a box of tissues by your side, as this practice is known for clearing out your nasal passages!

HOW TO DO IT:

- Sit comfortably on the floor or a cushion in a cross-legged position.
- Inhale through your nose and sweep your arms up toward the ceiling, forming a wide V shape with your palms open and your fingers spread wide.
- Exhale through your nose as you curl your fingers on each hand in toward your palms, keeping your thumbs extended out. Hold this arm position for the duration of the breathing practice.
- To prep for breath of fire, open your mouth and visualize a puppy panting, simulating that rapid rhythm with your own breath. It may feel a little silly, but this will help you establish a rhythm for your breath of fire practice.
- Once your rhythm is set, close your mouth and breathe only through your nostrils at the same pace. Your inhalations should match the length of your exhalations. As you breathe, feel your stomach pumping in and out rapidly at the same pace, with your belly gently pushing out as you inhale and drawing in as you exhale.

- Practice for 1 to 3 minutes.
- To close your practice, take a full, deep breath in through your nose and slowly exhale through your nose. Release your arms down, place your palms on your lap, and take a few moments in stillness.
- Observe any sensations in your body and notice how you feel.

USE BREATH OF FIRE TO:

- energize your body and mind, especially during periods of fatigue or depression
- release anger and other deeply buried emotions
- improve mental alertness and wake up your brain
- improve lung capacity
- relieve congestion

Cautions and Contraindications

Activating breathing techniques like Breath of Fire can cause emotional flooding, agitation, anxiety, or overwhelm in some people who have experienced severe trauma or stress. Do not practice breath of fire if you are pregnant, have high blood pressure, a history of seizures, glaucoma, retinal detachment, asthma, or psychiatric conditions like bipolar disorder, psychosis, or paranoia. If you feel light-headed or dizzy, stop immediately.

Bellows Breath

Bellows breath quickly oxygenates your body and stimulates your sympathetic nervous system. Remember that, although the sympathetic nervous system is the home of our fight-or-flight response, it is also the home for emotions like joy, elation, excitement, and arousal. Bellows breath can be particularly helpful with depression, as it momentarily activates your arousal system and helps energy flow through your body.

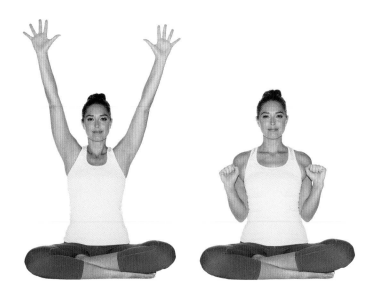

HOW TO DO IT:

- Sit on the floor or a cushion in a cross-legged position with your spine erect. If sitting cross-legged is uncomfortable, you may also sit on a chair with both feet planted on the ground.

- Bend your elbows and hug them into your ribs. Keeping your elbows bent, raise your hands to shoulder height and make tight fists.

- Inhale through your nose as you powerfully reach both arms straight up over your head, with palms open and fingers spread wide.

- Exhale through your nose as you powerfully draw your arms back down to your starting position with fists clenched and elbows next to your rib cage.

- Practice 10 rounds to start at the rate of 1 inhalation and 1 exhalation per second.

USE BELLOWS BREATH TO:

- combat sluggishness, fatigue, or depression
- quickly oxygenate your body
- invigorate your body and mind

Cautions and Contraindications

Do not practice bellows breath if you are pregnant, have high blood pressure, have asthma, are currently experiencing panic attacks, have been diagnosed with bipolar disorder, or have a history of manic episodes. If you feel light-headed or dizzy, stop immediately.

Chapter 9

Movement Sequences for Physical and Emotional Healing

The body is a multilingual being. It speaks through its color and
its temperature, the flush of recognition, the glow of love, the ash
of pain, the heat of arousal, the coldness of nonconviction. It speaks
through its constant tiny dance, sometimes swaying, sometimes
a-jitter, sometimes trembling. It speaks through the leaping of the
heart, the falling of the spirit, the pit at the center, and rising hope.
—Clarissa Pinkola Estés

The following Primal Yoga sequences were designed to help ground and center you to move through any challenge you may be facing. Each sequence is intentionally created to help you find relief from some of the most common symptoms of trauma, including depression, anxiety, fear, anger, chronic pain, chronic fatigue, digestive issues, and more.

Flip to the sequence your body, mind, and spirit needs the most on any given day. Like any form of exercise, the sequences are best used as preventative measures, but they are also very effective in helping you relieve unpleasant and uncomfortable symptoms, thoughts, and sensations in the moment. While nothing is a miracle cure, many of my students constantly express their amazement at how simple and effective these techniques are for easing their anxiety, lifting their energy, boosting their mood, relieving pain, and creating a sense of empowerment—all in less than an hour.

Even if you don't get through every movement in each sequence or decide to simply start with your breath and leave the rest for another day, know that you are taking powerful steps toward reclaiming your health and vibrancy. Have patience with and compassion for yourself during the process.

Take a moment to acknowledge the courage it took to get here. If you are holding this book in your hands, you are already showing up for yourself in a powerful way. May these sequences provide you with continued inspiration to keep showing up for yourself. You are so very worth it.

It is always best to consult with a doctor for medical clearance before starting any exercise program. Stop if you experience any pain, shortness of breath, or dizziness.

Yoga Props to Support Your Practice

Many of the sequences to follow include the optional use of yoga props. Common props like blocks, bolsters, and blankets are used to help support a practitioner in creating more stability, better alignment, and greater comfort or deepening in any given posture.

Blocks: A block is one of the most common and useful yoga props. They are usually made of cork, wood, or firm foam and resemble a large brick with general dimensions of 9 by 6 by 4 inches. They can be used in an infinite number of ways, including supporting people with injuries or tight muscles, refining postures, and helping create better balance and stability. Choosing which block is right for you is simply a matter of personal preference. Wooden blocks are incredibly durable, but are often slippery with sweaty hands or feet, may slide on wooden floors, and are generally more expensive. Cork blocks are a sturdy and aesthetically pleasing option offering great grip and durability. The downside is that they absorb sweat, which can result in an unpleasant odor over time. They are also heavier, which makes them less travel friendly. Foam blocks are the cheapest, softest, most lightweight, and most travel-friendly option. The downside is that they show dirt and sweat easily and aren't as sturdy as cork. My favorite blocks are the cork or recycled foam blocks from Manduka Yoga (available online at www.manduka.com), but more affordable options are easily found online.

Bolsters: A yoga bolster is a common prop that looks similar to a firm body pillow (though it is usually rectangular or cylindrical in shape). It provides support in restorative poses to create a gentle opening in your body. You can purchase yoga bolsters online or simply use a stack of firm pillows as an alternative.

Blankets: Yoga blankets provide greater comfort and support in many seated and restorative postures. They are made of thickly woven material and come in many sizes and colors. You can purchase them online, or simply use your own thickly woven, folded blankets from home.

Moving Through Depression

The universe works in mysterious ways and always seems to deliver the lessons we need to learn at just the right moment. As I write these words, I am currently witnessing someone very close to me struggle to emerge from one of the darkest pits of depression I have ever seen.

Depression is dangerous because it can sneak up so slowly that you often don't recognize it until it's too late. Despite my great personal interest, research, and work in the subject, it embarrasses me to say that I missed the most telltale signs. Or perhaps I chose not to see the signs because, up until that point, this person was one of the most positive, upbeat people I had ever met. After introducing this person to my dad, I asked, "Have you ever met someone so freaking positive all the time?"

My dad responded, "Yes, but where does he put the rest of it?"

It was an astute observation by someone who would know. My father struggled with clinical depression for much of his adult life. When I was a teenager, he would skip work, lock his bedroom door, and sleep all day. As he slept away what felt like weeks and months, my family tiptoed around him, knowing that something was wrong but not knowing how to help. We lived a mile away from the beach, and when I was in my twenties, my father confided in me that he once swam out as far from the shore as possible and contemplated what it would be like to simply stop swimming—to sink and never resurface.

I'm happy to say that my dad now manages his depression with a combination of medication and exercise. While his diet could certainly use a little help—okay, *a lot* of help (sorry, Dad!)—he is in good spirits.

Sleep disturbances are one of the first signs of depression, and it was the sign that I, unfortunately, missed with my friend. Sleep disturbances can show up in different ways for different people—some sleep too much and simply can't seem to get up and out of bed, while others can't sleep at all. My friend complained of insomnia, but I chalked it up to stress. When I checked in on him a few weeks later, the positive person I once knew had completely vanished and been replaced by a severely depressed man who was barely eating, working, or functioning.

Had I fully grasped what was happening, I would have encouraged him to get moving as soon as the first signs of depression appeared. As Dr. John Ratey says, "At its core, depression is defined by an absence of moving toward anything, and exercise is the way to divert those negative signals and trick the brain into coming out of hibernation."[1]

Depression is a classic symptom of trauma. It drains you of your life force energy. The telltale signs of depression are symptoms that persist for a prolonged period of time (at least two weeks or more) and can include one or more of the following:

- feelings of hopelessness
- persistent sadness or feelings of "emptiness"
- persistent anxiety
- irritability
- lack of motivation
- loss of interest in activities that were once pleasurable
- low energy and chronic fatigue
- difficulty concentrating and making decisions
- foggy memory
- difficulty sleeping
- loss of appetite and/or weight gain or loss
- suicidal thoughts or attempts
- chronic pain with no clear cause
- digestive issues

If you are experiencing any of the symptoms above, practice natural prevention now, so you don't require medical intervention later.

The following Primal Yoga sequence enlivens your body on a cellular level through energizing breathing techniques and uplifting yoga postures designed to clear physical or emotional blockages and reconnect you with your vital life force energy.

Quick Tip:
Bouncing Qigong

While a full sequence to combat depression follows on page 87, I would like to begin by offering a single, simple movement to alleviate depression. If you're having a hard time getting up and moving, begin with this baby step. Here's an exercise you can do right here, right now. No sneakers, sweatbands, or workout gear required. The beauty of bouncing qigong is its simplicity. Unlike other forms of qigong, it doesn't require you to learn a sequence, breath pattern, or any other set of rules.

HOW TO DO IT:

- Clear a small space, making sure you have enough room to swing your arms without bumping into anything. Stand with your feet slightly wider than hip-width distance apart. Gently bend your knees and let your arms hang loosely down by your sides.

- Allow your body to relax and begin to softly bounce. Your feet don't need to leave the floor—bounce by simply bending your knees.

- After a few moments, experiment with lifting your heels off the floor as you bounce. Bounce with a little more vigor while still keeping your limbs relaxed. Let yourself wiggle and jiggle. Shake your wrists, wiggle your fingers, and let your arms flop and flap as you bounce.

- Let your intuition guide you. Explore jumping up and down. Explore closing your eyes and keeping them open. Relax your neck and let your head nod yes and shake no. Let your arms swing and shake up in the air or shake them down low. Wiggle your hips. Bounce in a circle. Bounce silently or let yourself laugh, cry, or howl.

- There is no time limit. When you feel like stopping, stop. Pause for a moment standing still. Let your arms rest gently down by your sides without touching your body or your clothing. Close your eyes or keep them open—whatever feels most comfortable to you.

- Take a moment to tune into your body. Observe what you are feeling. Notice any and all sensations. Do you feel a rush of heat? A tingling in your palms or fingers? An increase in your heart rate? Track these sensations without any judgment or mental commentary. Observe any emotions that may have arisen and welcome them all with curiosity.

- Take a slow, deep inhale through your nose and audibly sigh it out of your mouth to close your practice.

- Repeat this practice daily and any time you are feeling low on energy. It's a wonderful way to get moving first thing in the morning to bring vibrancy to your day.

Why It Works: Shaking Off Your Stress

Need more motivation to bounce? While bouncing qigong is inspired by ancient wisdom, modern trauma research backs it up. Researchers have discovered that, unlike humans, animals in the wild don't display symptoms of PTSD, although they are exposed to traumatic situations on a regular basis. Remember our discussion about how animals shake off their trauma by literally shaking and trembling from head to toe? That shaking helps rid their nervous system of stress hormones, allowing them to go back to homeostasis moments later.

Bouncing qigong works to much the same effect. It allows you to begin shaking off stored trauma and releasing stuck emotions. Welcome any and every emotion as a success on your path to healing.

Primal Yoga Sequence for Releasing Depression

1. Bouncing Qigong *(see instructions on page 85)*

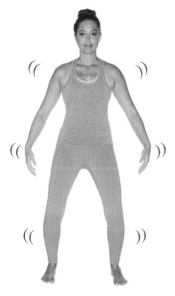

Begin with 3 minutes of bouncing qigong to warm up your body. Depression can numb us to emotions and sensations. Bouncing energizes your body, gets your blood flowing, and connects you to your vital life force energy.

Once you've finished bouncing, let your arms rest gently down by your sides without touching your body. Close your eyes or keep them open—whatever feels most comfortable to you. Take a moment to tune into your body. Observe what you are feeling. Track all sensations with curiosity.

2. Heart Taps

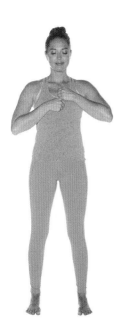

Stand with your feet hip-width distance apart. Make light fists with both hands. Bring your fists to the center of your chest, one fist above the other, and begin lightly tapping your heart with both fists simultaneously. Continue tapping for 1 minute.

Benefits: In Chinese medicine, it is believed that our spirit (called shen) is housed in the heart. If our heart is not being cared for, our spirit gets lost and confused. The heart is ruled by the element of fire, and if we are deficient in heart qi, our inner fire can burn out. This leads to depression, lack of animation, loss of creativity, and low energy. Tapping our heart awakens our heart chakra, enlivens our lungs, and brings energy and sensation to a place we may have closed off or kept numb.

3. Lung Taps

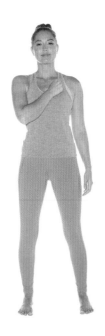

Stand with your feet hip-width distance apart. Make a light fist with your right hand, bend your right elbow, and bring your right fist to the left side of your chest just below your collarbone. Begin gently tapping the left side of your chest, below your collarbone and over your heart. Tap back and forth from your left shoulder to the center of your chest. Increase your tapping to a pressure that feels firm yet comfortable. As you continue tapping, raise your left arm out in front of you, palm facing up. Tap from your chest down your left arm. Tap your biceps, your forearm, your wrist, your thumb, and the palm of your hand, then tap back up your arm until you end up back at your chest.

Repeat the tapping sequence on the opposite side. When you have finished tapping, release your arms down by your sides and observe how you feel. Notice any sensations in your body. Do you feel more energized?

Benefits: Tapping is an ancient self-healing practice that moves energy in the body. According to traditional Chinese medicine, we have twelve main meridians (or energy pathways) in the body. The meridians run symmetrically on both sides of the body. Each meridian corresponds to a different organ system, and each organ system is paired with a particular emotion. Grief is stored in the lungs, and can be accompanied by depression and fatigue. The lung meridian starts in the upper chest near the collarbones and shoulder and runs down the arm into the thumb. In this tapping practice, we bring vibrancy to the lung meridian to start moving stagnant energy like grief and depression.

4. Joyful Breath *(see instructions on page 76)*

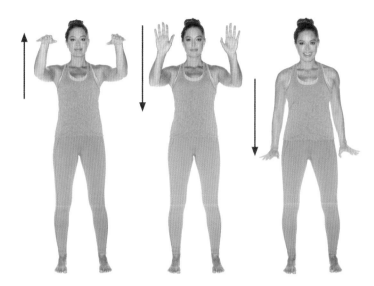

Do 5 to 10 rounds of joyful breath to energize your body and uplift your mood.

5. Mountain Pose Stretch

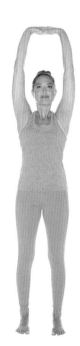

Stand with your feet hip-width distance apart, feet parallel. Plant your feet firmly, spread your toes, activate the inner arches of your feet, and engage your thigh muscles, drawing energy up from the earth. Inhale and sweep your arms overhead. Bring your palms together, interlace your fingers, and press your palms open toward the ceiling as you elongate through your spine. Keep the base of your neck soft and your shoulders relaxed away from your ears.

Benefits: This pose stretches your abdomen; opens your chest and shoulders; and energizes your body.

6. Joyful Crescent

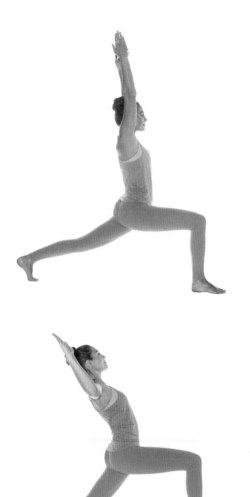

Start standing with your feet hip-width distance apart, holding your spine tall. Step your left foot back approximately one leg length, and bend your right knee to a 90-degree angle to come into a crescent lunge. Lengthen your tailbone toward the floor and press your left heel toward the back of the room. Inhale and sweep your arms up toward the ceiling with your palms facing each other. Lengthen your torso and draw your front ribs in to engage your core. Exhale to deepen the pose.

On your next inhale, turn your palms to face forward and bend your elbows out to the side at a 90-degree angle, creating a goal-post shape with your arms. Send your elbow tips slightly forward as you lift your heart up toward the ceiling and gaze softly up, without straining your neck. Put a gentle bend in your back knee, lengthen your tailbone toward the floor, and continue to hug your front ribs in to engage your core and support your lower back. Exhale and return to crescent lunge.

Do 3 rounds, synchronizing your movement with your breath, then repeat on the opposite side.

Benefits: This movement stretches your legs and hip flexors; opens up your chest and shoulders; strengthens your back, thighs, and butt; improves your balance; increases energy and stamina; and reduces fatigue.

7. Bridge Pose

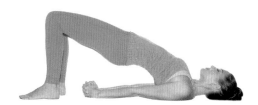

Lie on your back, bend your knees, and place your feet flat on the floor hip-width distance apart. Inhale and drive your heels down as you lift your hips up off the floor. Engage your inner thighs and glutes and lengthen your tailbone toward the back of your knees. Interlace your fingers beneath you and wiggle your shoulders closer together to create more expansion in your chest. Press the back of your head gently into the floor, keeping your neck neutral and your gaze softly lifted. Hold the pose for 5 full cycles of breath.

Benefits: This pose stretches your chest, neck, and hips; strengthens your back and legs; opens up your spine; energizes your body; helps relieve mild depression; reduces fatigue; and relieves backache.

8. Supported Bridge

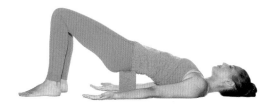

Lie on your back, bend your knees, and place your feet flat on the floor hip-width distance apart. Inhale and drive your heels down as you lift your hips up off the floor. Place a block under your sacrum (the triangular bone at the base of your spine) and let your pelvis rest down on the block. Adjust the height of the block to what feels most comfortable and best supports your body. Rest your arms down on the floor to either side of you, palms facing up. Stay in supported bridge pose for 5 to 8 cycles of breath.

Benefits: This pose stretches your chest, neck, and hips; opens up your spine; helps relieve mild depression; calms your brain; and relieves backache.

9. Supported Half Shoulderstand

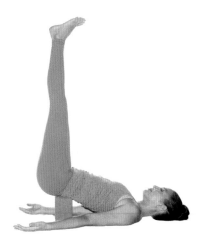

From supported bridge pose, bring one knee into your chest at a time, staying balanced on the block as you move. Slowly reach both legs straight up toward the ceiling and flex your feet. Your heels should stack directly above your hips. Adjust the block higher up toward your hips if you feel unsupported or unsteady. Rest here with your arms down by your sides for 5 to 8 cycles of breath.

Benefits: This pose reduces fatigue; calms your mind and eases anxiety; helps relieve mild depression; alleviates insomnia; relieves tired legs; and stretches your shoulders and neck.

10. Supported Rest Pose with Heart Opening Variation

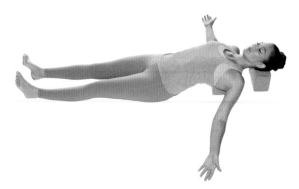

Lie down on your back and place a block horizontally underneath your shoulder blades. Place a second block beneath your head for support. Adjust the height of the blocks so you feel a gentle stretch in the front of your chest without straining your neck or back. Rest your arms on the floor, away from your torso with palms up. Release any muscular tension in your body and allow your chest to expand. Stay in the pose anywhere from 5 to 10 minutes.

Benefits: This pose stretches the front of your chest; supports your upper back; supports the release of any sadness, heaviness, or numbness stored in your heart; helps lower blood pressure; deeply calms your body and soothes your mind; helps relieve stress, anxiety, and mild depression; reduces insomnia; and promotes a sense of well-being.

Moving Through Anxiety and Stress

According to the Anxiety and Depression Association of America (ADAA), anxiety disorders are the most common mental health issue in the United States today, affecting 40 million adults. That's 18 percent of our entire population! Not only that, but despite the fact that anxiety is treatable, only one-third of those who suffer from it receive treatment. This may well have to do with the fact that dealing with anxiety from a Western point of view is expensive: a full one-third of the United States' total mental health bill of $148 billion goes toward anxiety—that's *$42 billion per year.* Anxiety is often accompanied by depression, the latter of which is the leading cause of disability among American adults between the ages of fifteen and forty-five.[2]

Anxiety makes it hard to concentrate on tasks, be present with our loved ones, and feel safe within ourselves and our surroundings. It rapidly shrinks our world and may prevent those afflicted with it from attending social gatherings, meeting new people, and creating new experiences.

The following sequence helps you shake off stress and anxious energy before moving into a series of restorative postures that are effective for calming your mind and balancing your nervous system.

1. Bouncing Qigong *(see instructions on page 85)*

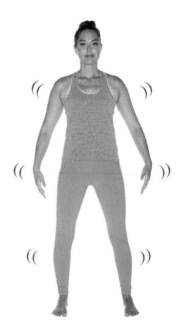

Before we begin, take a moment to rate your anxiety on a scale of one to ten. Then begin with 3 minutes of bouncing qigong to warm up your body and shake off any anxious energy. Bouncing qigong is as effective for anxiety as it is for depression. Anxious energy gets trapped in our body and can create a host of unpleasant physical sensations. To calm our nervous system, we must first release this pent-up nervous energy, and bouncing is a great way to let it go!

Once you've finished bouncing, let your arms rest gently down by your sides. Close your eyes or keep them open—whatever feels most comfortable to you. Take a moment to tune into your body. Observe what you are feeling. Notice any and all sensations without any judgment. Check in with yourself and rate your anxiety again. Where does it fall now on a scale of one to ten?

2. Energy Gathering

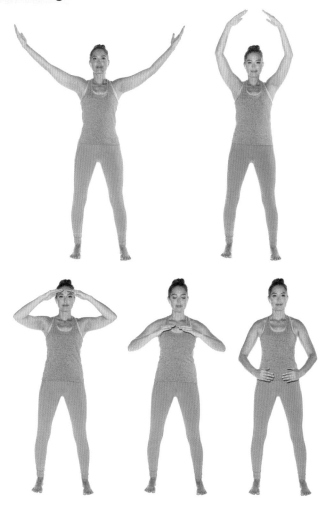

Stand with your feet hip-width distance apart, arms resting down by your sides. Inhale and sweep your arms out and up over your head as if you were holding a giant beach ball. As you exhale, slowly lower your arms down in front of your forehead, continuing down the center line of your body past your navel, as if you were pressing the ball down toward the floor. Visualize pulling any nervous or anxious energy down from your head and releasing it out through the soles of your feet, where it is neutralized and absorbed by the earth. Release your arms down by your sides and take a few moments to root down through your feet, feeling centered and grounded.

Benefits: In qigong, this energy-gathering movement is sometimes referred to as "pulling down the heavens." Anxiety often takes up residence in our head, creating racing thoughts and fears. This simple, gentle movement encourages agitated energy to move out of your head and be released out of your body, leaving you grounded and calm.

3. Returning *Qi*

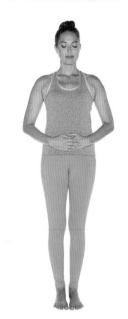

Step your feet together and place one hand on top of the other on your lower belly, just below your navel at your lower abdomen. Visualize sending yourself healing energy through your palms into your lower *dantian* (your body's lower energy center or "elixir field") and see this energy radiating out from your center, nourishing every cell in your body.

Benefits: This movement gathers and guides any excess qi *back to your lower* dantian *to help neutralize any energy imbalances and prevent energy from being scattered.*

4. Supported Standing Forward Fold

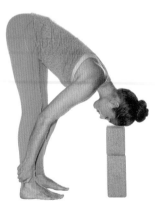

Start standing with your feet parallel, hip-width distance apart. Inhale and sweep your arms up toward the ceiling with palms facing each other, elongating through your spine. Exhale and fold forward from your hips, allowing your spine and head to drape forward toward the floor. Rest your forehead gently on two blocks in front of you. You may use more or fewer blocks, depending on how open your hamstrings feel. If you don't have blocks, stack up a pile of pillows instead.

Lightly catch your ankles with your hands as you release your spine to gravity. If your hands don't reach your ankles, you can place them down on additional blocks to either side of you. Bend your knees slightly and engage your quadriceps, lifting your kneecaps. Shift your weight slightly forward toward the balls of your feet so your hips stack over your ankle bones. Feel your sitting bones drawing up as you continue to drape your torso down, creating a stretch through the backs of your legs. Breathe deeply in and out through your nose. Hold the pose for 1 minute.

Benefits: This pose increases flexibility in your hamstrings and calves, creates suppleness in your spine, relieves tension in your neck and shoulders, calms your brain and soothes nerves, helps relieve anxiety and mild depression, and helps ease headaches and insomnia.

5. Supported Seated Forward Fold

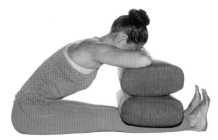

Sit down with your legs straight out in front of you, feet flexed. Inhale and sweep your arms up toward the ceiling, elongating through your spine and reaching through the crown of your head. Exhale and fold forward from your hips. Place one or two bolsters or pillows gently on your shins and rest your forehead down on the bolsters. You may fold your arms on top of the bolsters and rest your forehead on your forearms if you need more support. Soften the base of your neck as you breathe deeply in and out through your nose. Hold the pose for 1 minute.

Benefits: This pose stretches your spine, hamstrings, and calves; calms your mind and helps relieve anxiety and mild depression; reduces fatigue; and helps ease headaches and insomnia.

6. Legs up the Wall

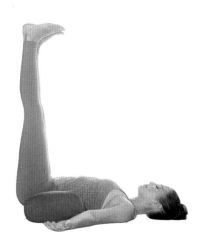

Place a bolster parallel to the wall and a few inches away from it. Sit parallel to the wall on the bolster. Gently roll onto your back as you swing your legs up the wall. Press your heels into the wall and lift your hips slightly off the bolster, allowing your hips to wiggle forward so your sitting bones gently release into the space between the bolster and the wall. Rest your arms down on the floor, palms up. Stay in the pose for 3 to 8 minutes.

Note: A pillow or stacked and folded blankets may be used in place of a bolster.

Benefits: This pose helps relieve anxiety and mild depression, helps relieve headaches and migraines, eases menstrual cramps and premenstrual symptoms, soothes tired legs, and promotes restful sleep.

7. Supported Rest Pose

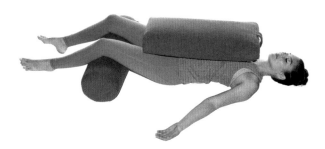

Lie down on your back and place a bolster under your knees to ease tired legs and help support your lower back. If you don't have a bolster, you can use pillows or a rolled blanket. As an option, place a second bolster on your torso and chest. The gentle weight of the extra bolster acts like a weighted security blanket, providing a deeper sense of security as you rest. Rest your arms on the floor, away from your torso with palms up and fingers soft. Release any muscular tension in your body as you soften into the floor. Stay in the pose anywhere from 5 to 15 minutes.

Benefits: This pose helps to lower blood pressure; deeply calms your body and soothes your mind; helps relieve stress, anxiety, and mild depression; reduces insomnia; and promotes a sense of well-being.

8. Alternate Nostril Breath *(see instructions on page 71)*

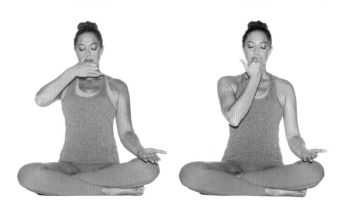

End your practice with 5 to 10 cycles of alternate nostril breath to deeply calm your nervous system and create a sense of balance and well-being.

9. Seated Heart Hug

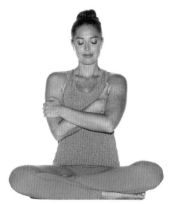

After you have completed a few rounds of alternate nostril breath, breathe naturally and sit comfortably with your legs crossed. Fold your arms across your chest and tuck the fingers of one hand into your opposite armpit, leaving your thumb out. Place your opposite hand on your opposite upper arm with a gentle squeeze. One side usually feels more comfortable and comforting than the other, so experiment to determine which side feels most nurturing to you. Take a few moments to hold yourself in this warm and loving embrace. You can mentally affirm: *I am safe. I am grounded.*

Benefits: This simple posture is a grounding, self-soothing technique that nurtures your body, mind, and spirit and creates a sense of safety and security.

Quick Tip:
Anxiety Antidote: Wash Away Your Worry

If you're feeling anxiety creeping up on you but don't have time to practice the full sequence above, try splashing cold water on your face from your scalp line to your lips. This stimulates your vagus nerve and slows down your heart rate, essentially tricking your brain into feeling less stressed. You can also try taking a cold shower.

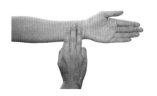 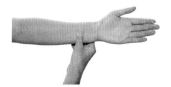

Anxiety can strike at the most inopportune moments, like when you're sitting in the middle of a meeting about to give a big presentation. If you don't have time to run to the bathroom to splash cold water on your face or aren't chummy enough with your coworkers to show off your bouncing qigong skills, try this acupressure technique that is discreet enough to do in public without anyone being any the wiser.

Nei guan, or "inner gate," is an acupressure point located three finger-widths below your wrist crease in between the two tendons of your forearm. It's effective for easing anxiety and is also used for relieving nausea, motion sickness, and headaches.

To find it, turn your left palm open and measure three fingers down from your wrist using your right hand. Using your right thumb, find the two tendons located here and press firmly down between the tendons. Hold this downward pressure for 5 seconds.

Moving Through Fear

Our culture teaches us to see fear as a sign of weakness. As a fearful child who grew into a fearful adult, I always felt like I was failing at life because everything scared me. When I was a teenager, my mom gave me a book called *The Gift of Fear*, by Gavin de Becker. Unfortunately, I parked it on my bookshelf to collect dust. Had I actually read it, I would have saved myself a lot of unnecessary suffering by learning to trust my intuition and use fear not as my enemy, but as my ally.

In the book, de Becker, who is a leading expert in the prediction and prevention of violence, talks about the difference between true fear, which is a gift, versus unwarranted fear, which can be a curse. True fear is our body's best warning system. True fear is what caused me to break into a full sprint when I heard heavy breathing and a stranger's footsteps quickening behind me as I walked home alone in the dark a few years ago. Maybe the stranger was completely harmless, but it's also very possible I saved my own life that night by not rationalizing and just running.

There is a place for fear. Our body reacts (for example, the hairs on the back of our neck stand up) and our gut knows when we're in the presence of someone who doesn't feel safe or a situation that just feels off. Yet, when we've been through trauma, our internal alarm system can malfunction, making it hard to determine the difference between a real threat and an imagined one.

Fear can get trapped in our body and make a home in our muscles and connective tissues. Our work is to release old fear so our nervous system can find its way back into balance.

The following sequence targets the specific muscles in our body where fear most often gets trapped. The psoas is our biggest muscle of fight or flight. It is a deep core and hip flexor muscle with many functions: it helps stabilize our spine; propels us forward when we walk or run; and allows us to bend at our hips and bring our legs toward our chest. It is the only muscle in the body that connects our spine to our legs. Interestingly enough, this important muscle also has fascial connections to our diaphragm (our primary muscle of breathing), and, as a result, has a direct impact on our fight-or-flight response.

The psoas instinctively contracts when we're under stress or in fear. Chronic tightness or weakness in this muscle can create a host of physical issues, ranging from lower back pain to hip pain. It can also be a dumping ground for emotional stress.

In this sequence, we will work on stretching, strengthening, and stabilizing this muscle to provide physical and emotional release. This sequence also targets our hamstrings and quadriceps, which are secondary muscles of fight or flight. Our legs are what we use to run or kick when faced with danger. Our legs also both physically and metaphorically move us forward in life. So if you are feeling stuck or frozen in fear, this is the perfect sequence to help move you forward.

Primal Yoga Sequence for Releasing Fear

1. Kidney Taps

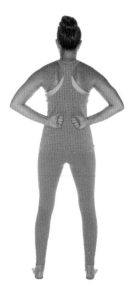

Stand with your feet slightly wider than hip-width distance apart with your knees gently bent. Make light fists with your hands, bring your fists behind you, and begin gently tapping the middle of your lower back just below your ribs. This is where your kidneys and adrenal glands sit.

Tap with light pressure and observe how your body responds. Notice any sensitivity or tenderness. If your kidneys feel tender, switch from tapping to gentle massaging, moving your hands in a circular motion. If there is no tenderness, you can increase the pressure of your taps. Tap for 30 seconds to 1 minute.

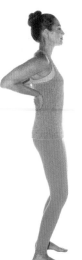

Benefits: Our adrenal glands sit on top of each kidney and are key players in our stress-response system, producing fight-or-flight stress hormones like adrenaline and norepinephrine.

Chronic stress depletes our adrenals, which can lead to adrenal fatigue and symptoms like mild depression or anxiety, the inability to handle stress, a lack of energy, low blood sugar, food cravings, reliance on stimulants like caffeine for energy, and a weakened immune system.

In traditional Chinese medicine, the kidneys are ruled by the element of water, and the emotion associated with the kidneys is fear. If your kidney qi is out of balance, it can lead to intense fear, anxiety, and panic attacks. Tapping and massaging the kidneys is an ancient Eastern self-healing practice that helps bring blood flow and vitality back to the area to help improve kidney and adrenal function, while calming fears and anxiety.

2. Leg Taps

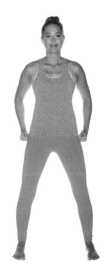

Stand with your feet slightly wider than hip-width distance apart, feet parallel. Make light fists with your hands, bend your elbows slightly, and tap your outer hips with your fists. Bend at your hips, leaning your torso slightly forward and pushing your hips slightly back as you tap your outer legs and thighs. Bring your fists behind you and continue tapping the backs of your legs and hamstrings. Bend your knees deeper, folding forward even more to tap your outer shins, calves, and ankles. Continue tapping your inner ankles, inner calves, and inner thighs.

As you are tapping, observe any tender spots and spend a little extra time there. You can increase or decrease the pressure of your taps according to what feels most comfortable to you. As you are tapping, visualize any fears or nervous energy flowing out of your body and releasing out through the soles of your feet. Spend 1 to 2 minutes on this tapping sequence, then roll gently back up to a standing position, release your arms down by your sides, take a few slow, deep breaths, and observe how you feel.

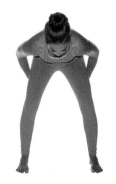

Benefits: Our legs are our first responders during fight or flight. In traditional Chinese medicine, our kidney and bladder meridians run down our legs, and both organ systems are associated with the emotion of fear. The bladder channel has points that run down the backs of our legs, while the kidney channel starts in the soles of our feet and runs up our inner leg and inner groin into our torso. Tapping our legs and hips is a self-healing energy practice that stimulates these energy pathways in our body to help us release fear, doubt, worry, and anxiety.

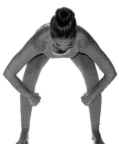

Note: When practicing the following leg sequence, perform instruction numbers 3 through 8 on your right side first. Then switch and repeat on your left side before moving on.

3. Low Crescent Lunge

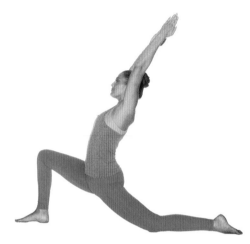

Start in downward facing dog (see instructions on page 120) and inhale your right leg up to the ceiling. On an exhale, draw your right knee toward your nose and step your foot between your hands. Release your back knee to the floor. On an inhale, lift your chest and reach your arms up toward the ceiling, wrapping your triceps forward. Lengthen your sides up out of your pelvis to prevent sinking into your hip joints. Visualize energy rising up from your pubic bone to your navel. Gently hug in your front ribs to engage your core. Hold the pose for 5 cycles of breath.

Benefits: This pose stretches your psoas muscle, which is part of our hip flexor group and our biggest muscle of fight or flight, and your quadriceps (our secondary muscles of fight or flight); opens your chest, back, and shoulders; and lengthens your spine.

4. Half Split

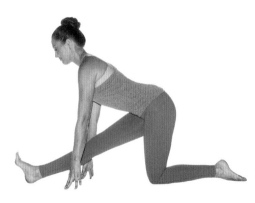

From low crescent lunge, release your hands down to the floor to either side of your right leg. Shift your weight back toward your left leg as you press your right leg straight and flex your right foot to come up onto your heel, pulling your toes back toward you. Keep your hips stacked over your left knee. Inhale and lengthen your spine, reaching your heart forward toward your right toes. Exhale to fold deeper into the stretch, drawing your shoulders down and back, away from your ears. Hold the pose for 5 cycles of breath.

Benefits: This pose stretches your hamstrings and calves; helps relieve sciatica pain; and stretches your lower back.

5. Crescent Lunge

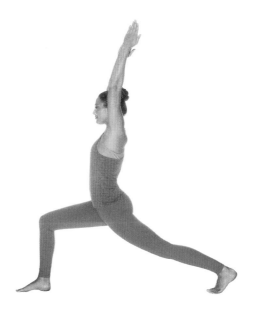

Start standing with your feet hip-width distance apart, spine tall. Step your left foot back approximately one leg length and bend your right knee to a 90-degree angle to come into a crescent lunge. Lengthen your tailbone toward the floor and press your left heel toward the back of the room. Inhale and sweep your arms up toward the ceiling with palms facing each other. Lengthen your torso and draw your front ribs in to engage your core. Exhale to deepen the pose. Hold the pose for 5 cycles of breath.

Benefits: This pose stretches your legs and hip flexors; opens up your chest and shoulders; strengthens your back, thighs, and butt; improves your balance; increases energy and stamina; and reduces fatigue.

6. Front Kick

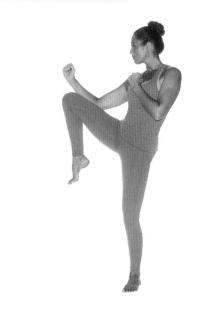

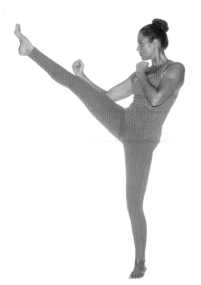

From crescent lunge, shift your weight into your right leg (front leg) and step your left foot forward about 6 inches in front of your right foot with your toes turned out about 45 degrees. On an inhalation, transfer your weight into your left foot as you draw your right knee in toward your chest with your heel pulled back toward your body (this is called a *chambered position*).

As your knee lifts, make fists with both hands and draw your elbows in toward your ribs. On an exhalation, extend your right leg straight out into a front kick. Press through the ball of your foot as you curl your toes back (the striking surface is the ball of your foot). Re-chamber your leg by drawing your knee back in toward your chest (this helps you find stability and balance after throwing the kick). Keep the majority of the weight on your left leg, as you place the ball of your right foot down next to your left to reset for a second kick.

The height of the kick may be low (aiming for knee level), mid-level (aiming for rib height), or high (aiming for head height), depending on your individual range of motion and flexibility. Practice the chamber and the kick slowly at first to work on control and stability, for at least 3 rounds. Then experiment with adding a little more speed and power. Practice 3 to 5 kicks at the speed that feels best in your body. As you are practicing your kicks, visualize taking a stand for yourself and kicking through any physical and mental barriers that have prevented you from moving forward in your life.

Benefits: This movement strengthens your hip flexors (including your psoas muscle) of your kicking leg while stretching your psoas muscle of your standing leg; creates core strength, balance, and stability; and empowers you to break through physical and emotional barriers.

7. Warrior II

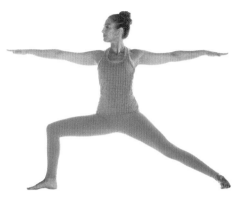

From your front kick, step back to your original crescent lunge with your right leg forward and left leg back. From crescent, spin your back heel flat and open up your hips and torso to face the side of the room. Make sure your right knee is stacked directly over your right anklebone, with your thigh parallel to the floor and your back leg pressing straight with your toes angled slightly in. Your right heel should be in a straight line with the arch of your back foot. Exhale and open your arms out toward either side of you at shoulder height. Hug your right outer hip in, lengthen your tailbone down toward the floor, and hug your front ribs in as your elongate your spine and lift through the crown of your head. Gaze over your front fingertips. Hold the pose for 3 to 5 cycles of breath.

Benefits: This pose strengthens your legs; stretches your groin; opens up your hips, chest, and shoulders; builds concentration; and increases stamina.

8. Triangle

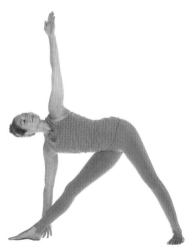

From warrior II, inhale to press your right leg straight. Engage your quadriceps and lift your kneecaps to prevent locking out your knee joint. Exhale and press into your back foot as you shift your weight into your left hip, tilting forward at your right hip crease while keeping your chest open to the side of the room. Continue exhaling as you reach your right arm forward, extending through the right side of your waist, and slowly reach your right hand down to the floor outside your right ankle. If your hand doesn't comfortably reach the floor, you may place it on your shin or on a block placed either right next to the inner arch of your right foot or just outside the outer edge of your foot.

Inhale and send your left arm straight up toward the ceiling as you revolve your torso open. Lengthen evenly through both sides of your waist. Gently shift your gaze up toward your top hand. If this feels uncomfortable for your neck, keep your gaze lowered toward the floor. Hold the pose for 3 to 5 cycles of breath.

Benefits: This pose stretches your legs, inner thighs, outer hips, and ankles; opens your chest and shoulders; strengthens your thighs, knees, ankles, obliques, and back muscles; relieves stress and anxiety; and stimulates your abdominal organs to aid with digestion.

9. Supported Bridge with Hip Flexor Stretch

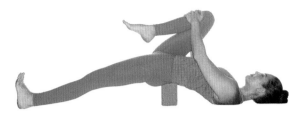

Lie on your back, bend your knees, and place your feet flat on the floor hip-width distance apart. Inhale and drive your heels down as you lift your hips up off the floor. Place a block under your sacrum and let your pelvis rest on the block. Adjust the height of the block according to what feels most comfortable and best supports your body. Rest your arms down on the floor to either side, palms facing up. Stay here for 3 to 5 cycles of breath, then draw your right knee into your chest and interlace your fingers over your right shin. Slowly slide your left leg out toward the front of the room until it is straight, keeping your heel on the floor and your foot flexed, toes pointing up. Hold the stretch for 5 cycles of breath. Return your right foot to its starting position and repeat on the left side.

Benefits: This pose stretches your primary hip flexors, chest, and neck; opens up your spine; helps relieve mild depression; calms your brain; and relieves backache.

10. Constructive Rest Pose

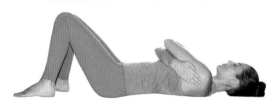

Lie down on your back, bend your knees, and place your feet flat on the floor, parallel and slightly wider than hip-width distance apart. Gently knock your knees in toward each other until they touch. Inhale and reach your arms open, as if you were about to give someone an embrace. Exhale and embrace yourself into a loving hug, crossing your arms over your chest and gently holding both shoulders with your opposite hands. Send yourself loving kindness and mentally affirm: *I am safe. I am loved.*

Benefits: This pose neutralizes your spine after backbends; relieves back, hip, and leg tension; and creates a sense of calm, safety, and well-being.

11. Pigeon Pose

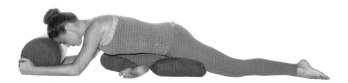

Start in a tabletop position: your hands shoulder-width distance apart on the floor and knees hip-width distance apart. Bring your right knee forward toward your right wrist and your right ankle forward toward your left wrist, so your shin is parallel to the front of the room. Keep your right foot flexed to help support your knee joint. If you experience any knee discomfort or sensitivity, bring your shin away from parallel and into more of a diagonal, with your heel drawing closer to your body. Slide your left leg straight back as you lower your hips toward the floor. Keep your spine tall and your chest lifted as you slide your left leg back. Inhale and expand your chest while squaring your hips forward. Exhale and fold over your front leg. Rest your forehead on the floor and hold the pose for 5 to 8 cycles of breath. Return to tabletop position and repeat this pose on the left side. For added support, place a bolster under your front hip and a second bolster under your forehead.

Benefits: This pose opens your hips; stretches your hip flexors, including your psoas; helps alleviate sciatic pain; helps release fear and other emotions stored in your hips; and calms your nervous system.

12. Seated Forward Fold

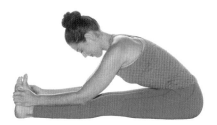

Start seated with your legs extended straight out in front of you, feet flexed. Inhale as you lift through your sternum and reach the crown of your head toward the ceiling to lengthen your spine. Exhale and hinge from your hips with your spine lengthened to fold over your legs. Be mindful not to round your lower back, which can strain your muscles. Reach for the outer edges of your feet with your hands. If your hands don't reach your feet, rest them on your shins instead. Rest your gaze down and breathe. Hold the pose for 5 cycles of breath.

Benefits: This pose stretches your hamstrings, calves, and spine; calms your mind; alleviates anxiety and stress; and promotes healthy digestion.

13. Alternate Nostril Breath *(see instructions on page 71)*

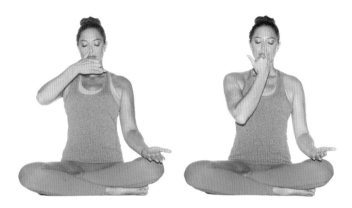

Find a comfortable seat after your forward fold and do 5 to 10 cycles of alternate nostril breath to deeply calm your nervous system and create a sense of balance and well-being.

14. Supported Rest Pose with Open Hip Variation

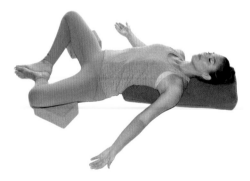

Sit down with a bolster behind you, its shorter end pressed up against your buttocks. Bend your knees, bring the soles of your feet together, and slide your heels in toward your body. Allow your knees to gently fall open and place a block under either knee for support. Gently lean back onto the bolster with the length of the bolster supporting your entire spine from your hips to your head. Place a folded blanket under your head if you need more support for your neck. Rest your arms down on the floor away from the sides of your body, palms facing up. Close your eyes if that feels safe and comfortable in your body. You are welcome to keep your eyes open with a soft gaze if you do not feel comfortable with them closed. Stay in this pose for 3 to 5 minutes.

Benefits: This pose calms your nervous system, opens your hips and stretches your inner thighs, opens your chest, supports digestion, and creates a sense of well-being.

Moving Through Anger

One of the biggest pieces of my healing was making peace with my anger, a necessary process that was, unfortunately, stunted by all the spiritual bypassing I encountered within the yoga community where I sought healing.

I was searching for ways to find peace within myself and was consistently told that anger was bad and forgiveness and love were the true answers. Well intentioned as this advice may be, it's bullshit. You can't bypass anger and skip ahead to forgiveness. Anger is a necessary and appropriate response to situations in which we've been physically or emotionally harmed, manipulated, or deceived. To deny ourselves the right to feel angry when we've been hurt is to deny part of our humanness. Anger needs to be felt before it can be released.

As of the writing of this book, more than 400 high-profile executives and employees across various industries have been outed for sexual assault and harassment as a result of the #MeToo movement, leading to resignations, firings, suspensions, and arrests.[3] It is a collective sense of outrage that is opening up a global conversation about sexual violence and helping to create a safer future for women around the world. Healthy anger helps us create necessary boundaries, empowers us into action and activism, and helps us stand up against injustice.

However, anger can easily turn toxic without a healthy outlet. My anger has been a major source of guilt and shame in my life. While I have generally avoided conflict and confrontation, the rage that would spill out of me when I was triggered left me shocked, scared, and deeply ashamed. As someone who has been through abuse, I couldn't reconcile how any part of me could be good if I carried the same seething anger within me as those who had abused me. In my mind, only abusive people got angry, so I created a shadow belief that I was inherently bad.

I was terrified that if people only knew how angry I really was, no one could possibly love me. So I did everything in my power to push it away, hide it, and deny its existence. That never works. Suppressing our emotions creates a toxic buildup that leads to an inevitable implosion (collapsing in on ourselves) or explosion (lashing out at others). To keep our anger from turning toxic, we must allow ourselves to feel and express it constructively.

Working with our anger in a constructive way means meeting it with awareness and compassionately listening to what it has to say. Anger always has an underlying message. When we peel back the curtain, there's usually another emotion hiding behind it like disappointment, fear, grief, or shame. Listening to our anger without lashing out or lashing in lays the foundation for healthy communication, assertiveness, and empowerment.

The following sequence was created to honor your anger and give it sacred space to be felt, moved, and released. It opens with an invigorating breath of fire practice to help reveal latent anger. The sequence then moves into heating core work, martial arts, and deep twists, all of which activate our third chakra, the solar plexus or *manipura* chakra. It is here that unresolved anger and frustration reside. I encourage you to breathe into your emotions and let anything you have been suppressing rise to the surface. We close with a cooling breathwork technique to bring our body and mind back to balance.

Primal Yoga Sequence for Releasing Anger

1. Breath of Fire *(see instructions on page 78)*

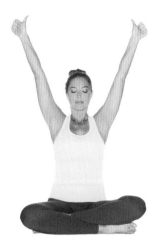

Find a comfortable seated position and practice breath of fire for 3 minutes. Set the intention to release any anger or frustration that you have been holding on to. Allow any repressed anger to rise up from your lower belly and release as you exhale.

At the end of your breath of fire practice, open your palms, reach your arms straight up toward the sky, and allow yourself to give voice to your anger. Scream at the top of your lungs for a few seconds to release any remaining emotion. Then slowly release your arms down by your sides and take a few moments to sit quietly and observe how you feel. Has anything shifted? Do you feel lighter? Do you feel more empowered? What did it feel like to give yourself permission to scream?

2. Boat Pose

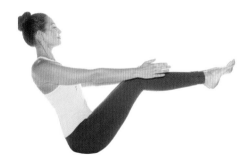

Begin in a seated position. Lengthen your spine and lift through your chest. Lean back slightly as you bend your knees and lift your feet off the floor. Continue lengthening your spine as you press your knees together and lift your shins parallel to the floor. Reach your arms forward and soften your shoulders away from your ears. Hold for 5 cycles of breath. If you're in the mood for more of a challenge, engage your thigh muscles to straighten your legs out in front of you.

Benefits: This pose strengthens your core, hip flexors, quadriceps, and back muscles; creates confidence; and connects you to your center.

3. Bicycle Crunches

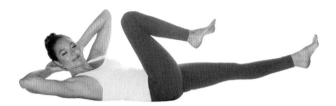

Lie on the floor on your back. Bring your hands behind your head with your elbows wide. On an exhale, lift your head and shoulder blades off the floor, being careful not to pull or strain your neck, and draw your knees in toward your chest. Inhale and straighten your left leg out, hovering just a few inches off the ground. Keep your lower back flat on the ground and your front ribs hugging in. Exhale as you revolve your upper body to the right and draw your left elbow toward your right knee. Switch sides fluidly (as if you're pedaling a bicycle with your legs) to complete one rep. Do 2 sets of 10 reps.

Benefits: *This pose strengthens your abdominal muscles, specifically your rectus abdominis, or "six-pack" abs, and your obliques; helps improve blood circulation to your internal organs; aids digestion; and creates a sense of strength and confidence.*

4. Horse Stance Punches

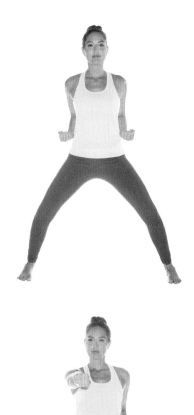

Stand tall and step your feet apart about two times wider than hip-width distance. Exhale as you bend your knees to drop down into a wide-leg squat, also known as horse stance. Keep your spine elongated by lifting through the crown of your head while lengthening your tailbone toward the floor. Stack your shoulders directly on top of your hips and hug your front ribs in to engage your core.

Make fists with both hands, knuckles facing up, and hug your elbows in tightly against your body. Inhale and draw your elbows back, squeezing your shoulder blades together, and pull your fists to your body just below your bottom ribs. Exhale and extend your right arm forward into a straight punch position keeping your arm at shoulder height. Your forearm and hand rotate as you punch, so your knuckles end up facing down. Keep your left arm in a tight fist at your left hip. On your next exhale, send your left arm straight out with power into a straight punch, pivoting your knuckles down. Simultaneously retract your right arm back to the bent elbow position at your hip. Exhale forcefully out through your mouth, with an audible *shhhhh* sound. Do 3 sets of 10 punches.

OPTION

In martial arts, horse stance is traditionally performed with your feet parallel and toes pointing forward, but if this causes any discomfort in your knees, you may turn your toes slightly out and have your knees point in the same direction as your toes.

Benefits: This pose strengthens your legs, glutes, hips, knees, ankles, shoulders, arms, spine, and core; releases anger and frustration; and builds confidence and power.

5. Twisting Crescent

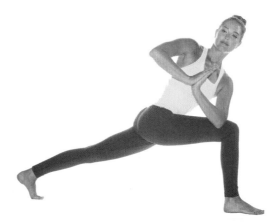

Start in a crescent lunge (see instructions on page 105). Exhale and bring your hands together at the center of your chest with your elbows wide. Revolve your torso to the right as you lean forward, keeping your spine lengthened. Hook your left elbow outside your right thigh, just above your knee. Press your elbow against your outer leg to create leverage to deepen your twist as you roll your chest open. Soften your shoulders away from your ears, reach through the crown of your head, and press your back leg straight, reaching through your left heel. Draw your lower abdomen in as you twist, lifting your torso off your thigh. Hold the pose for 5 cycles of breath, then repeat on the opposite side.

Benefits: This pose strengthens your legs, glutes, spine, and core; stretches your hip flexors; opens your chest and shoulders; creates mobility in your spine; improves balance; helps improve blood circulation to your internal organs; aids digestion; and helps release anger and frustration.

6. Seated Twist

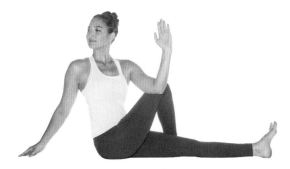

Start seated with your spine lengthened and both legs straight out in front of you. Bend your right knee and draw your right heel in toward your right sitting bone. Lift your right leg and cross your right foot over your left leg. Keep your right knee bent and place your right foot flat on the floor just outside of your left outer thigh. Inhale and reach your left arm straight up toward the ceiling. Exhale, revolve your torso to the right, bend your left elbow, and bring your left elbow outside your right thigh with your fingers pointing up. Place your right hand directly behind you, roll your shoulder open away from your ear, continue to lift through your spine, and expand your chest. Gaze over your right shoulder. Hold this pose for 3 to 5 cycles of breath as you visualize negative emotions wringing out of the body like water from a wet rag. Repeat on the opposite side.

OPTION

Instead of keeping your left leg straight, fold it in toward your right sitting bone. This is a slightly deeper variation that creates an additional gentle stretch in your left hip, knee, and ankle.

Benefits: This pose tones your abdomen; increases blood flow to your digestive organs, which improves digestion; creates strength and mobility in your spine; helps relieve some types of back pain; releases anger and frustration; and opens your chest.

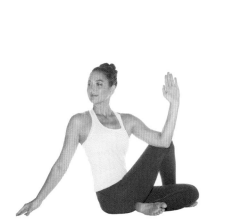

7. Seated Head to Knee Pose

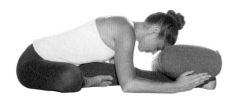

Sit on the floor with both legs straight out in front of you. If you need extra support, place a blanket under your buttocks. Bend your right knee and bring the sole of your right foot to your inner left thigh. Inhale, sit up tall, and expand your chest as you reach the crown of your head toward the ceiling. Exhale, gently revolve your torso toward your left knee, and fold your torso over your left leg. Reach your arms forward to your foot and interlace your fingers around the sole of your foot if possible. Relax your neck and drop your gaze down. Optional: Rest your forehead on a bolster for additional support and comfort. Hold the pose for 5 cycles of breath, then repeat on the opposite side.

Benefits: This pose stretches your hamstrings, calves, hips, inner groin, and spine; calms your mind; relieves anxiety and stress; eases mild depression; helps with fatigue; improves digestion; and helps alleviate insomnia.

8. Cooling Breath *(see instructions on page 74)*

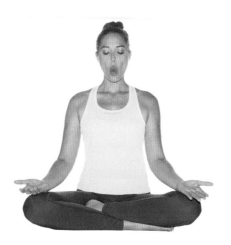

Close your practice with 5 rounds of cooling breath to balance and cool your body after a very heated practice. As you breathe, visualize any remaining anger, frustration, or agitation gently leaving your body. Finish by sitting quietly for a few moments and observe how you feel.

Moving Through Grief

Grief is a natural and necessary emotion that helps us process and move through loss. But that doesn't mean it doesn't hurt like heck. The pain of grief can manifest physically in our body, causing us to collapse in on ourselves and close off our heart. Grief's posture is protective and collapsed. It rounds our shoulders, tightens our chest, and can literally take our breath away.

In Chinese medicine, grief is housed in our lungs. If our lung *qi* is deficient, the grip of grief can feel unrelenting, turning into despondency and depression. When working with clients who are deeply grieving, I've noticed that their chest muscles (more specifically their pectoralis minor muscle, which attaches our shoulders to our ribs) are often chronically tight—a physical manifestation of an energetic defense to protect our heart from pain. Stretching this muscle by opening up our chest can release a healthy wave of suppressed emotion.

The sequence on the following pages is designed to strengthen and harmonize our lung *qi* while stretching our chest and strengthening our upper back to support the physical and emotional opening of our heart.

Primal Yoga Sequence for Releasing Grief

1. Lung Taps *(see instructions on page 88)*

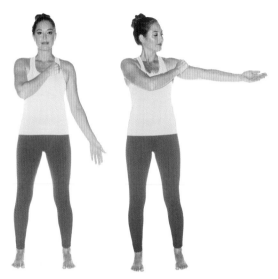

Begin with 1 to 3 minutes of tapping the lung meridians in your chest and arms. As you're tapping, set your intention to allow any grief or sadness to move through you and release during your practice. When you have finished tapping, release your arms down by your sides and observe how you feel. Notice any sensations in your body.

2. Downward Facing Dog

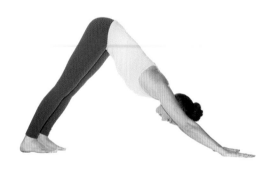

Start in a tabletop position with your knees hip-width distance and your hands shoulder-width apart. Spread your fingers wide and stack your shoulders over your wrists and your hips over your knees. Exhale, tuck your toes, lift your hips up and back, and press your legs straight as you root down into your hands. Lengthen your spine, roll your shoulders open away from your ears, and press the floor actively away, rooting through your thumb and index fingers. Reach your heels toward the floor and gaze gently back toward your toes. Hold the pose for 5 cycles of breath.

Benefits: This pose strengthens your wrists, shoulders, arms, and legs; stretches your hamstrings and calves; elongates your spine; calms your brain; and helps relieve stress and mild depression.

3. Plank

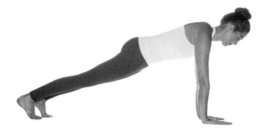

Start in downward facing dog. Inhale and shift your weight forward, lowering your hips and stacking your shoulders over your wrists. Actively engage your core by hugging your front ribs in, firm your thighs, and lengthen your tailbone toward your heels. Be mindful of not allowing your hips to sink too low or your lower back to collapse. Your body should be in one straight line from your heels through the crown of your head. Hold the pose for 5 full cycles of breath

Benefits: This pose strengthens your chest, arms, shoulders, wrists, legs, back, and core; helps improve posture; builds strength and stamina; and creates confidence.

4. Low Push-Up

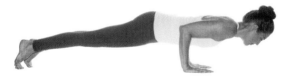

From plank pose, inhale deeply as you shift your weight forward on the balls of your feet. Feel your shoulders moving slightly forward past your wrists. As you exhale, press firmly through your hands, bend your elbows to a 90-degree angle, hug them in tightly to the sides of your rib cage, and lower your body in a straight line into a low push-up position. Stack your elbows over your wrists and keep your shoulders at the same height as your elbows. Hug your front ribs in to engage your core and lengthen your tailbone toward your heels. Maintain a straight line with your body as you slowly lower to your belly.

Benefits: This pose strengthens your shoulders, wrists, legs, chest, back, and core; creates full-body stabilization; and energizes the body and mind.

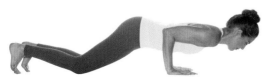

OPTION

If it feels too challenging to lower your body down in a straight line while maintaining proper form, release your knees to the floor.

5. Cobra

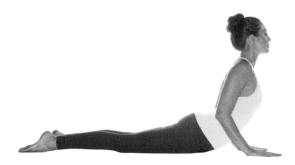

Lie flat on your stomach with your legs reaching back and toes pointed behind you. Plant your palms under your shoulders and spread your fingers. Hug your elbows in toward your rib cage. Press into the tops of your feet, firm your thighs, and press your pubic bone down into the floor. On an inhale, press into your hands and lift your chest off the floor as you begin to straighten your arms. Keep a bend in your elbows as you extend through your spine and draw your chest forward. Hold for 3 to 5 breaths.

Benefits: This pose strengthens your spine, upper back, arms, and shoulders; stretches your chest and abdomen; opens up your lungs; creates space in your heart; and energizes your body.

6. Locust

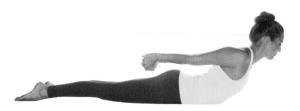

Lie flat on your stomach with your arms down by your sides, your legs reaching back, and toes pointed behind you. Keeping your arms straight, interlace your fingers behind your back. On an inhalation, press into the tops of your feet, squeeze your shoulder blades together, reach your knuckles toward the back of the room, and engage the muscles along your spine to lift your chest. Press your pubic bone down toward the floor and lengthen your tailbone toward your heels. Gaze softly down without dropping your head forward. Hold the pose for 3 to 5 cycles of breath.

Benefits: This pose strengthens your back muscles, buttocks, legs, and arms; opens your shoulders and chest; stretches your abdomen; helps improve your posture; improves digestion by stimulating your abdominal organs; energizes your body; and has an antidepressive effect on your mind.

7. Prone Chest Stretch

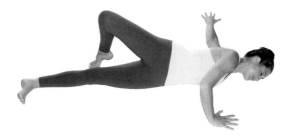

Lie flat on your belly. Send your left arm straight out to the side in a half-T formation, and turn your left cheek down. Plant your right palm outside your right ribs. Bend your right knee and fold your right heel toward your butt. On an inhalation, press into your right palm, roll onto your left hip, and gently place your right foot down behind your left leg. Adjust the placement of your right foot so there is no strain on your lower back. Stay here for your exhalation. On your next inhalation, press into your right palm firmly and roll your right shoulder open, expanding across your chest to deepen the stretch. Hold for 5 cycles of breath, then release back onto your belly. Repeat on the opposite side.

Benefits: This pose stretches your chest, specifically your pectoralis minor muscle, which is an emotional storehouse for grief, sadness, and resignation; creates mobility in your spine; opens your hips; and helps release difficult emotions that are held in your heart and chest.

8. Rest Pose with Heart Opening Variation

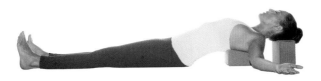

Lie down on your back and place a block horizontally underneath your shoulder blades. Place a second block beneath your head for support. Adjust the height of the blocks so you feel a gentle stretch in the front of your chest without straining your neck or back. Rest your arms on the floor, away from your torso with palms up. Release any muscular tension in your body and allow your chest to expand. Stay in the pose anywhere from 5 to 10 minutes.

Benefits: This pose stretches the front of your chest; supports your upper back; supports the release of any sadness or heaviness stored in your heart; helps lower blood pressure; deeply calms your body and soothes your mind; helps relieve stress, anxiety, and mild depression; reduces insomnia; and promotes a sense of well-being.

9. Sound Meditation

Lying in supported rest pose, inhale deeply through your nose and exhale slowly through your mouth making an *sssssss* sound, similar to letting the air out of a tire. Visualize golden light filling you as you inhale and any sadness leaving you as you exhale. Continue for as many cycles of breath as needed until you feel complete.

Quick Tip:
Let Go of Sadness and Grief—
Pec Minor Release with a Rubber Ball

The pectoralis minor is located in your upper chest under your pectoralis major, and is a muscle that tends to be chronically tight on most people. A tight pectoralis minor muscle pulls your shoulders forward, which contributes to a slumped and rounded posture. Not only that, but the pec minor is also a storehouse for grief, sadness, and depression. This targeted stretch will help release your pec minor. Releasing this muscle can often release a flood of emotion. Welcome any tears and allow them to flow. The only way to heal is to allow ourselves to feel.

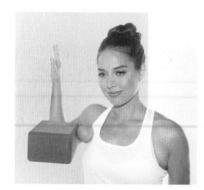

HOW TO DO IT:

- Stand sideways with your right shoulder a few inches away from the wall. Using your left hand, place a block against the wall and place a tennis ball against the block at shoulder height.

- Position the ball just under your right collarbone against your pectoralis minor muscle, which originates from the third to fifth ribs and inserts in your scapula (shoulder blade).

- Place your right hand against the wall. Apply pressure into the ball and gently cross-fiber the muscle by rolling back and forth for 5 to 8 breaths, then release and switch sides.

Moving into Self-Worth and Empowerment

I have an inner critic in my head that keeps a running list of all the reasons I suck. She tells me to play it small because life is safer when you don't take risks. She tells me that the world will judge. Yet she judges me more harshly than anyone else ever could.

Most of us have an inner critic. That voice of doubt that tells us we're not enough. Trauma creates the myth that we are separate, and in our separateness, the seeds of unworthiness are planted. Our stories of unworthiness are often programmed within us before we're even old enough to know what self-worth is. As a child, you may have been shamed for wetting the bed, scolded for sucking your thumb, or yelled at for being a "bad boy (or girl)!" These may seem like trivial things, but these negative messages have a way of weaving into our subconscious, creating toxic beliefs that we are inherently bad, stupid, or unlovable.

Unworthiness takes on many shapes. It can shift into the shape of depression, fan into the flames of anger, constrict into the knot of fear, sharpen into the tongue of criticism, or coil into the snake of jealousy. Too often in my own life, I have torn down other people behind their backs out of my own deep sense of lack. My inner critic *loves* when I do that because it gives her a chance to make me feel even smaller. She whispers, "If people only knew who you *really* are . . ."

Stepping into our self-worth means telling our inner critic to go shove it. We're human, so that judgmental voice may never completely go away, but we can certainly turn down the volume until eventually it just becomes background noise we can choose to tune out.

There's a beautiful quote I love from an unknown source: "Maybe the journey isn't so much about becoming anything. Maybe it's about unbecoming everything that isn't really you so you can be who you were meant to be in the first place." Stepping into self-worth is an act of faith that asks us to dismantle the myth of not being enough and to have the courage to allow ourselves to be seen and heard. When we own our worth, we are able to see the worth of others. When we stand in self-love, we are able to witness others with loving eyes.

Owning who we are and showing up *as we are* shines a light on the darkness of doubt, fear, jealousy, gossip, criticism, and scarcity, and creates a space of belonging where everyone thrives.

The following sequence was created to connect you to your authentic voice and power and incorporates poses to help you embody your expansiveness. As you move into these poses, allow yourself to spread your arms wide and take up space in the room. Witness yourself with love and let your voice be heard.

Primal Yoga Sequence for Self-Worth and Empowerment

Note: *When practicing this leg sequence, perform instruction numbers 1 through 3 on your right side first. Then switch and repeat on your left side before moving on.*

1. Primal Warrior

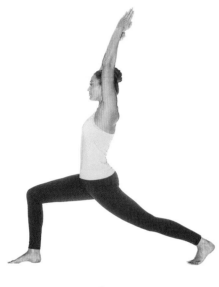

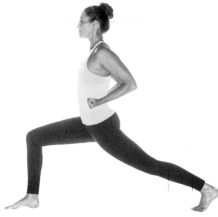

Start in a crescent lunge (see instructions on page 105). Take a deep, full inhalation, with your arms reaching up toward the ceiling. Exhale powerfully through your mouth, making a loud *ha* sound as you create fists and forcefully pull your arms down, bending your elbows and drawing your fists to your waist. As you pull your fists down, send your elbows behind you and squeeze your shoulder blades together to open your chest. Keep your front ribs hugging in to engage your core and support your lower back. On an inhalation through your nose, sweep your arms back toward the ceiling, then exhale powerfully with an audible *ha* sound as you pull your fists back to your waist. Repeat the dynamic motion for 5 rounds.

Benefits: This movement stretches your legs and hip flexors; opens up your chest and shoulders; strengthens your back, thighs, and butt; improves your balance; increases energy and stamina; reduces fatigue; opens up your throat chakra; and builds confidence.

2. Triangle

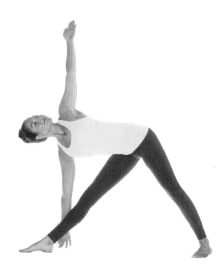

From crescent, open up into warrior II (see instructions on page 107). From warrior II, inhale to press your right leg straight. Engage your quadriceps and lift your kneecaps to prevent locking out your knee joint. Exhale and press into your back foot as you shift your weight into your left hip, tilting forward at your right hip crease, while keeping your chest open to the side of the room. Continue exhaling as you reach your right arm forward, extending through the right side of your waist, and slowly reaching your right hand down to the floor outside your right ankle. If your hand doesn't comfortably reach the floor, you may place it on your shin or on a block. Inhale and send your left arm straight up toward the ceiling as you revolve your torso open. Lengthen evenly through both sides of your waist. Gently shift your gaze up toward your top hand. If this feels uncomfortable for your neck, keep your gaze lowered toward the floor. Hold the pose for 3 to 5 cycles of breath.

Benefits: *This pose stretches your legs, inner thighs, outer hips, and ankles; opens your chest and shoulders; strengthens your thighs, knees, ankles, obliques, and back muscles; relieves stress and anxiety; and stimulates your abdominal organs to aid with digestion.*

3. Half Moon

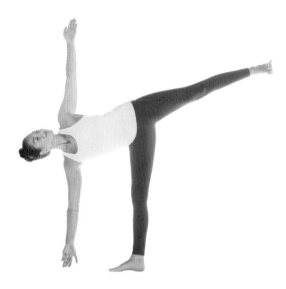

Start in triangle. Take a deep, full inhalation. Exhale as you drop your gaze down, bend your right knee, and shift your weight forward into your right leg, reaching your right hand toward the floor about 8 inches in front of your right toes. Press your right leg straight as you float your left leg straight out and up, flexing your left foot and pushing through your heel as if you were doing a side kick through a wall. Inhale and reach your left arm up toward the ceiling, fingers pointing up, and roll your chest open, stacking your left shoulder on top of your right. Your hips should stack open as well. Lengthen evenly through both sides of your waist. Exhale as you turn your gaze up toward the ceiling. If this feels uncomfortable for your neck, either turn your gaze halfway up to face the side of the room or keep your gaze down. Hold the pose for 5 cycles of breath.

Benefits: *This pose tones your buttocks, hips, and thighs; stretches your groin and hamstrings; cultivates balance; opens your chest, shoulders, and spine; and creates an empowered sense of expansion.*

4. Blooming Horse

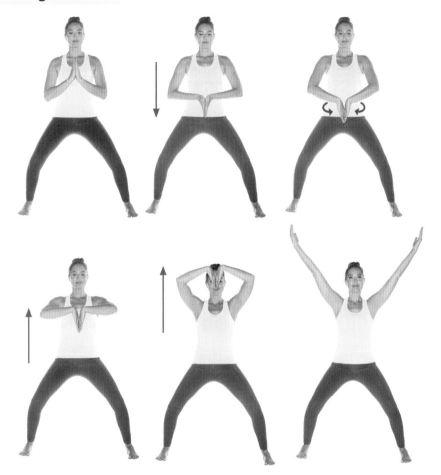

Start in horse stance (see instructions on page 115). Bring your palms together at the center of your chest, fingers pointing up. Keeping your palms together, rotate them down toward the floor, and slowly lower your arms down toward your lower energy center, or *dantian*, just below your navel. Keeping your thumbs touching, spin your palms outward until the backs of your hands touch, fingers still pointing downward. On an inhalation, slowly start to draw your hands up the center line of your body with the backs of your palms touching, wrists and elbows bent. Continue pulling your palms up past your heart and toward your forehead. At the level of your third eye chakra (the home of your intuition, according to the chakra system), allow the backs of your hands to slowly draw apart, expanding your arms out and open to the sky, fingers pointing up. Sit deeper into your horse stance as you softly shift your gaze up. Visualize yourself blossoming open like a flower. Release any feelings of smallness and allow yourself to sit in the beauty of your own expansiveness and power. Hold this pose for 5 cycles of breath. You may choose to mentally affirm to yourself: *I am worthy. I am loved.*

Benefits: This movement strengthens your legs, glutes, hips, and back; stretches your wrists; opens your chest and shoulders; and creates a sense of empowerment.

5. Forearm Plank

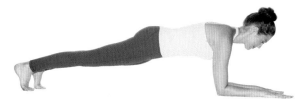

From a tabletop position, come down onto your forearms. Place your hands shoulder-width distance apart, keeping your elbows in line with your wrists. Step one foot at a time back to forearm plank. Actively push down through your forearms as you draw your front ribs in. Keep your hips low without collapsing your lower back. Lengthen your tailbone toward your heels. To strengthen your core connection in the pose, visualize trying to draw your toes forward toward your elbows and your elbows back toward your toes. Hold the pose for 5 cycles of breath.

Benefits: This pose strengthens your core, including your erector spinae muscles (located along your spine), rectus abdominis, and transverse abdominis (one of the deepest layers of core musculature that helps stabilize your spine); sculpts your shoulders; strengthens your chest, glutes, thighs, and calves; energizes your body; and builds confidence.

6. Sphinx Pose

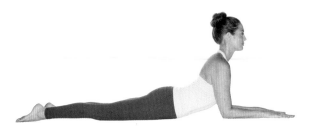

From forearm plank, release your hips and legs down to the floor. Point your toes straight back and press your pubic bone down into the floor. Keep your forearms down, with your elbows stacked under your shoulders and your hands spread. Inhale, press down into your palms, and lift through the crown of your head, lengthening your upper spine. Expand your chest and pull your heart forward and up, while keeping your shoulders drawing away from your ears. Be careful not to sink into your lower back. Keep your front ribs gently hugging in while you expand your chest. Hold the pose for 5 cycles of breath.

Benefits: This pose tones your arms and shoulders; opens your chest; strengthens your back; creates mobility in your spine; stretches your hip flexors; improves digestion; energizes your body; and wards off fatigue.

7. Seated Lotus Mudra

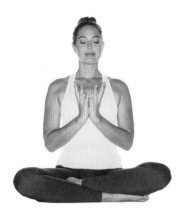

Find a comfortable cross-legged seat. Bring your palms together at the center of your chest with your fingers pointing up. Keep the heels of your palms, your thumbs, and your pinkie fingers together, then inhale and open all your other fingers like a lotus flower blossoming out of the mud. Hold your lotus blossom open at the center of your heart. Mentally repeat the affirmation: *I am worthy. I love and accept myself unconditionally. I am the one I have been waiting for.*

Benefits: This pose soothes your nervous system, creates a sense of calm and well-being, connects you with your divine nature and highest self, and cultivates self-worth and self-love.

Symbolism of the Lotus Flower

In many cultures, the lotus flower is a revered symbol that represents rebirth, purity, and the strength to overcome adversity. The lotus rises from mud and murk to blossom into beauty. Buddha is often depicted sitting in meditation on a lotus, as its muddy origins make it a symbol of spiritual awakening and enlightenment.

Moving Through Sexual Trauma

The impact of sexual trauma is best told by the courageous voices of those who have lived through it and emerged more resilient on the other side. I am honored to share a powerful story of healing from sexual trauma through the voice of Susan Alden, a graduate of the United States Military Academy, a Certified Yoga Therapist, and the executive director for the nonprofit organization Warriors at Ease (www.warriorsatease.org). Susan served as a logistics officer in the 82nd Airborne and 3rd Infantry Divisions and first began teaching yoga in the military in 1997 as a second lieutenant, sharing the practice with her own soldiers as part of the unit fitness program. Married for the past nineteen years to a recently retired Army Special Forces soldier (Green Beret), she has been especially involved in serving the Special Operations Forces community and Gold Star Families and continues to dedicate her life to bringing the power of yoga and meditation to the military community. The healing work she does to support the health, resiliency, and posttraumatic growth for active duty members, veterans, and military families was informed by her own experience of Military Sexual Trauma (MST) over two decades ago. In her own words:

> Over twenty years ago I was raped by a West Point upperclassman a few months before I raised my right hand and entered the academy. Three more incidents of sexual assault and repeated sexual harassment would follow by three different perpetrators throughout my time at West Point and in the military. I was certainly affected by all the incidents, but the rape has been the single most transformational experience of my life.
>
> Initially, I was shocked that such a thing could happen to me. This was followed by a whirlwind of confusion, sadness, anger, shame, disbelief, rage, and even guilt over not having been stronger, wiser, or able to see it coming and prevent it. This whirlwind evolved into a secret depression that I hid from everyone, perhaps even myself. I didn't have time for depression. I was a new cadet at West Point, just trying to survive the summer so I could officially become a member of the USMA Corps of Cadets.
>
> What was perhaps even more traumatic than the rape itself was the perpetrator's sadistic presence in my life, which was unavoidable given that I was his subordinate. I had no voice by nature of the traditional structure and rigors of the academy. My roommate was privy to my rapist's sly and threatening visits, which, though not harmful physically, were surely an attempt to further assert his power over me. Eventually it was my roommate—who had more presence of mind than I at the time—who said, "This has to stop. If you don't tell someone about it all, I will."

Though I did not formally report the rape for various reasons, I did speak to a very compassionate and concerned senior officer who was serving as a cadet counselor. I told her about the rape and threatening sexual harassment that ensued. In that moment, I felt heard and supported. My perpetrator was banned from interacting with me further.

There are some important things to understand about Military Sexual Trauma. One must understand that, first and foremost, survivors are warriors, even those who are very new to the military. Regardless of branch of service or how they might have come into the military, a new recruit raises his or her right hand and swears to "support and defend the Constitution against all enemies, foreign and domestic," a commitment that potentially requires one to fight to his or her death. Conversely, sexual trauma makes you feel weak, unworthy, and disempowered, and is a detriment to the warrior ethos that has been cultivated from early military indoctrination.

Second, I think it's helpful to realize that Military Sexual Trauma is most likened to incest. The military is like a close-knit family. Senior leaders may be viewed as elders, mentors or even parent-like. We commonly refer to our comrades as our brothers- and sisters-in-arms. Subordinates could be likened to children, as leaders are charged with their subordinate's health, safety, and well-being. In addition, members of the military community generally live and work in close proximity to one another. Sexual violations, particularly those occurring where the perpetrator and survivor are in the same unit, tear at the very fabric of the military family.

For the nine years I was a card-carrying member of the Department of Defense, I largely focused on maintaining my unbreakable warrior spirit and not causing waves in the family I'd grown to love. During my time in service, the ratio of men to women was slightly less than ten to one. I had a fierce drive to succeed as a woman in a man's world. I was intent on being a hard-core airborne soldier, and I'd be damned if I was going to admit to what I believed was a crack in my armor. It wasn't until I got out of the military and began my journey into the healing arts that I finally took my body armor off, realized that true strength was found in vulnerability, and began healing.

I always say, we can't heal what we can't feel. When I began feeling, I began healing. Deepening my yoga and meditation practice was the first step in the journey.

Once I learned to no longer resist vulnerability and hide my pain, I was blessed by much support from my family, close friends, and some extraordinary healers, teachers, and mentors. Most important, I learned to tune into and truly embrace the healer-teacher within me, who is my most intimate and beloved support.

During a time when I felt very raw from trauma, I also practiced a lot of ecstatic dance, specifically Gabrielle Roth's 5Rhythms. I sweat my prayers, danced till I puked, and at times, felt like I was ripping the Band-Aid off of a deep wound. It wasn't always pretty, but I needed to feel the freedom to move my body with reckless abandon, to reengage my spirit that had been caged, and to reignite my voice that had been silenced. I would dance to the 5Rhythms, and then take my blistered feet and blissed-out soul back to my mat, returning to my old faithful friend, yoga, in order to reground and restore.

Susan's story is a powerful illustration of how movement heals. She now devotes her time to bringing awareness to the impact posttraumatic stress has on individuals and families and works to empower those in the military community to find health and healing on a yoga mat.

It is said that "our issues are in our tissues." Connecting to our bodies after a violation can feel uncomfortable and scary, but, as Susan so eloquently stated, we can't heal what we can't feel.

This sequence is designed to ground you in your body and connect you to your personal power. Within the physical postures, you will have the opportunity to assert your personal boundaries and bring breath and awareness to the places in your body (such as your hips) where sexual trauma often gets trapped.

Primal Yoga Sequence for Healing Sexual Trauma

1. Heart Taps

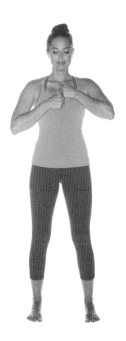

Stand with your feet hip-width distance apart. Make light fists with both hands. Bring your fists to the center of your chest, one fist above the other, and begin to simultaneously lightly tap both fists on your chest over your heart. Continue tapping for 1 minute.

Benefits: In traditional Chinese medicine, it is believed that our spirit, or shen, *is housed in the heart. If our heart is not being cared for, our spirit gets lost and confused. The heart is ruled by the element of fire, and if we are deficient in heart qi, our inner fire can burn out, which leads to depression, lack of animation, loss of creativity, and low energy. Tapping your heart awakens your heart chakra, enlivens your lungs, and brings energy and sensation to a place you may have closed off or kept numb.*

2. Leg Taps

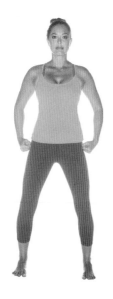

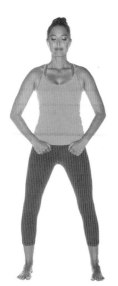

Stand with your feet slighter wider than hip-width distance apart, feet parallel. Make light fists with your hands, bend your elbows slightly, and simultaneously tap your outer hips with your fists. As you tap, say, "These are my hips."

Continue tapping down your upper and lower legs, saying out loud, "These are my legs." Once you reach your ankles, start to tap back up your inner calves, inner thighs, and inner groin. Keep declaring out loud ownership of whatever body part you are tapping. *This is my body.*

Take a few moments to tap your groin—if you were wearing jeans, this would be the place where your pockets sit. Notice any sensations or emotions that arise. Notice if you feel like detaching or feel very little at all. There is no right or wrong, just keep tapping.

After you have spent a few moments here, spend some time on any other parts of your body that you feel guided to. Are there any parts that feel numb or disconnected? Tap there. As you tap, continue to claim ownership of your own body. *These are my arms. This is my heart. This is my body.* When your tapping feels complete, release your arms down by your sides, take a few slow, deep breaths, and observe how you feel.

Benefits: Tapping is an ancient practice that stimulates our body's own natural healing energy to help us move through blockages and release fear, doubt, worry, and anxiety. It physically grounds us in the here and now.

3. Immovable Horse Stance

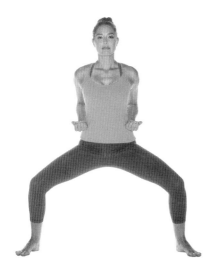

Start in horse stance (see instructions on page 115).

Keep your spine elongated by lifting through the crown of your head while lengthening your tailbone toward the floor. Stack your shoulders directly on top of your hips and hug your front ribs in to engage your core. Make fists with both hands' knuckles facing up, and hug your elbows in tightly against your body. Inhale and draw your elbows back, squeezing your shoulder blades together and pulling your fists to your body just below your bottom ribs. As you exhale, bring your hands to chest height and cross one wrist in front of the other, forming an X shape with your arms while opening your fists. Keep your elbows bent and push your arms forward away from your chest, creating space between your hands and your heart. Sit deeper into your horse stance as you push your palms forward. Hold the pose for 5 cycles of breath.

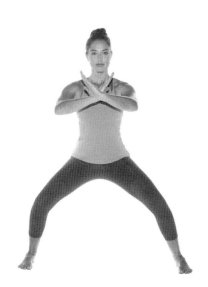

We're often taught that to get ahead in life, we need to say yes to everything, even if saying yes drains us physically, emotionally, mentally, and spiritually. Addiction expert, speaker, and best-selling author Dr. Gabor Maté says that when we continually say yes to things, people, or situations that we don't really want to say yes to, eventually our body will say no. Perhaps you have felt this in your own life or health. Visualize yourself creating an invisible boundary. Perhaps it's an invisible force field, a wall, or your own fortress. When we have experienced sexual trauma, someone has physically and emotionally crossed our boundaries without our consent. Use this exercise to reestablish your boundaries for yourself. You might say "No!" or "Stop!" out loud each time you push your palms forward. Once you have completed 5 reps, straighten your legs, release your arms down by your sides, and take a few moments to notice how you feel.

Benefits: This pose strengthens your legs, glutes, hips, knees, ankles, shoulders, arms, spine, and core; releases anger and frustration; helps create boundaries; and builds confidence and power.

4. Warrior II

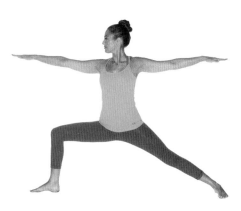

From horse stance, straighten your legs to rise to standing, pivot your right foot 90 degrees to the right, and bend your right knee. Make sure your right knee is stacked directly over your right anklebone, with your thigh parallel to the floor and your back leg pressing straight with your toes angled slightly in. Your right heel should be in a straight line with the arch of your back foot. Adjust your back foot as needed. Exhale and open your arms out toward either side of you at shoulder height. Hug your right outer hip in, lengthen your tailbone down toward the floor, and hug your front ribs in as you elongate your spine and lift through the crown of your head. Gaze over your front fingertips. Hold the pose for 3 to 5 cycles of breath, then repeat on the other side.

Benefits: This pose strengthens your legs; stretches your groin; opens up your hips, chest, and shoulders; builds concentration; and increases stamina.

5. Tree Pose

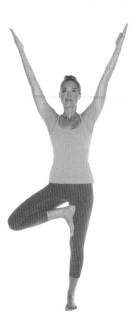

Start in mountain pose (see instructions on page 142). Draw your right knee into your chest, reach down, and catch your right ankle with your right hand. Externally rotate your right knee out to the right as you place your right foot against your left inner thigh. Firm your right foot against your left inner thigh and your inner thigh against your foot. If placing your foot on your inner thigh doesn't feel comfortable or accessible, try placing your foot against your right inner ankle or calf. On an inhalation, sweep your arms up toward the ceiling and spread your fingers wide. Hug your front ribs in to engage your core as you lengthen your spine and lift through the crown of your head.

My soul sister Kate Berlin, founder of Purple Dot Yoga Project, affectionately refers to tree pose as her "manifesting pose." Visualize yourself opening your arms toward the universe and calling in your heart's greatest desire. What do you want to manifest in your life right now? We've already practiced saying no. Now give yourself permission to say "Yes!" to manifesting your dreams in this lifetime. Hold this pose for 5 cycles of breath, then repeat on the other side.

Benefits: This pose opens your hips; strengthens your legs and ankles; tones your core, back, and arms; stretches your thighs and inner groin; improves balance; and creates confidence and empowerment.

6. Pigeon Pose

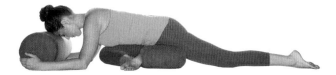

Start in a tabletop position with your hands shoulder-width distance apart on the floor and knees hip-width distance apart. Bring your right knee forward toward your right wrist and your right ankle forward toward your left wrist, so your shin is parallel with the front of the room. Keep your right foot flexed to help support your knee joint. If you experience any knee discomfort or sensitivity, bring your shin away from parallel and into more of a diagonal with your heel drawing closer to your body. Slide your left leg straight back as you lower your hips toward the floor. Keep your spine tall and your chest lifted as you slide your leg back. Inhale and expand your chest while squaring your hips forward. Exhale and fold over your front leg. Rest your forehead on the floor and hold the pose for 5 to 8 cycles of breath. Repeat on the other side. For added support, place a bolster under your front hip and a second bolster under your forehead.

Benefits: This pose opens your hips; stretches your hip flexors, including your psoas, which is the biggest muscle of fight or flight; helps to alleviate sciatic pain; helps release fear and other emotions stored in your hips; and calms your nervous system.

7. Supported Rest Pose with Open Hip Variation

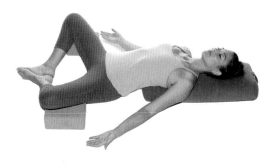

Sit down with a bolster behind you, its shorter end pressed up against your buttocks. Bend your knees, bring the soles of your feet together, and slide your heels in toward your body. Allow your knees to gently fall open, then place a block under either knee for support. Gently lean back onto the bolster with the length of the bolster supporting your entire spine, from your hips to your head. Place a folded blanket under your head if you need more support for your neck. Rest your arms down on the floor away from the sides of your body, palms facing up. Close your eyes if that feels safe and comfortable in your body. You are welcome to keep your eyes open with a soft gaze if you do not feel comfortable with them closed. Stay in this pose for 3 to 5 minutes.

Benefits: This pose calms your nervous system, opens your hips and stretches your inner thighs, opens your chest, supports digestion, and creates a sense of well-being.

Moving Out of Dissociation

Dissociation often accompanies sexual trauma, especially trauma experienced at an early age. But it can also appear in adults who have lived through any type of life-threatening event. Dissociation is often described as a feeling of separateness from our body. It is a survival mechanism that shields us from feeling intense physical sensations, such as pain. However, dissociation can become a maladaptive strategy that prevents us from feeling the full spectrum of sensations and emotions that life has to offer. Yoga is a safe and effective way to help individuals learn to tolerate intense emotions and sensations without checking out physically or mentally.

This grounding sequence creates a safe space for you to reinhabit your body, connect to your breath, and orient you into the present moment.

Quick Tip:
Dry Brushing to Reduce Dissociation

Dry brushing is a self-care practice that exfoliates our skin and helps stimulate our lymphatic system, which supports immune function. While dry brushing is often touted as a way to reduce cellulite and create softer skin, what's far more impressive is its effectiveness in helping reduce dissociation. Dry brushing helps ground you back into your body, connect you with gentle sensations, and define your physical boundaries.

HOW TO DO IT:

- Buy a natural-bristle body brush. You can buy one for $10 or less at most local pharmacies or beauty supply stores or online. I use Earth Therapeutics Purest Palm Body Brush.

- Dry brushing should be done on completely bare and dry skin. I like to do it first thing in the morning and again in the evening before showering. Start at your feet and make long sweeping motions up your legs toward your heart. Reach as many areas on your lower body as possible—ankles, calves, inner and outer thighs, and buttocks.

- Once you've brushed your legs, move to your arms. Lift your arm overhead and begin sweeping from your wrist down toward your chest, making several passes over your inner arm, armpit, and outer arm. Then switch sides.

- Next, brush from your lower back up toward your heart, and, finally, your abdomen up toward your heart. When you have finished brushing your entire body, take a few deep breaths and observe any sensations.

1. Mountain Pose

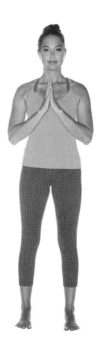

Stand with your feet parallel and hip-width distance apart. Spread your toes wide; root down through your big toe mound, pinkie toe mound, and heel; and engage the inner arches of your feet. Put a micro-bend in your knees, engage your thighs, and visualize yourself grounded and immovable like a mountain. Lengthen your spine, hug your ribs softly in, and bring your palms together at the center of your heart. Take a moment to feel the connection of your feet to the floor and the sensation of your hands pressing together. Hold this pose for 3 to 5 cycles of breath. As you breathe, mentally repeat the affirmation: *I am grounded.*

Benefits: This pose grounds you when you are feeling ungrounded; strengthens your thighs, knees, and ankles; tones your abdomen; improves your posture; and connects you to the present moment.

2. Leg Taps

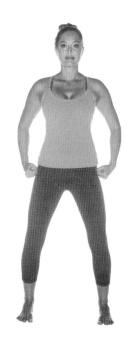

Stand with your feet slighter wider than hip-width distance apart, feet parallel. Make light fists with your hands, bend your elbows slightly, and simultaneously tap your outer hips with your fists. As you tap, say out loud, "These are my hips." Continue tapping down your upper and lower legs, saying out loud, "These are my legs."

Once you reach your ankles, start to tap back up your inner calves, inner thighs, and inner groin. Keep declaring out loud ownership of whatever body part you are tapping. *This is* my *body.* Take a few moments to tap your groin—if you were wearing jeans this would be the place where your pockets sit. Notice any sensations or emotions that arise. Notice if you feel like detaching or feel very little at all. There is no right or wrong, just keep tapping.

After you have spent a few moments here, spend some time on any other parts of your body that you feel guided to. Are there any parts that feel numb or disconnected? Tap there. As you tap, continue to claim ownership of your own body. *These are my arms. This is my heart. This is my body.* When your tapping feels complete, release your arms down by your sides, take a few slow, deep breaths, and observe how you feel.

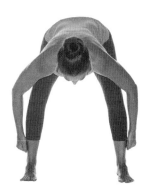

Benefits: Tapping is an ancient practice that stimulates our body's own natural healing energy to help us move through blockages and release fear, doubt, worry, and anxiety. It physically grounds us in the here and now.

3. Breathing Horse

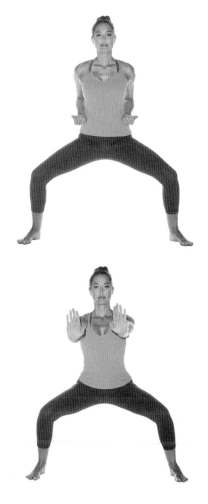

Stand tall and step your feet about two times wider than hip-width distance apart. Exhale as you bend your knees, dropping down into a wide-leg squat, known as horse stance. In martial arts, horse stance is traditionally performed with feet parallel and toes pointing forward, but if this causes any discomfort in your knees, you may turn your toes slightly out and have your knees point in the same direction as your toes.

Keep your spine elongated by lifting through the crown of your head while lengthening your tailbone toward the floor. Stack your shoulders directly on top of your hips and hug your front ribs in to engage your core. Make fists with both hands, knuckles facing up, and hug your elbows in tightly against your body. Inhale and draw your elbows back, squeezing your shoulder blades together and pulling your fists to your body just below your bottom ribs. As you exhale, push both arms straight forward to chest height with your palms open and fingers pointing up. Sit deeper into your horse stance as you push your palms forward. Inhale, pull your fists back to your waist as you straighten your legs slightly, then exhale and push your palms out, again sitting deeply into your legs.

Continue for 5 full cycles of breath. Each time you exhale and push your arms forward, visualize yourself creating an invisible boundary. Perhaps it's an invisible force field, a wall, or your own fortress. Use this exercise to reestablish your boundaries for yourself. You might say "No!" or "Stop!" out loud each time you push your palms forward. Once you have completed 5 reps, straighten your legs, release your arms down by your sides, and take a few moments to notice how you feel.

Benefits: This pose strengthens your legs, glutes, hips, knees, ankles, shoulders, arms, spine, and core; releases anger and frustration; helps create boundaries; and builds confidence and power.

4. Chair Pose

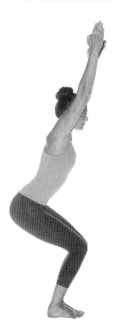

Start standing with your feet together. Inhale and sit deeply back, as if you were sitting in a chair. Reach your arms up toward the sky. Feel your shins moving back as your weight shifts away from your toes, which will help prevent undue stress on your knees. Lift through the inner arches of your feet and feel your inner thighs rolling down as you lift through your chest. Hold for 5 cycles of breath, then release to standing.

Benefits: This pose strengthens your hip flexors, glutes, adductors, and quadriceps; tones your core; strengthens your back; connects you to your legs; grounds you in the present moment; and creates a sense of empowerment and confidence.

5. Supported Standing Forward Fold

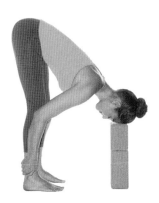

Start standing with your feet parallel, hip-width distance apart. Inhale and sweep your arms up toward the ceiling with palms facing each other, elongating through your spine. Exhale and fold forward from your hips, allowing your spine and head to drape forward toward the floor. Rest your forehead gently on two blocks in front of you. You may use more or fewer blocks depending on how open you feel in your hamstrings. Lightly catch your ankles with your hands as you release your spine to gravity. If your hands don't reach your ankles, you can place them on additional blocks to either side of you. Put a slight bend in your knees and engage your quadriceps, lifting your kneecaps. Shift your weight slightly forward toward the balls of your feet so your hips stack over your ankle bones. Feel your sitting bones draw up as you continue to drape your torso down, creating a stretch through the backs of your legs. Breathe deeply in and out through your nose. Hold the pose for 1 minute.

Benefits: This pose increases flexibility in your hamstrings and calves, creates suppleness in your spine, relieves tension in your neck and shoulders, calms your brain and soothes nerves, helps relieve anxiety and mild depression, and helps ease headaches and insomnia.

6. Seated Butterfly

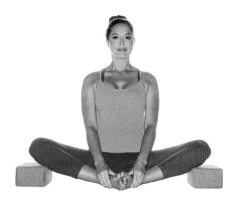

Start seated with your legs straight out in front of you. Bend your knees and bring the soles of your feet together. Draw your heels in closer toward your body and allow your knees to open to either side of you. Place a block or pillow under each knee for added support. Hold on to the outer edges of your feet with your hands. Inhale, lift your chest, then exhale and gently fold forward as far as feels comfortable. As you're holding the pose, you can use your thumbs to gently massage the soles of your feet.

There are many therapeutic acupressure points in your feet to help relieve anxiety, depression, fatigue, insomnia, anger, and more. Don't worry about specific points; just massage in a circular motion until you find a point that feels tender and spend a few extra moments applying gentle pressure there. Hold the pose for 8 to 10 breaths.

Benefits: This pose opens your hips; stretches your inner thighs, groin, and knees; is therapeutic for sciatica; soothes menstrual cramps, premenstrual symptoms, and symptoms of menopause; eases stress; and relieves mild depression and fatigue.

7. Supported Rest Pose

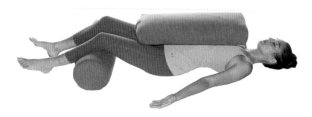

Lie down on your back and place a bolster under your knees to ease tired legs and help support your lower back. If you don't have a bolster, you can use pillows or a rolled blanket. As an option, place a second bolster on your torso and chest. The gentle weight of the extra bolster acts like a weighted security blanket, providing a deeper sense of security as you rest. Rest your arms on the floor away from your torso with palms up and fingers soft. Release any muscular tension in your body as you soften into the floor. Stay in this pose anywhere from 5 to 15 minutes.

Benefits: This pose helps lower blood pressure, deeply calms your body and soothes your mind, helps relieve stress, anxiety, and mild depression, reduces insomnia, and promotes a sense of well-being.

Moving into Intimacy and Connection

One of the most devastating effects of trauma is the loss of connection to ourselves and others. Trauma often occurs within the context of relationships—a wife or a husband abused by their spouse, a child molested by a parent, or an employee assaulted by a superior.

Interpersonal trauma deeply damages our trust in the people around us and impacts our ability to develop healthy relationships, which can lead to social isolation. This is no small thing. In fact, science says that social isolation can be deadly. According to the AARP's Loneliness Study, approximately 42.6 million adults over the age of forty-five in the United States are suffering from chronic loneliness. Social isolation is linked to lowered immunity, higher stress, sleep disturbances, cognitive decline, and early death.[4]

In the aftermath of trauma, it's crucial to find a therapist, mentor, life coach, friend, family member, loved one, or support group that will assist you in beginning to create safe and healthy connections. The key word is *safe*. A safe person is someone who holds your thoughts and feelings with the utmost care, provides a nonjudgmental space for you to share difficult emotions, respects your boundaries, and honors confidentiality.

This sequence is designed to be practiced with a safe person in your life who can support you in building trust and connection. It does not have to be practiced with an intimate partner. Connection can be found equally in intimate and platonic relationships.

Primal Yoga Sequence for Intimacy and Connection

1. Shared Breath

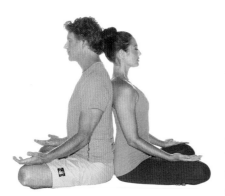

Sit back-to-back with a partner in a comfortable cross-legged position. Prop yourself up on a blanket or cushion if necessary. Place your palms open on your knees, signifying your openness to receive the gift of intimacy and connection.

Lengthen your spine and allow your shoulders to soften away from your ears. Begin to breathe in and out deeply through your nose. Take a few moments to experience the sensation of breath in your own body. Then begin to shift your awareness to your partner. Notice their pattern and rhythm of breathing. Feel the rise and fall of breath in their body as their spine connects with yours. Begin to synchronize your breathing with your partner, creating one fluid union of breath.

Benefits: This breathing exercise relieves anxiety, stress, and mild depression and creates connection and intimacy.

2. Partner Twist

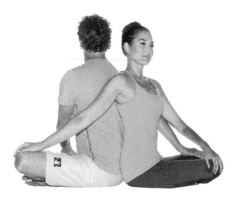

Sit back-to-back with a partner in a comfortable cross-legged position. Inhale as you both reach your arms up toward the ceiling and lengthen your spine. Exhale as you both revolve your torso to the right and place your left hand on your own right knee and your right hand on your partner's left knee. Keep your arms straight, your spine lifted, and your shoulders drawing away from your ears. Hold the pose for 5 cycles of breath, then switch sides.

Benefits: This pose tones your abdomen, increases blood flow to your digestive organs for improved digestion, creates strength and mobility in your spine, helps relieve some types of back pain, opens your chest, and creates connection and intimacy.

3. Partner Stretch

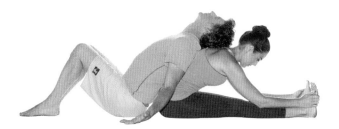

Sit back to back with your partner in a comfortable cross-legged position. One partner will extend their legs straight out as the other partner bends both knees and places both feet flat on the floor, hip-width distance apart. Inhale through your nose. As you exhale, the partner with both legs extended will fold forward, while the other leans back onto their partner and releases their arms down toward the floor with palms open. Hold the pose for 5 cycles of breath, then switch.

Benefits: This pose stretches your hamstrings and calves, opens your chest, creates mobility in your spine, balances your nervous system, and creates trust and connection.

4. Eye Gazing

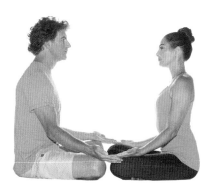

Sit in a cross-legged position, knee to knee with your partner. Rest your palms open on your knees. Close your eyes and take a few deep cycles of belly breath. Notice how you feel in your body. Gently open your eyes and gaze softly at your partner. Hold each other's gaze in silence for 5 minutes. Observe what it feels like to truly see your partner and observe what it feels like to be seen.

Eye gazing is incredibly intimate and can make you feel very vulnerable and uncomfortable at first. When I facilitate this exercise during workshops and trainings, it's very common for people to laugh or giggle uncontrollably at the start. Allow all reactions, thoughts, and feelings to be perfectly okay. While it may be tempting to drop your gaze or look away, challenge yourself to hold your gaze steady without words. If you break your gaze, close your eyes for a moment, take a full deep grounding breath, then simply open your eyes and continue the exercise. Notice any sensations and emotions that may arise without judgment.

Benefits: This pose creates trust, intimacy, and connection and can release oxytocin, known as the "love" or "cuddle" hormone, which promotes bonding.

5. Heart-to-Heart

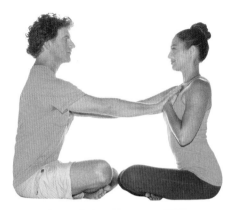

Sit in a cross-legged position, knee to knee with your partner. Place your left hand on your heart. Reach your right arm out and place your right hand over your partner's hand on their heart. Hold this heart-to-heart connection and take a few deep breaths. Once you've finished, thank your partner for creating a safe space for you and thank yourself for having the courage to be vulnerable.

Benefits: This pose creates trust, intimacy, and connection and can release oxytocin, known as the "love" or "cuddle" hormone, which promotes bonding.

Moving into Restful Sleep

I have suffered with bouts of insomnia during various times in my life and have been driven to the brink of insanity when sleep has eluded me. Sleep disturbances rarely occur on their own. They are almost always accompanied by other life disrupters, such as depression, anxiety, chronic pain, serious illness like cancer, or PTSD.

In many cases, insomnia can be the first sign of a more serious underlying issue, such as depression, but sleep disturbances can also occur simply as a result of stress. Whatever your reason may be for not being able to get your quality *zzzz's*, yoga can help. Several clinical trials have shown that yoga may help improve insomnia and other sleep difficulties among cancer patients.[5] Yoga was also linked to reduced frequency of use of sleep medication and an overall improved quality of life for cancer patients. Another small study, by researchers at Harvard Medical School, found that eight weeks of daily yoga can help improve sleep efficiency, duration of sleep, the amount of time it takes to fall asleep, and wake time after the onset of sleep.[6]

This gentle, restorative yoga sequence is designed to help your body and mind wind down in preparation for a restful night's sleep.

Primal Yoga Sequence for Restful Sleep

1. Self-Massage

Find a comfortable sitting position and bring your palms together at the center of your heart. Rub your palms vigorously together until they feel palpably warm. Once you've activated healing energy in your palms, you will use your own healing touch to massage your hands, feet, forehead, and ears. This will deeply calm your nervous system and prepare your body for restful sleep.

Hands

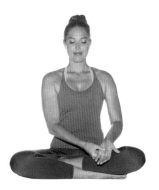

Rest your left hand on your lap and begin massaging the palm of your hand with your right thumb. Apply firm downward pressure with circular motions. Spend a little extra time on any spots that feel tender to your touch. Switch sides.

Feet

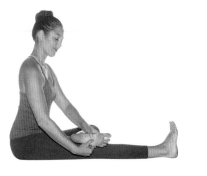

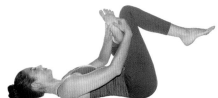

Sit tall with your right leg straight out in front of you. Bend your left knee and cross your left ankle over your right thigh. Use both hands to massage the sole of your foot. Massage in a circular motion, applying firm downward pressure. Spend a little extra time on any spots that feel tender to your touch. Observe any physical sensations or emotions that arise as you hit certain acupressure points. Switch sides.

You may also practice a variation on your back. Lie flat on your back with both feet firmly planted hip-width distance apart. Cross your left ankle above your right knee and draw your right knee in toward your chest. Use both hands to gently massage your left foot. This supine variation offers you the added benefit of a deep outer hip stretch. Switch sides.

Forehead

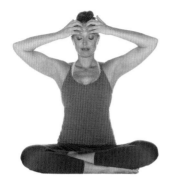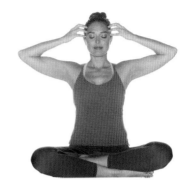

Place the fingertips of both hands on your forehead with your elbows open wide to either side of you. Apply firm and even pressure to the center of your forehead and gently pull your fingertips across your forehead toward your ears, massaging the skin across your brow. Continue this motion for a few cycles of breath.

Ears

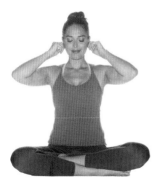

Use your fingers to gently massage your ears. Use your thumb and forefinger to massage both the cartilage of your upper ear and your earlobes in a circular motion.

Benefits: *This massage sequence stimulates self-healing acupressure points to help with a variety of symptoms, including anxiety, depression, and insomnia; improves circulation; relieves muscular and joint pain; relieves arthritis in your hands; deeply calms your nervous system; releases tension and stress; and creates a sense of well-being.*

2. Seated Straddle Forward Fold

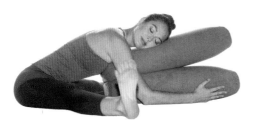

Sit in a wide-leg straddle position with toes point-ing straight up. You may sit on a folded blanket if you need more support. Place one or two bolsters or stacked pillows directly in front of you. Inhale and sit tall to lengthen your spine. Exhale as you fold your torso forward, resting your chest and cheek on the bolsters. Release your arms to the floor, bend your elbows, and gently hug the bolsters as you soften into the pose. Hold for 5 cycles of breath, then turn your cheek to the opposite side and hold for 5 more cycles of breath.

Benefits: This pose stretches your hips, hamstrings, inner thighs, and groin; calms your mind; alleviates anxiety and stress; promotes healthy digestion; and promotes restful sleep.

3. Legs up the Wall

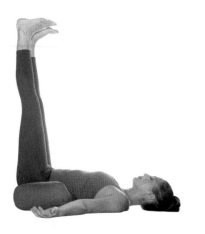

Place a bolster a few inches away from the wall. Sit parallel to the wall on the bolster. Gently roll onto your back as you swing your legs up the wall. Press your heels into the wall and lift your hips slightly off the bolster, allowing your hips to wiggle forward so your sitting bones gently release into the space be-tween the bolster and the wall. Rest your arms down on the floor, palms up. Stay in the pose for 3 to 8 minutes.

Benefits: This pose helps relieve anxiety and mild de-pression, helps relieve headaches and migraines, eases menstrual cramps and premenstrual symptoms, soothes tired legs, and promotes restful sleep.

4. Rest Pose with Progressive Muscle Relaxation

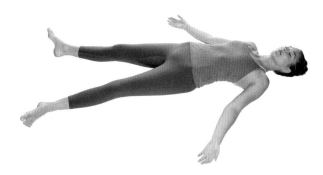

Progressive muscle relaxation involves tensing specific muscle groups in different parts of the body, then releasing the tension, which allows your muscles to relax. Since insomnia can often involve racing thoughts and the inability to "turn off your brain," it is helpful to start with your feet first (the body part farthest away from your noisy brain) and slowly make your way up through each muscle group, finishing with your forehead last.

Lie flat on your back with your arms and legs outstretched. Squeeze each muscle group for approximately 5 seconds, then release all the tension from that body part and allow the muscle to stay relaxed for a minimum of 10 to 15 seconds before moving onto the next muscle group.

- **FOOT**
  Curl the toes of your right foot downward toward the balls of your feet. Hold for 5 seconds, then release.

- **LOWER LEG**
  Flex your right foot by pulling your toes toward your shinbone, and contracting your calf muscle and shin. Hold for 5 seconds, then release.

- **UPPER LEG**
  Engage your thigh muscles on the right side, tightening and drawing your kneecap up, and engaging all the muscles surrounding your knee all the way up to your hip. Hold for 5 seconds, then release.

  Repeat the entire leg sequence on the left side starting with your left foot.

- **BUTTOCKS**
  Squeeze your glutes together. Hold for 5 seconds, then release.

- **ABDOMEN**

  Hug your ribs in and brace your abdominals as if you were doing a crunch. Hold for 5 seconds, then release.

- **HAND**

  Clench your right fist and tighten your forearm. Hold for 5 seconds, then release.

- **UPPER ARM**

  Engage your right biceps by doing a slow bicep curl with a clenched fist. Hold the bicep curl for 5 seconds. Keep the tension in your arm as you slowly straighten your elbow and lower your arm, creating tension in your triceps as the elbow extends. Hold the tension for 5 seconds, then release.

- **SHOULDERS**

  Tense your right shoulder up toward your ear. Hold for 5 seconds, then release.

  Repeat the entire arm sequence on the left side starting with your left hand.

- **EYES AND CHEEKS**

  Squeeze your eyelids shut and scrunch up your cheeks. Hold for 5 seconds, then release.

- **FOREHEAD**

  Furrow your brow. Hold for 5 seconds, then release.

Benefits: *This sequence is therapeutic for insomnia, relieves anxiety, eases chronic pain, calms your brain, and soothes your nervous system.*

Moving Out of Chronic Pain and Fatigue

Chronic pain and chronic fatigue often go hand in hand. Living in unrelenting pain drains us of our life force energy. Similarly, living with chronic fatigue can lead to the development of pain. Movement is like oil for our muscles, joints, and connective tissues, and when we're too tired to get and up get moving, our body pays the price.

Unfortunately, Western medicine doesn't offer many nonpharmacological interventions for chronic pain and fatigue relief. The good news is that emerging research is showing that natural, drug-free interventions like yoga can be effective at relieving pain from chronic conditions such as fibromyalgia, rheumatoid arthritis, chronic back pain, and more. A 2013 meta-analysis of randomized controlled trials involving 743 patients found that yoga had a medium to large effect as a treatment for chronic low back pain (CLBP) and was also effective as a treatment for functional disability.[7]

Research is also showing that yoga works to alleviate chronic pain by bolstering an individual's pain tolerance within the brain. Catherine Bushnell, scientific director of the National Center for Complementary and Integrative Health (NCCIH) at the U.S. National Institutes of Health (NIH), says, "Practicing yoga has the opposite effect on the brain as does chronic pain."[8] Yoga appears to increase the gray matter of our brain in certain key areas relating to how we process and regulate pain. It also appears to strengthen white matter in the same regions. In one study, researchers found that experienced yoga practitioners were able to tolerate the pain of having their hand immersed in cold water more than twice as long as the non-yoga group.[9]

In addition to yoga, other successful Eastern medicine approaches to relieving both chronic pain and chronic fatigue include the use of herbs, acupuncture, and dietary and lifestyle changes. A review of randomized clinical trials published in *Complementary Therapies in Medicine* found that traditional Chinese medicine appears to be effective at alleviating the fatigue symptom for people with chronic fatigue syndrome (CFS).[10]

In the Chinese Five Elements Theory, protecting our kidney energy is extremely important to our health and vitality. As we've discussed, our kidneys are associated with fear. Conscious or subconscious fears can deplete our life force energy, leading to anxiety, depression, muscle and joint pain, insomnia, and severe exhaustion.

This sequence nourishes your kidney energy and introduces gentle stretches to relieve muscle tension, calm your nervous system, and help provide physical relief and an emotional buffer against the stress of living with both chronic pain and chronic fatigue.

Primal Yoga Sequence for Releasing Chronic Pain and Fatigue

1. Seated Kidney Massage

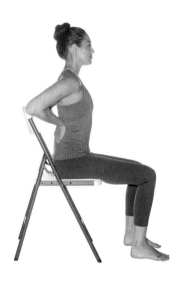

Sit at the edge of a chair with your spine long and your feet planted firmly on the ground, hip-width distance apart. Bring your hands behind you and begin gently massaging the middle of your lower back, just below your ribs. This is where your kidneys and adrenal glands sit. Massage in a circular motion. Notice any sensitivity or tenderness. Massage for 30 seconds to 1 minute.

Benefits: Our adrenal glands sit on top of each kidney and are key players in our stress-response system, producing hormones like adrenaline and norepinephrine. Chronic stress depletes our adrenals, which can lead to adrenal fatigue and symptoms like mild depression or anxiety, an inability to handle stress, lack of energy, low blood sugar, food cravings, reliance on stimulants like caffeine for energy, and a weakened immune system. Tapping and massaging the kidneys is an ancient Eastern self-healing practice that helps bring blood flow and vitality back to this area to help improve kidney and adrenal function while calming fears and anxiety.

2. Seated Shoulder Rolls

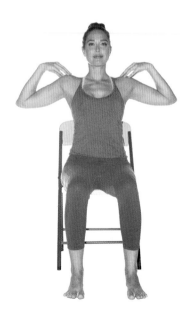

Sit at the edge of a chair with your spine long and your feet planted firmly on the ground, hip-width distance apart. Bring your fingertips to the tops of your shoulders with your elbows wide. Begin slowly drawing circles with your elbows in one direction as you breathe in and out deeply through your nose. Circle 3 to 5 times in one direction, then reverse directions.

Benefits: This movement opens your shoulders, chest, and upper back and helps to relieve tension and stress.

3. Seated Neck Stretch

You can do this stretch either on a chair or seated in a cross-legged position on the floor.

Position 1

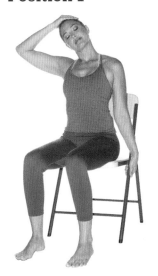

Sit at the edge of a chair with your spine long and your feet planted firmly on the ground, hip-width distance apart. Reach your left hand down and grab the edge of the chair or chair leg. Draw your left shoulder down, away from your left ear. Inhale, sit up tall, and reach your right arm straight up overhead. Exhale, gently place your right hand to the left side of your head, and softly draw your right ear toward your right shoulder. Hold the stretch for 3 to 5 cycles of breath.

Position 2

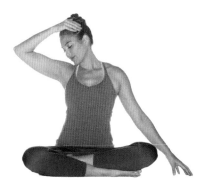

If performing this stretch on the floor rather than a chair, start in a cross-legged seated position. Reach your left arm out to the side, touching your fingertips to the floor. Keeping your right hand on your head, slowly turn your chin down toward your right armpit, dropping your gaze down. Hold the stretch for 3 to 5 cycles of breath. Release your hand from your head, gently roll your chin down toward your chest to stretch the back of your neck, and then release back to a neutral position, sitting up tall.

Benefits: *This movement stretches the muscles in your neck, including your scalenes and levator scapulae; releases tension in your shoulders, neck, and upper back; calms your mind; and relieves headaches.*

4. Seated Spinal Opening

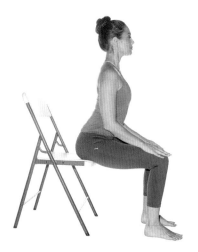 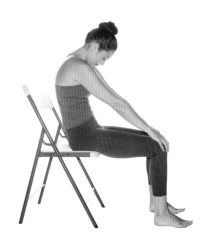

Sit at the edge of a chair with your spine long and your feet planted firmly on the ground, hip-width distance apart. Place your palms down on your knees. Inhale, bend your elbows, extend through your spine, and pull your chest forward. Allow your chest to expand and your lower back to gently arch. Exhale, press your arms straight, draw your chin toward your chest, and round your upper back as your tailbone tucks under. Repeat for 5 cycles of breath.

Benefits: This movement creates mobility in your spine, opens your chest and shoulders, stretches your neck, relieves back pain, and releases tension in your shoulders and neck.

5. Spinal Twist

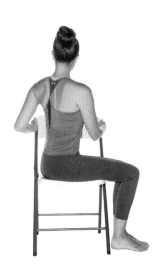

Sit sideways on a chair with your spine long and your feet planted firmly on the ground, hip-width distance apart. Inhale and lift through the crown of your head, sitting up as tall as you can. Exhale and revolve your torso toward the back of the chair, twisting from the base of your spine first. Place your hands on either side of the seat back and inhale to lift your chest while keeping your shoulders drawing away from your ears. Exhale and use your hands on the chair for added leverage to deepen your twist. Hold the twist for 5 cycles of breath. Repeat on the other side.

Benefits: This movement tones your abdomen; increases blood flow to your digestive organs, which improves digestion; creates strength and mobility in your spine; helps relieve some types of back pain; and opens your chest.

6. Seated Hip Stretch

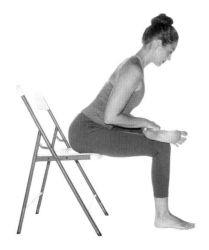

Sit at the edge of a chair with your spine long and your feet planted firmly on the ground, hip-width distance apart. Lift your left foot off the floor, bend your left knee, and place your left ankle on your right thigh. Allow your left knee to open up toward the left side of the room, creating a gentle stretch in your outer hip. Inhale, lift through the crown of your head, and lengthen your spine. Exhale and fold forward over your left shin to deepen the stretch. Hold the pose for 5 cycles of breath, then repeat on the other side.

Benefits: This movement opens your hips, inner thighs, and groin; lengthens your spine; is therapeutic for sciatica; and improves digestion.

7. Chest and Shoulder Opener

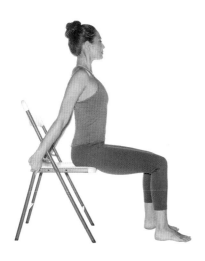

Sit at the edge of a chair with your spine long and your feet planted firmly on the ground, hip-width distance apart. Reach both arms behind you and grab the back of the chair. Inhale, press your elbows straight, squeeze your shoulder blades together, and expand your chest toward the front of the room. Feel your heart lifting toward your chin as you elongate through your neck and draw your shoulders away from your ears. Hold the pose for 5 cycles of breath.

Benefits: This movement opens your chest and shoulders, strengthens your upper back, improves posture, relieves back pain, and energizes your body.

8. Bridge Pose

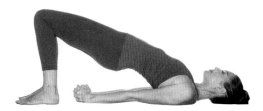

Lie on your back, bend your knees, and place your feet flat on the floor, hip-width distance apart. Inhale and drive your heels down as you lift your hips up off the floor. Engage your inner thighs and glutes and lengthen your tailbone toward the backs of your knees. Interlace your fingers beneath you and wiggle your shoulders closer together to create more expansion in your chest. Press the back of your head gently into the floor, keeping your neck neutral and your gaze softly lifted. Hold the pose for 5 full cycles of breath.

Benefits: *This pose stretches your chest, neck, and hips; strengthens your back and legs; opens up your spine; energizes your body; helps relieve mild depression; reduces fatigue; and relieves backache.*

9. Starfish Stretch

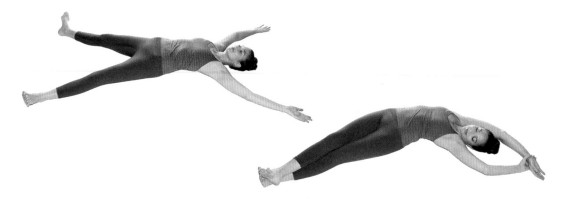

Lie flat on your back and spread your arms and legs wide like a starfish. Take a full deep inhalation, then exhale and swing your right leg over to your left, crossing your right ankle over your left. Keep both legs straight. Inhale and sweep your right arm over toward your left arm. Catch your right wrist with your left hand and gently pull to deepen the stretch in your side body. Hold the stretch for 5 cycles of breath, then repeat on the other side.

Benefits: *This pose stretches your abdomen, side body, lower back, spine, lats, and outer hips; opens your shoulders; relieves back pain; opens your lungs; and improves breathing capacity.*

10. Knee-to-Chest

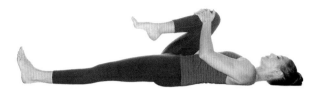

Perform exercises 10 and 11 on the right side first, then repeat both on the left. Lie flat on your back with your legs straight out in front you, toes pointing up and feet hip-width distance apart. Inhale slowly through your nose. As you exhale, draw your right knee into your chest and interlace your fingers over your shin as you hug your knee in. Stay in the pose for 5 cycles of breath.

Benefits: *This pose relieves lower back pain; stretches your buttocks, hamstrings, and hip flexors; improves digestion; and calms your mind.*

11. Reclined Hamstring Stretch

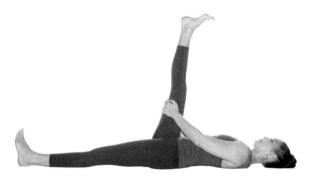

Start in knee-to-chest pose. Interlace your fingers at the back of your knee. Inhale and straighten out your right knee as you stretch your right leg up toward the ceiling. Flex your right foot, drawing your toes down toward your chest. Exhale as you hold the stretch. Stay in the pose for 5 cycles of breath.

Benefits: *This pose relieves lower back pain; stretches your buttocks, hamstrings, calves, and hip flexors; is therapeutic for restless legs; and calms your mind.*

12. Supported Rest Pose

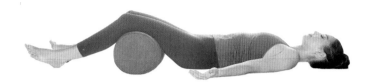

Lie down on your back and place a bolster under your knees to ease tired legs and help support your lower back. If you don't have a bolster, you can use pillows or a rolled blanket. Rest your arms on the floor away from your torso, with palms turned up and fingers soft. Release any muscular tension in your body as you soften into the floor. Stay in the pose anywhere from 5 to 15 minutes. For a deeper release of tension from the body, use the progressive muscle relaxation technique on page 155.

Benefits: *This pose eases chronic pain and relieves fatigue; helps to lower blood pressure; deeply calms your body and soothes your mind; helps relieve stress, anxiety, and mild depression; reduces insomnia; and promotes a sense of well-being.*

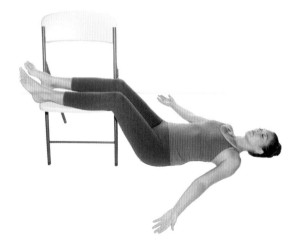

OPTION

Instead of a bolster, rest your legs on the seat of a chair. This is a deeply restorative pose that is therapeutic for your lower back. Your comfort in this pose depends on the height of the chair. Ideally, you want your knees bent at a 90-degree angle, with your calves resting evenly on the seat of the chair. For additional support and comfort, you can place a blanket on the seat of the chair, a folded blanket under your hips, and a folded blanket under your neck.

Releasing Trauma from Our Body

Quick Tip:
Earthing to Relieve Pain and Inflammation

Earthing (also known as grounding) is one of the simplest, most accessible and natural methods to alleviate pain, inflammation, sleep disorders, and free radical damage. Best of all, it's as easy as kicking off your shoes and walking barefoot in the grass, dirt, or sand. Seriously. It's that easy.

Earthing is based on the discovery that our body is a conductor of electricity and we can absorb negative-charged free electrons from the earth. Put simply, this means we all have the ability to connect to the earth's natural healing energy. But many of us are cut off from this abundant natural energy source because of modern conveniences like rubber-soled shoes, multistory homes, and high-rises, which disconnect us from actually touching, sitting, or sleeping in contact with the earth.

If you can't get outdoors, there are a number of earthing products available that allow you to easily ground indoors, including earthing mats (which can be placed under your desk), sheets (which have been successful at treating insomnia), patches, body and knee pads for chronic pain and injuries, and even earthing pet pads to help your four-legged friends relieve symptoms of anxiety and stress, ease joint pain, and more.

For more information on earthing and the science behind it, check out the groundbreaking book *Earthing: The Most Important Health Discovery Ever!*, by Clinton Ober, Stephen T. Sinatra, and Martin Zucker, or shop for earthing products at www.earthing.com.

Moving into Digestive Health

All health begins in the gut. While nutrition is naturally the biggest piece to keeping our gut healthy and happy, exercise can play a supporting role in the process. Regular exercise improves digestion and supports healthy elimination. However, certain types of exercise are better than others for digestive health.

Prolonged high-intensity exercise can temporarily shut down digestion, as blood flow is redirected away from our gut to our muscles (remember fight or flight?). Researchers out of Monash University in Australia found that after two hours of continuous endurance exercise (like vigorous running and cycling) at a 60 percent maximum intensity level, actual damage to the gut can occur.[11]

Low-impact exercise like yoga, on the other hand, can benefit our gut, as yoga is one of the few forms of exercise to stimulate our parasympathetic nervous system, which enables digestion to switch on.

This sequence emphasizes core work and twisting postures to increase blood flow to our digestive system and massage our abdominal organs.

Primal Yoga Sequence for Digestive Health

1. Knee-to-Chest

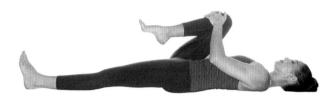

Lie flat on your back with your legs straight out in front of you, toes pointing up, and feet hip-width distance apart. Inhale slowly through your nose. As you exhale, draw your right knee into your chest and interlace your fingers over your shin as you hug your knee in. Stay in the pose for 5 cycles of breath, then repeat on the other side.

Benefits: *This pose relieves lower back pain; stretches your buttocks, hamstrings, and hip flexors; improves digestion; and calms your mind.*

2. Windshield Wipers

Lie flat on your back and send your arms wide to either side of you, palms facing down. You have two options for this movement.

Bent Knee Variation

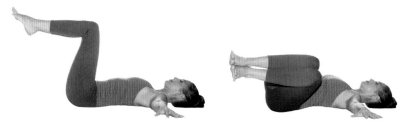

Bend your knees and pull them in toward your chest as you lift your feet off the floor. Stack your knees directly over your hips with your shins parallel to the floor. Keep your knees together and take a full, deep inhalation. As you exhale, rotate your lower body to the left, letting your knees hover a few inches off the floor. Keep your shoulder blades flat on the floor and your neck neutral, eyes gazing softly toward the ceiling. Inhale and use your abdominal muscles to draw your knees back to center, then exhale your knees over to the opposite side. This completes one cycle. Repeat for 5 cycles.

Straight Leg Variation

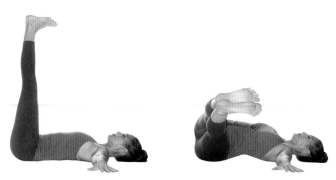

To increase your strength, challenge yourself to try this straight leg variation. Start flat on your back with your knees drawn into your chest. On an inhalation, straighten out your knees and send both legs straight up toward the ceiling. Keeping your legs firmly together, exhale and rotate your lower body to the left, letting your legs hover a few inches off the floor. Keep your shoulder blades flat on the floor and your neck neutral, eyes gazing softly toward the ceiling. Inhale and use your abdominal muscles to draw your legs back to center, then exhale your legs over to the opposite side. This completes one cycle. Repeat for 5 cycles.

Benefits: *This movement strengthens your core muscles, hip flexors, and back; stretches your outer hips and tensor fasciae latae (TFL); increases blood flow to your digestive organs; and improves digestive function.*

3. Seated Twist

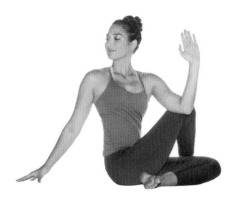

Start seated with your spine long and both legs straight out in front of you. Bend your right knee and draw your right heel in toward your right sitting bone. Lift your right leg and cross your right foot over your left leg, placing your right foot flat on the floor outside your left thigh. Fold your left leg in toward your right sitting bone. Inhale and reach your left arm straight up toward the ceiling. Exhale, rotate your torso to the right, bend your left elbow, and bring your left elbow outside your right thigh with your fingers pointing up. Place your right hand directly behind you, roll your shoulder open away from your ear, continue to lift through your spine, and expand your chest. Gaze over your right shoulder. Hold the pose for 3 to 5 cycles of breath, then repeat on the other side.

Benefits: *This pose tones your abdomen; increases blood flow to your digestive organs, which improves digestion; creates strength and mobility in your spine; helps relieve some types of back pain; releases anger and frustration; and opens your chest.*

4. Seated Forward Fold

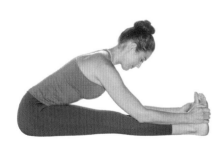

Sit down with your legs straight out in front of you, feet flexed. Inhale and sweep your arms up toward the ceiling, elongating through your spine and reaching through the crown of your head. Exhale and fold forward from your hips. Reach your arms forward and grab the outer edges of your feet as you soften your gaze down. If you need more support, place a bolster or pillow gently on your shins and rest your forehead down. Hold the pose for 1 minute.

Benefits: *This pose stretches your spine, hamstrings, and calves; calms your mind and helps relieve anxiety and mild depression; reduces fatigue; helps ease headaches and insomnia; and improves digestion.*

5. Abdomen Massage

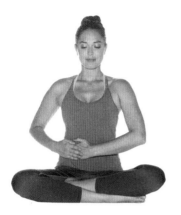

Sit comfortably and bring your palms together at the center of your heart. Rub your palms vigorously together until your palms feel palpably warm. Once you've activated your own healing energy in your palms, place your hands on your lower abdomen (lower *dantian*), with one hand on top of the other. Begin to slowly massage your entire abdomen with your entire hand in a circular motion. Circle 9 times in one direction, then 9 times in the opposite direction. Close by resting your palms over your lower *dantian*. Visualize sending healing energy to your internal organs, bathing them in white or golden light.

Benefits: *This movement improves blood flow to your abdomen and improves digestion, and your own nurturing touch creates a sense of comfort and healing.*

6. Rest Pose

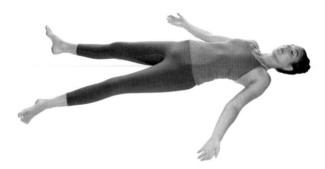

Lie flat on your back with your arms and legs outstretched. Feel the support of the floor beneath you as you release all muscular tension. Offer yourself the space to let go of any worries, thoughts, or emotions. Give yourself the gift of pure presence and offer yourself gratitude for taking the time to practice self-care. Stay in the pose for 5 minutes.

Benefits: *This pose calms your mind, releases muscular tension, and activates your parasympathetic nervous system ("rest and digest").*

Stop and Smell the Citrus

If you've been under a lot of stress or anxiety and your digestive system is paying the price, slice open a fresh orange or lemon and breathe in its citrus scent. The strong citrus scent of a lemon will help turn on your salivary glands and kick-start your digestive system back into action—not to mention help alleviate anxiety on the spot! Our digestive system is ruled by our parasympathetic nervous system, which brings us back into a calmer state.

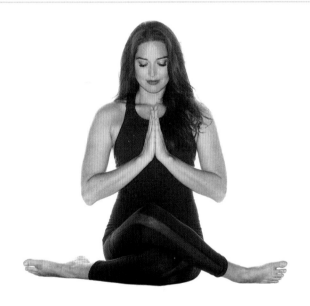

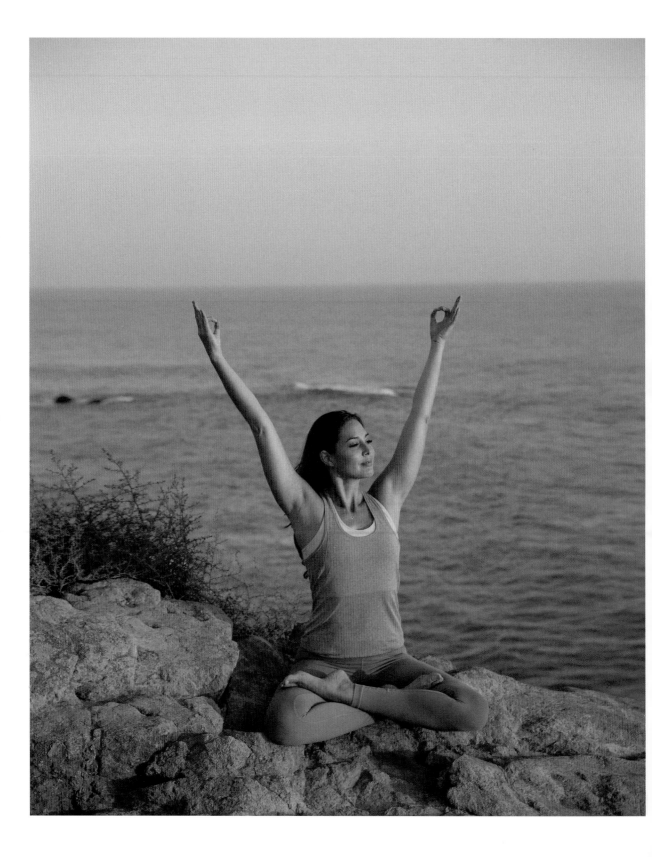

Part III

Using Mindfulness to Rewire Our Brain for Resiliency

Chapter 10

Wired to Wander

If it weren't for my mind, my meditation would be excellent.
—Ani Pema Chödrön

Have you ever pulled into your driveway after a long day at work, turned off your car, and realized you have no recollection of how you got home? Thankfully you made it back in one piece, but you have no memory of getting off at your exit. Who knows? Maybe you missed your exit altogether because your mind was elsewhere. The first time this happened to me, I remember thinking, *Shit. Where the heck was my brain for the last hour? This can't be safe!* This experience got me thinking about how many other tasks I floated through on autopilot every single day.

It's the nature of our mind to wander. Think about it. How many moments during your day are you here, but not really *here*? You're out to dinner with friends but instead of enjoying your meal, you're taking a photo of your food to post on Instagram. Or you're at your daughter's soccer game and miss her winning goal because you're thinking about that big presentation you have at work on Monday.

The ancient yogis call this constant mind chatter *chitta vritti*, or our "monkey mind." The first verse of Patanjali's *Yoga Sutras*, a seventeen-hundred-year-old tome that is widely regarded as the definitive text on yoga philosophy, reads "Atha Yoganusasanam," or "Now, the teachings of yoga." *Atha* means "now" in Sanskrit, and it is no coincidence that *now* is the very first word in the very first line of this ancient text. Yoga happens in the here and *now*. At its core, yoga is a practice of presence.

Patanjali's second verse, "Yogas-citta-vritti-nirodhah," goes on to tell us that the primary goal of yoga is "to still the patterning of consciousness" or "restrain the modifications of the mind." In other words, we practice yoga to quiet our mind.

Within the *Yoga Sutras*, Patanjali outlines an eight-limbed path to reaching enlightenment. The physical postures of yoga (known as *asana*) are the third limb on the eightfold path that ultimately serves as a vehicle to prepare the body to sit still for long periods of time in deep meditation. The last three limbs relate to the practice of meditation itself, including concentration of the mind (*dharana*) and the uninterrupted flow of concentration or steadfast meditation known as *dhyana*. According to Patanjali, when a yogi is finally able to master *dhyana* and the six preceding limbs, he reaches the eighth limb, a state of enlightenment known as *samadhi*. In *samadhi*, a state of bliss is obtained due to transcendence over the Self.

While meditation has been a revered practice in world religions including Hinduism for thousands of years, the good news is you don't have to be a yogi, speak Sanskrit, subscribe to any particular tradition or religion, or even sit for hours on end in full lotus posture to achieve many of the benefits the ancient texts espoused.

Mountains of research continue to uncover the numerous benefits that meditation and mindfulness reap for our body and mind, including reduced stress, lowered blood pressure, alleviation of anxiety and depression, pain reduction, reduced inflammation, improved digestion, reduced cravings, improved sleep, strengthened immune function, improved concentration and learning, and even a slowing down of diseases like Alzheimer's.

A 2013 study conducted by the University of Pittsburgh and Carnegie Mellon University revealed that mindfulness can shrink gray matter volume in the amygdala, our brain's fight-or-flight center, which has been correlated to a decrease in stress levels and less reactivity to potentially frightening stimuli. MRI scans of meditators have also shown that as our so-called stress center shrinks, the prefrontal cortex—the center of executive functions in the brain including attention, awareness, and complex planning—increases in volume. Essentially, mindfulness gives us the ability to stress less and focus more.

Mindfulness meditation has been my saving grace in my own battle with anxiety and panic attacks. I credit my meditation practice for keeping me from ever having to pop a single antianxiety pill. Even though my panic attacks are a thing of the past, I still consistently practice mindfulness to defuse everyday stress and build emotional resiliency.

Beyond its ability to reduce stress, perhaps one of the most exciting prospects of mindfulness is its effectiveness in treating pain. Chronic pain is a leading cause of disability in the United States. According to the National Center for Health Statistics, a staggering 76.2 million people in the United States have suffered from pain that lasts longer than 24 hours—that's one in every four Americans.[1] It's no wonder the United States is currently facing a devastating opioid epidemic that was recently declared a national emergency. More than ninety Americans die every day from overdoses of opioids, which include common prescription pain relievers such as OxyContin, Vicodin, and morphine. Addiction to painkillers and synthetic drugs tragically took the life of my high school sweetheart. He was a star athlete whose career was ended by injuries, which led to years of both prescription and nonprescription drug use to cope with the pain.

A former yoga student recently sent me his mother Nancy Shappell's brave and haunting self-published memoir *A Voice in the Tide*, which chronicles her years of horrific childhood trauma and abuse that resulted in what she describes as a "life of shame in a body fighting against itself."[2] The excruciating chronic pain she lived with ultimately led to an OxyContin addiction and a resulting near-death experience. In her book, she recalls asking the nurse who handed her a prescription for the powerful opioid, "Well, how long would I take it, and what happens when I need to stop?" The nurse replied, "Don't worry about that now. When it's time, you will simply cut back and stop, that's all." Desperate for relief, Nancy accepted the prescription against her better judgment. As she put it, her gut said no, but her pain said yes.

Nancy describes in heart-wrenching detail the debilitating pain she endured that almost killed her while detoxing from the dangerous drug two years later:

> My stomach burns. Diarrhea blasts into every filthy toilet I find myself on. Every inch of skin crawls. Drugs seep rancid out of every pore. Lightning bolts crack where my nerves used to run. I am out of my mind crazy with pain. It grows worse as time ticks. I rock and kick and gulp for breath. I do not drink. I do not eat. I do not sleep. . . . There is nothing lower than lying on the cold dirty floor of a mental ward with your privates smeared in feces, and begging someone you love to save you.

Fortunately, Nancy's story ends triumphantly. Today she helps people consciously heal from their own trauma using holistic tools like mindfulness. But for so many others, addiction and pain are a daily battle. The encouraging news for people suffering from pain is that meditation can offer profound relief. A 2011 study published in the *Journal of Neuroscience* showed that meditation reduces pain by 40 to 57 percent, which is double the pain-relieving strength of morphine![3]

As an athlete, I've had to deal with many injuries, including torn ligaments and broken bones. When I had knee surgery in 2016, the doctor sent me home with a prescription for painkillers that I was instructed to take every four hours. I took half a pill that first night, then threw the rest of the bottle away. I knew the painkillers would simply mask the pain and give me the false confidence to jump back into my yoga and martial arts practice before my knee had actually recovered. It was important for me to *feel*, so I could track my real healing. I won't lie. The pain wasn't pleasant, but deep breathing and mindfulness techniques made it manageable.

The Disease of Stress

Beyond helping to alleviate pain, new research suggests that both yoga and meditation can actually change your genes and reverse stress-related conditions on a cellular level. *Whoa!* Imagine being able to suppress the genetic pathways that promote inflammation in your body and to actually decrease the production of inflammatory proteins simply by sitting still, breathing deeply, and being present. Sounds pretty radical in its simplicity, but that's exactly what meditation can do.

An article entitled "Yoga and Meditation Can Change Your Genes, Study Says" in *Time* magazine recently pointed to an analysis of eighteen previously published studies that took a look at how meditation, yoga, breathwork, qigong, and tai chi affect us on a biological level. It was concluded that these types of mind-body practices could lead to "the reversal of the molecular signature of the effects of chronic stress."[4]

Chronic stress, as we know, wreaks havoc on our physical, mental, and emotional health. It affects everything from our mood to our metabolism, our digestion, our immunity, and even our libido and fertility. To put the gravity of today's epidemic of stress into perspective, another *Time* article, "Save Yourself from Stress," notes the negative impact stress can have on our fertility—or lack thereof. Stress can negatively impact a woman's ability to release eggs and also adversely affects GnRH, the primary reproductive hormone.[5] In other words, stress literally damages our biology and the proliferation of our species.

I should also point out that there actually *is* such a thing as good stress. Take exercising, for example. When we exercise, we put our bodies under physical stress. Healthy structural stress on our bones (like holding a yoga posture for two minutes) actually makes our bones stronger and can help increase bone density.

This same idea applies in a figurative way, as well. Some degree of emotional stress is also healthy because it teaches us resiliency. We need to fall to learn we can pick ourselves back up again. Without many of life's greatest challenges, we wouldn't learn and hone valuable skills like courage, confidence, and perseverance.

But of course there is a tipping point where stress is no longer useful and becomes harmful. So what is the line between healthy stress and traumatic stress? Stress shouldn't include uncomfortable or painful symptoms that don't fade. Yes, your muscles may ache after a great workout, but that burn goes away after a day or two. Yes, your heart may ache after a breakup, but a few weeks later you're back on Match.com.

The stress of trauma is a different kind of stress that takes over our lives. It can be tricky to identify, because this sort of stress often initially presents itself in seemingly small ways. Maybe you're always getting sick or you're tired all the time. Perhaps you constantly have headaches, body aches, stomachaches, digestive issues, or brain fog. Strangely, many of us have become accustomed to accepting most of these physical symptoms as normal. Are they common? Yes. Are they *normal*? No. These are all signs that our body is in distress! And these smaller disruptions can signal bigger issues down the road, such as chronic diseases and autoimmune disorders, which many people with trauma and childhood abuse or neglect end up developing.

There's an old parable about a religious man who was stranded in his home during a flood. He climbed to the roof and trusted that God would save him. A neighbor came by in a canoe and said, "The waters are rising; jump in my canoe so we can get to dry land."

"No, thanks," replied the religious man. "I know God will save me."

Next, a police officer came by in a motorboat. "The waters are rising; jump in my boat and I'll take you to safety."

"No, thanks," replied the religious man. "I trust God will save me."

A little while later, a helicopter appeared and a rescue worker dropped down a rope ladder. "The waters are rising; climb up and I'll fly you to safety."

"No, thanks," replied the man. "I know God will save me."

The floodwaters continued to rise and the man drowned. When he arrived in Heaven, he was upset at God. "I held my faith in you to save me, but you let me drown. I don't understand why!" he exclaimed.

God replied, "I sent you a canoe, a motorboat, and a helicopter! What more did you expect?"

What does this have to do with stress? Our body rarely—if ever—shuts down without warning. It sends us loud and clear signals when we are not well or off-balance, but unfortunately, most of us tend to ignore or dismiss these signals.

Dr. Gabor Maté, renowned addiction expert, childhood trauma researcher, speaker, and author, says, "When we have been prevented from learning how to say no, our bodies may end up saying it for us."[6] Think about all the times in your life you've said yes to something because you felt obligated or feared the consequences of saying no. *Yes, I'll take on that extra shift at work, even though I'm so tired I can barely stand. Yes, I'll get that business report finished tonight, even though it means I won't sleep. Yes, I'll go on a date with you, even though my intuition says no.* Now think of how much stress saying yes has inflicted upon you.

All our collective yeses eventually lead our body to say no. And sometimes our "no" is stripped cruelly away from us by force. A child in an abusive household has no chance of saying no. A woman raped in a dark alley doesn't get to exercise her "no." But that child and that woman will likely experience their "no" in the form of some internal physiological rebellion later on in life. Your body's "no" can be your greatest gift. It's the canoe rescuing you from the flood. Don't wait until you need a helicopter, and certainly don't wait until you drown to listen to what your body is trying to tell you.

Bolster Your Stress Immunity

1. *Connect with others.* Research shows that having a support system reduces stress and strengthens resiliency. At our core, we all yearn for connection and a sense of belonging. As Bessel van der Kolk puts it, "Study after study shows that having a good support network constitutes the single most powerful protection against becoming traumatized."[7] Recovery from trauma involves (re)connecting with our fellow human beings.

   Strengthen your connections by scheduling face time with family, phoning a friend, or joining a support group, religious community, or meet-up group.

2. *Get out in nature.* Researchers in Japan have studied a practice called *shinrin-yoku,* more commonly known as "forest bathing." Essentially, this involves the art of mindfully walking through a forest. A study published in 2010 found that walking in forest environments reduced stress hormones such as adrenaline and noradrenaline and significantly reduced blood pressure.[8]

   Don't have access to a forest? Don't sweat it. The key here is to find a serene, natural environment that will remove you from the busyness of your daily environment. This might include the shoreline of a body of water, a nature trail, or even a tranquil tree-lined street.

3. *Start a gratitude journal.* Gratitude is one of the quickest ways to shift our emotional state. Studies have confirmed that gratitude is an effective way to boost our mood, reduce depression, and improve overall psychological health.

   When you wake up in the morning, write down five things you're grateful for; do the same again in the evening before bed. When you're coming up with your gratitude list, remember that the little things count. Maybe you love the way the sunlight pours in through your window or your morning cup of coffee. Whatever it is, gratitude naturally attracts the energy of abundance and shifts our lens to focus on the beauty in our lives. When we focus on what's right instead of what's wrong, we begin to fundamentally change our relationship with the world around us.

4. *Adopt a furry friend.* Hands down, my two rescue dogs are two of the biggest blessings in my life. I always say *they* rescued *me.* Sharing a life with a pet has proven health benefits, including lowered blood pressure, reduced anxiety and depression, boosted immunity, and even a decreased risk of heart attack and stroke.

   If you're an introvert like me, owning a pet can also help pull you out of isolation. Walking your dogs or taking them to the park is a great way to socialize with other dogs—and humans, too!

Multitasking Our Way to Stress

What I've always found fascinating is our human tendency to glorify stress. We talk about it with a measure of pride, as if the more stress we have and the more daily tasks we manage, the more effective and high performing we are. In corporate culture, multitasking is praised and comes as a standard requirement of the job. Yet research shows that multitasking can actually decrease productivity by up to 40 percent.[9]

According to research out of the University of California, Irvine, not only do we tend to switch activities at an astounding rate of once every three minutes during the course of a typical workday, but multitasking also makes it take us a significantly longer time to get back to the original task because our brain has to "toggle" back and forth.[10] It's also an illusion that we're saving time by doing multiple things at once. A University of Michigan study showed that participants who multitasked writing a report and checking email took one and a half times longer to finish than those who did one task and then the other.[11]

The bottom line is that stress makes us less effective in our jobs, on the athletic field, and in our lives. Mindfulness can help. In its simplest form, mindfulness is all about mono-tasking. It's about being present in each moment and observing whatever the moment holds without judgment. If you are washing dishes, be fully immersed in the experience. Notice the weight of the dish in your hand. Note its color and texture. Feel the temperature of the water on your skin. Turning mindless tasks into mindful moments can rewire our brains for more efficiency, clarity, and calm.

Combat Multitasking with a Digital Detox

A few years ago I had a sobering realization: I was an iPhone addict. My phone was the first thing I checked when I woke up in the morning and the last thing I saw before I went to bed at night. I took it everywhere with me—to the grocery store, to the beach, and even into the bathroom when nature called. I would go into a panic if I left the house without it.

One day, I was out walking my dogs with my nose predictably buried in my phone, when one of my dogs unexpectedly stopped and wouldn't budge. With my face still buried in Facebook, I tugged on her leash, annoyed at her disobedience. When she still didn't move, I turned around to find that she had stopped to smell a flower. Literally, she had stopped to smell the roses. I felt like an asshole and realized in that instant how unhealthy my addiction to technology had become.

Think about it. How often do you check your phone, email, iPad, computer, or social media feed throughout your day? A 2017 study by Deloitte found that, on average, Americans check their phones forty-seven times per day. This adds up to us collectively checking our phones more than 8 billion times per day as a nation. That's an *absurd* amount of screen time.[12]

Child development specialists also note that our addiction to our devices is negatively impacting our children and the way they learn and interact in the world. Pediatrician and child development specialist Dr. Jenny Radesky told NPR that children "learn by watching us how to have a conversation, how to read other people's facial expressions. And if that's not happening, children are missing out on important development milestones."[13] How many moments of crucial attachment bonding are you missing out on when your baby looks up at you from their stroller, only to find that Mom or Dad is busy watching a funny cat video compilation on YouTube? And what message is that sending to your child?

Challenge yourself to go on a digital detox. You don't have to quit cold turkey. Use the tips below to help you cut down your screen time. You'll soon realize that you don't need Wi-Fi to connect. The best connections are made face-to-face.

- Declutter your smartphone by deleting all unnecessary apps.
- Turn off all social media notifications from your devices.
- Create designated phone hours. For example, you can use your device for social media or emails from 9:30 to 10:00 A.M. only. Commit to having your phone off for the remainder of the day.
- Limit the temptation to check your phone every five minutes by keeping it out of sight. Place it in a drawer or in a different room.
- When you have to have your phone on you, turn off the ringer and place it in airplane mode.

Chapter 11

Cultivating a Mindfulness Practice

Do practice while you can. You'll need it when you can't.
—Krishna Das

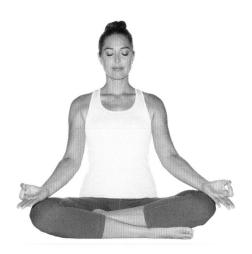

The words *meditation* and *mindfulness* are often used interchangeably, although they are not the same thing. (However, as we'll discuss, there *is* some overlap.) What both practices have in common is that they have been shown to improve physical and mental health.

Meditation is a formal practice in which practitioners intentionally dedicate time to practice techniques to help develop concentration, clarity, equanimity, and a focused state of mind. When I meditate, I carve out a set time in my day, create a peaceful space free of distractions, set a timer for twenty minutes, and then pick one meditation practice to sit with that day. There are many different types of meditation, including Zen meditation, mantra meditation, Transcendental Meditation, Kundalini meditation, *metta* meditation (also known as loving-kindness meditation), and, yes, mindfulness meditation.

Mindfulness can also be a formal meditation practice, with its roots in traditional Buddhist meditation practices that have been adapted over time. One of the most popular and research-backed mindfulness practices in the West today is mindfulness-based stress reduction (MBSR), which was developed in 1979 by Dr. Jon Kabat-Zinn. MBSR is used in hospitals, health clinics, and even psychotherapy practices to help people with depression, anxiety, addiction, chronic pain, and various medical conditions.

Unlike meditation, *mindfulness* can also refer to an informal practice that can be done anytime, anywhere, and during any activity or interaction. In this sense, mindfulness is simply being aware. It's about bringing awareness to each moment by noticing and observing thoughts, feelings, sensations, colors, textures, sights, sounds, and behaviors without judgment. It's the art of being present to whatever is going on around and inside you. Mindfulness can be practiced in line at the grocery store, while washing dishes, walking your dog, or having a conversation with a friend.

Still confused? Just think of *meditation* as a formal practice wherein you set a timer for a specific amount of time or attend a dedicated class. *Mindfulness meditation* is another form of meditation (you can also set a timer or go to a class). And *mindfulness* itself is simply being aware. The practices that follow are a combination of all three.

The Importance of Mindfulness

We now know that mindfulness has the power to help banish anxiety, depression, chronic pain, and even addiction. But how exactly does it accomplish these things?

- *Mindfulness anchors us in the present moment.* This frees us from the pain of the past and fear of the future and helps us stop obsessive thoughts in their tracks. Have you noticed that when you're really anxious about something, it's usually tied to an event or person from the past or linked to fear about how something will turn out in the future? For example, you wake up on Sunday morning, and instead of enjoying the weekend with no obligations or plans, you stress about that big presentation you have to give at work on Monday. You run through imaginary worst-case scenarios, such as forgetting your speech and standing there like a deer in the headlights in front of your boss and colleagues. Before you know it, your day off has passed you by and you've wasted it thinking about work. Or perhaps you're spending your Sunday overanalyzing how your blind date went last night. What did she mean when she said, "I have a busy week ahead, but we'll touch base?" Was that her way of blowing you off? Why didn't he go in for a kiss? Was he being a gentleman or was he not attracted to you?

We can't predict the future, and worrying about the past only takes away from what's right in front of us. As it says in the *Yoga Sutras*, "Heyam duhkham anagatam." Pain that has not yet come is avoidable. If we allow our present to be filled with the fear of future suffering, we needlessly suffer twice.

- *Mindfulness helps us recognize and separate our thoughts from our emotions and physical sensations.* It's difficult to make clear, levelheaded decisions when our emotions are running the show. The skills we cultivate through mindfulness allow us to recognize when our emotions are in control and can help pull us out of the dizzying irrational spiral that often accompanies them. Mindfulness can also help us handle overwhelming sensations. If you've ever experienced a panic attack, you know that sensations like feeling your heart beat quickly can trigger intense emotions such as fear that ultimately land you in the emergency room thinking you're in the midst of a heart attack. When we can observe our heartbeat without attaching any dire predictions or fear-based meaning to it, we begin to free ourselves from the clutches of panic.

  Mindfulness teaches us that sensations are temporary and feelings are not facts. Write that on a Post-it note and tape it to your bathroom mirror. *Sensations are temporary and feelings* are not *facts.*

- *Mindfulness helps us be less reactive and more in control of our emotions, thoughts, and behaviors.* Have you ever been on the receiving end of criticism and instantly retaliated by hurling back an insult you later regretted? That's *reacting.* Mindfulness creates the space for us to *respond* rather than react. For example, you first notice the emotion of anger arising. Next you pause and take a deep breath. You ask yourself where the other person is coming from. You then choose to respond with thoughtfulness rather than defensiveness.

Putting Mindfulness into Practice

Take a few minutes to practice mindfulness right now. To get started, read the following instructions all the way through, then set this book down and put your mindfulness skills to work!

1. *Settle in.* Find a comfortable seated position, or if you prefer, lie down. Set a timer for 5 minutes.

2. *Notice physical sensations.* Bring your attention to all the points where your body is in contact with the surface you are sitting or lying on. Does your body feel heavy,

light, tense, at ease? Are you experiencing pain, pressure, or discomfort? What is the texture of the surface you are sitting or lying on? Smooth, scratchy, hard, soft, warm, cold? Take a few moments to simply be curious and observe.

3. *Notice sounds.* Open your senses and begin paying attention to everything you hear around you. Notice sounds in the room as well as sounds off in the distance. If you're in a quiet environment, you might not hear any sounds at first. But even in the most quiet of settings, there is always sound present. Perhaps it's the gentle hum of your refrigerator or the breeze rustling through the trees. Can you hear the subtle sound of your own breath? Take a few moments to pay full focused attention to all sounds.

4. *Notice sights.* If your eyes are closed, open them and look at the environment around you with curiosity. Look at the floor. Is there a pattern, texture, or color? Is it tile, carpet, concrete, grass? Gaze up from the floor and explore the rest of the room. If you're indoors, notice the walls—take in their color and texture. Notice what's in the room with you. Look at the furniture, ceiling, and window. Be fully present as you observe.

5. *Notice when your mind wanders.* As you are exploring all the sensations, sights, and sounds around and within you, pay attention to the moments when your mind wanders off in thought or you become distracted. Observe these momentary breaks in presence with curiosity, and when you catch yourself wandering off, gently guide yourself back to the exercise. Remember that our minds are made to wander. You are not doing mindfulness "wrong" when you suddenly start thinking about what you're going to have for lunch. The practice is to notice *when* our mind has wandered and bring it back to the moment at hand. The more it wanders, the more opportunities you have to hone your skills!

Mindful Breathing Practices

Our breath is the quickest and most effective way to release ourselves from our obsessive thoughts, calm our nervous system, and tune into the present moment. You'll recall that conscious breathing techniques set the foundation for all of our movement sequences. So it is with our mindfulness and meditation techniques. Our breath is the way in.

Breath Labeling

Breath happens in the present moment, making it one of the most powerful ways to tune into the experience of *now*. Mentally labeling it—as we'll learn to do with this exercise—adds another layer of concentration, which helps keep your mind focused in the present.

- Find a comfortable seated or lying position. If it feels comfortable to you, close your eyes. Set a timer for 5 minutes.

- Begin to breathe in and out slowly through your nose.

- Place one hand gently on your belly and feel your abdomen softly inflating like a balloon as you inhale and naturally falling as you exhale. Notice any physical sensations as you breathe. Do you have any muscular tension or tightness? Do you feel expansive? Does your breath have any sensation of warmth or coolness?

- Continue breathing. Label your next inhale by mentally saying "in." As you exhale, mentally say "out." Continue silently repeating "in" and "out" in synchronization with each inhale and each exhale.

- If you lose track of the labels and find that your mind has wandered off, gently guide yourself back to your breath and begin your labels again.

Breath Counting

Breath counting is one of my favorite mindfulness practices. When I first decided to learn how to meditate, I had no real compass to guide me. I would set a timer for twenty minutes, scrunch my eyes shut, and pray that my mind would turn off. You can probably guess how well that went. My eyes would pop open thirty seconds later, by which point I was completely exasperated that my mental chatter had refused to silence itself. Learning to count my breath was a game-changer because it gave my monkey mind a point of focus.

- Find a comfortable position, either seated or lying down. If it feels comfortable to you, close your eyes.

- Begin to breathe in and out slowly through your nose. Place one hand gently on your belly and feel your abdomen softly inflating like a balloon as you inhale and naturally falling as you exhale.

- Continue breathing and begin to count each full cycle of breath mentally on each exhale. For example, inhale deeply, and as you exhale, mentally count "one." Take another full inhalation, and as you exhale, mentally say "two." Continue counting each exhalation all the way up to ten. Once you get to ten, count backward on each exhale until you reach one.

- If you are new to breath counting, you will inevitably find that you lose your count somewhere on your journey from one to ten. You may forget what number you were on or catch yourself counting all the way up into the twenties. When you notice you have lost count or counted beyond ten, simply bring your attention back to your breath and start your count over again from one.

- Set benchmarks for yourself. Your first benchmark is simply to make it from one to ten without your mind wandering. It may take a few sessions before you are able to reach ten breaths without being distracted. Once you are able to count from one to ten with full focused presence, challenge yourself to count backward down to one. Next, set a timer for 10 minutes and see if you can maintain continuous focused concentration counting from one to ten and ten to one until the timer rings. As always, be patient with yourself and approach the practice with curiosity rather than judgment.

Labeling Emotions

Developing mindful awareness of our emotions is a powerful tool that gives us more control over our thoughts and feelings. Labeling helps defuse emotional reactivity because the part of our brain that processes language is different from the one that serves as our emotional center. Giving our emotions a verbal label such as "anger" can help diminish the intensity of that emotion.

- Find a comfortable position, either seated or lying down. If it feels comfortable to you, close your eyes.

- Begin to breathe in and out slowly through your nose. Place one hand gently on your belly and feel your abdomen softly inflating like a balloon as you inhale and naturally falling as you exhale. Notice any sensations as they arise.

- After taking between 5 and 8 breaths, begin shifting your attention to any emotions you are experiencing. You might start by simply asking yourself, *How do I feel in this moment?* Happy, sad, nervous, anxious, calm, peaceful, agitated, angry, impatient? Sit with your emotions until you can truly identify what it is you're feeling. Give your emotion a label like "grief," "shame," "guilt," or "joy."

    You might feel a number of emotions shouting at you all at once. Identify the one with the loudest voice.

You might feel no emotion at all. If that's the case, I invite you to recall a situation in your life that carries an emotional charge—something that feels unresolved. It might relate to a particular person or event. Rather than getting caught up in the details of the story, simply draw your attention to whatever emotions arise when you recall this event.

- Once you have labeled the emotion, ask yourself where it lives. Where do you feel this emotion in your body? Does it show up as a clenching in your jaw? A tightness in your chest? A knot in your stomach? Tension in your shoulders? An ache between your shoulder blades? Get curious, tune in, and explore where the emotion is stored.

- If you can comfortably do so, once you have located the physical home of your emotion, place one or both hands over the part of your body where the emotion currently resides. You may place your hands over your heart or gently on your belly. Continue to breathe deeply with focused attention on the area where your hands are resting. Stay here for a few minutes. Notice if the sensation or emotion starts to shift or change. Does the emotion reach a crescendo? Once it peaks, does the intensity diminish? Are the edges of the emotion softening? Observe with curiosity and welcome all feelings as they rise and fall.

Labeling Thoughts

Our thoughts show up in two main ways: visual thoughts or mental images and auditory thoughts or our inner monologue. If I were to ask you to visualize a tree, you most likely would create a mental picture of a tree in your mind. You might visualize an oak tree or a palm tree, but whatever image you conjure up is an example of a visual thought.

An auditory thought is a thought that comes to us in the form of language. If you're standing in a crowded elevator and someone is wearing too much perfume, you might hear your own voice in your head saying, *Yuck. Someone needs to lay off the body spray.* Any time you hear your inner voice speaking up, that's an auditory thought.

Some people think mainly in pictures, others mainly in words, and some in a combination of both. The thought-labeling practices that follow help us recognize and separate out our thoughts so they no longer overwhelm, confine, or define us.

MINDFUL AWARENESS OF VISUAL THOUGHTS

- Find a comfortable position either seated or lying down. For this practice, it's helpful to close your eyes so you can focus on visual thoughts. Set a timer for 5 minutes.

- Begin to breathe in and out slowly through your nose. Take a few moments to anchor yourself into the sensation of your breath.

- Notice what you see with your eyes closed. You may be wondering, *How can I see anything when my eyes are closed?* (This, incidentally, would be an example of an auditory thought!) Even with our eyes closed, we still have a "mental screen." We might see shades of black, flickering spots, flecks of color, or light filtering in from our eyelids. Focus your attention on your mental screen and simply wait for your next mental image to appear.

- When a mental image does appear, mentally label it "see in," which is simply an abbreviated way of saying you *see* an image *in* your mind. The image may be a visual memory, a daydream, a mental picture of what you're going to have for dinner, your dog's furry face, a vision of a place that holds meaning to you, or a completely random place or object.

    Note that you don't have to label *what* it is that you are seeing, like "serene lake" or "spaghetti dinner." Just use the phrase *see in*. This will help prevent you from getting caught up in a story and keeps the focus on awareness of the thought itself. If no image comes, no problem. Continue breathing deeply and focusing on your mental screen, labeling any visual thought that arises with "see in."

- Notice what happens when you label your mental thought. Does the image go away? Does it stick around? Does it transform into another image? Do you go back to your mental screen? For most of us, the moment we become the observer of our thoughts, the thought itself momentarily evaporates. In that instant, we can experience total mental quietude.

- Once your timer goes off, open your eyes and sit with your experience for a few moments. Notice how you feel. Can you recall how many mental images arose for you within those 5 minutes?

MINDFUL AWARENESS OF AUDITORY THOUGHTS

- Find a comfortable position either seated or lying down. For this practice, it's helpful to close your eyes so you can focus on auditory thoughts, but I invite you to keep them open if that feels more comfortable to you. Set a timer for 5 minutes.

- Begin to breathe in and out slowly through your nose. Take a few moments to anchor yourself in the sensation of your breath.

- Set your intention to focus on your auditory thoughts. Sit quietly and wait for your next auditory thought to appear. Your next thought might be something like *What does she mean by wait for my next thought?* or *I don't know if I'm doing this right.* Those are both examples of auditory thoughts.

- When you hear your inner voice speak, label it "hear in," which is simply an abbreviated way of saying you *hear* a thought *in* your mind. There may be long or short periods of mental silence between thoughts, or your thoughts might be racing constantly. Remember, there is no right or wrong and there is no way to fail at this. We are simply practicing being the observer of our thoughts.

- After a few moments of using the label "hear in" any time an auditory thought pops in, you may experiment with adding a second label of "hear out." Hear out refers to any sound you hear outside of your inner experience—for example, a car passing by on the street, birds chirping in the trees, or a dog barking off in the distance. Sit quietly and mentally note any external sounds in your surrounding environment with the label "hear out" and any auditory thoughts in your internal environment with the label "hear in." In moments during which there is an absence of thought or sound, allow there to be quiet space without any labels.

- Once your timer goes off, open your eyes and sit with your experience for a few moments. Notice how you feel. Can you recall how many thoughts arose for you within those 5 minutes? Were you able to observe your thoughts rather than identify with them? With consistent practice, we become more easily able to extricate ourselves from the drama of our thoughts and simply witness them as a curious observer.

A Beginner's Guide to Meditation

If you've avoided meditation in the past because you "can't sit still" or your "mind never shuts off," or simply because you're "too busy," I have good news: meditation was made just for you. It's often the people who have the most resistance to meditation that benefit from it the most. I say this with authority, because I used to be one of those people who thought meditation was a complete waste of time. Just the thought of sitting still with my eyes closed, alone with my racing thoughts, made me agitated.

The meditation techniques in this book are designed to make meditation approachable, practical, and easy to fit into your busy life. Some techniques may resonate more than others. Use what works and leave what doesn't. Here are some basic guidelines to get you started.

Don't Worry About Doing It "Right"

Many people give up on meditation before they start because they feel like they're not doing it right. Let go of right and wrong. Your meditation practice will feel different each day. Some days your thoughts will be racing and you'll find yourself easily distracted. Other days you'll effortlessly drop into your practice. Let go of expectations and judgment. The most important thing is that you show up. Commit to flexing your meditation muscle, even if it's only for five minutes.

Consistency Is Key

Think of your meditation like a workout. The more you use your muscles, the stronger they become. It's the same with meditation. The more you practice, the more long-term benefits you'll reap. With regular practice, you can lower your baseline of emotional arousal. In other words, you will find yourself resorting less frequently to fear and more frequently to patience and equanimity.

Create a Sacred Space

Whenever possible, create a space that invites peace and tranquility. Designate a quiet corner in your home or office. Decorate it with candles, plants, or objects that create feelings of well-being for you. Turn off any distractions like your phone, computer, radio, or television when preparing for a formal meditation practice.

Although we're talking about meditation, it does bear mentioning that this doesn't necessarily apply to mindfulness. When you are practicing mindfulness, the more distractions, the better, because it gives you an opportunity to be present in a nonreactive, nonjudgmental way to whatever is around you.

Wear Comfortable Clothing

Wear soft, loose-fitting clothing that you can breathe in. When your physical body is at ease, your mind has the opportunity to follow suit.

Find Your Perfect Position

Many traditional forms of meditation are done seated on the floor or a meditation cushion with your spine upright and legs in a crossed position (or lotus posture). If this feels comfortable in your body, go for it. However, meditation can also be practiced standing, seated in a chair, or lying down. Support yourself with anything you need to create greater comfort and ease.

Practice on an Empty Stomach

This is not a hard-and-fast rule. In fact, there are no hard-and-fast rules in this book. There's only what works for you and what doesn't. However, I prefer to practice on an empty stomach because I find meditating after a heavy meal can make me feel drowsy. In a formal meditation practice, the idea is to create a calm yet alert state, not a sleep state. However, I never discourage my students from falling asleep during meditation. Many people I work with suffer from insomnia, and falling asleep during meditation is a gift their body may desperately need!

Common Questions and Misconceptions About Meditation

Is meditation a religion?

No. While meditation has roots in many of the world's major religions and many people do use it as a spiritual practice, you do not have to subscribe to any particular religion or tradition to meditate. It is a research-backed tool to help ease psychological distress and create greater health and well-being.

It still sounds a little too "hippie-dippie" for me.

I totally get it. I had an ex who proclaimed that every Sunday was to be "Silent Sunday," a day dedicated to meditation with no talking. If I wanted to communicate with him, I was instructed to do so via sticky notes. He's an example of what I call a "spiritual douchebag." That was enough to turn me off to meditation for a few years. But I'm so grateful that I rediscovered meditation again on my own terms, free of dogma or ego. There are so many different styles and techniques. If one style doesn't resonate with you, let it go and try another. My general rule of thumb is that if a teacher tells you their way is the only way or the right way, walk away.

I can't turn off my thoughts!

Neither can I. The goal is not to stop your thoughts. Our mind is wired to wander. Meditation is about observing when your mind has wandered off and catching yourself before it goes too far. The simple act of observing the fluctuations of our mind anchors us back into the present moment.

What happens if I fall asleep?

Great! Your body probably needed the rest. It's true that many traditional forms of meditation advocate a rigid upright posture with the aim of helping practitioners avoid falling asleep. The counterargument to that is that many combat veterans with PTSD report that meditation is one of the few times during their day when they are able to get so relaxed that they fall asleep.

Do I need to study with a teacher?

While I highly encourage you to study with a teacher who can show you the ropes and hold you accountable, it is perfectly fine to practice on your own. In addition to the practices offered below, there are thousands of free guided meditations available to download online. There are also a ton of great apps like Headspace or Insight Timer that offer guided meditations to get you started.

Chapter 12

Meditations and Mindfulness Practices for Healing

Thoughts, rest your wings. Here is a hollow of
silence, in which to hatch your dreams.
—Joan Walsh Anglund

The following meditations and mindfulness practices are meant to be companions to you in times of need. Reach for them whenever you need to get out of your racing thoughts and anchor into your heart. They are designed to comfort and ground you in times of stress, anxiety, anger, grief, numbness, pain, and fear.

The meditations that follow are organized in a way that allows you to easily flip to the practice you need the most based on whatever particular physical, mental, or emotional challenge you may be experiencing on any given day. They include a variety of both mindfulness practices and meditation techniques, offering you choice and freedom to use what works for you and to discard what doesn't. You may stick with just one technique or find multiple practices that ring true for you. Many of the meditations use mantras or affirmations. If the suggested mantras or affirmations don't resonate with you, feel free to create your own. *Remember, this is your practice.* While I sincerely hope this serves as a practical and powerful guide for you, trust that the answers are and always have resided within.

Last, note that meditation and mindfulness yield the best results when practiced consistently. When you incorporate these powerful tools of presence into your daily life, you will experience greater calm, clarity, focus, contentment, connection, intuition, emotional resiliency, empowerment, and well-being.

Meditation for Depression

Depression is marked by a lack of forward momentum, motivation, and energy. You may feel lethargic, numb, disconnected, discouraged, sad, or hopeless. Healing from depression requires reconnecting to your vital life force energy. This meditation has two phases, an active breathwork practice and a seated practice.

Phase 1: Joyful Breath

We covered this energizing and uplifting breathing technique in part II of this book and offer it again here as a powerful tool to enliven your body and mind when you're feeling low. Please refer to page 76 for instructions.

Phase 2: Seated Meditation

- Find a comfortable position either seated or lying down. Close your eyes or keep them open, depending on what feels most comfortable for you.

- Begin to breathe in and out slowly through your nose. Take a few moments to anchor yourself in the sensation of your breath.

- Raise your arms to chest height with your elbows softly bent and arms rounded, as if you were holding a giant ball. Visualize that this ball is now a boulder. Feel the weight of the boulder in your arms. Notice how the heaviness of this boulder affects your body, your posture, and your breath. Feel the energy it requires to simply hold up your arms. Notice any thoughts and emotions that arise from carrying this enormous weight. Breathe into whatever sensations, thoughts, and emotions arise.

- Allow yourself to gently put the boulder down and release the weight you have been carrying for far too long. This is not your weight to bear. As you let your hands gently rest in your lap, mentally repeat the following affirmation to yourself: *I release this weight. I choose to let it go.*

- Observe what it feels like to let this weight go. Notice any physical sensations. Do you feel lighter, taller, warmer, cooler, expansive, grounded? Notice any thoughts and emotions that are present. Welcome them all. Take a few moments to breathe into this new space of lightness.

- With your arms still gently resting in your lap, repeat the following affirmations silently to yourself or out loud:

    I am enough. I am more than enough.

    My life has meaning.

    I am worthy.

    I am loved.

    I love myself unconditionally.

- Take a few moments to sit quietly and feel the resonance of these affirmations in your body.

Mindfulness and Meditation for Anxiety and Panic

The accumulated trauma in my life left me wanting an escape hatch—anything to dampen the pain so I didn't have to feel all the emotions that threatened to overwhelm me on a daily basis. So I turned to drugs. Psychedelics, to be exact. Not surprisingly, this was a very bad call.

I had done drugs only a handful of times in my life, and nothing much harder than smoking the occasional joint while growing up in Hawaii. But at this particular period in my life, magic mushrooms seemed like an intelligent choice. The first few minutes of psychedelic euphoria quickly turned to dread. An hour in, I desperately wanted off the roller coaster. When the effects finally wore off, I was left exhausted and terrified. I had experienced my first panic attack, and unfortunately for me, though the mushrooms were gone, the anxiety remained.

It's like those mushrooms wove their way into my marrow, discovered the layers of trauma trapped in my bones, and decided the time had finally come to bring it all to the surface. After that night I started experiencing regular and debilitating panic attacks. I was terrified to go to sleep because I was convinced I wasn't going to wake up. The edges of reality blurred, my heart felt like it was going to explode, my arms and legs went numb, and I was one hundred percent certain that I was going crazy. I lived with an impending sense of doom, and the scope of life began to narrow. I was afraid to drive, get on an airplane, or go out in public. Plain and simple, I was afraid to live. The official diagnosis was panic disorder and agoraphobia (PDA). I was told by a very reputable and expensive therapist that I had a very long and challenging road ahead of me.

I desperately wanted a quick fix. Unfortunately, many "quick fixes" are prescribed in the form of antianxiety medications, despite their lengthy list of adverse side effects. My blessing in disguise was the fact that no matter how badly I wanted to take a magic pill, the thought of putting any kind of drug (even something as benign as aspirin) into my body instantly sent my nervous system into fight-or-flight mode. I wanted to crawl out of my skin, and for the first time ever, I understood with complete clarity how suicide could be the less painful option.

I knew I would have to find a natural solution for my anxiety and panic attacks. And not just a Band-Aid. I didn't want something to simply help me cope. What I needed was hope.

And so it was that I found mindfulness. It became the flashlight I needed to help me find my way out of the dark.

What Is Panic Disorder?

Think of panic disorder like a home alarm system. You're asleep in the middle of the night when suddenly your security alarm goes off without warning. Your fight-or-flight response kicks in—your eyes spring open, you jump out of bed, your muscles tense, and your heart starts racing as you grab your baseball bat, prepared to fight off a home invader. But let's say you have a faulty alarm system and instead of your alarm going off only when there's actual danger, it goes off *all the time*—even when no danger is present.

Regardless of whether you're experiencing an actual or imagined threat, your body responds the same. If that alarm continues to go off every night, pretty soon you'll be living in an anxious state of hypervigilance, afraid to close your eyes. It creates a self-perpetuating cycle of fear. One of the simplest definitions of panic disorder I've ever heard is "fear of panic." Wondering if you fit the bill? Here are some signs you might have a problem with anxiety or panic:

- Avoiding certain activities out of fear that they might trigger symptoms of anxiety.

- Avoiding certain places because you are afraid of having a panic attack in public.

- Using drugs or alcohol to reduce your anxiety.

- Using binge-eating, self-harm, or other unhealthy behaviors to reduce your anxiety.

- Avoiding leaving your home.

- Avoiding watching horror films or certain television shows because they cause anxiety.

- Extreme sensitivity to loud noises.

- Difficulty concentrating and the resulting concern that you won't be able to get important tasks done.

- Being afraid to go to sleep.

- Experiencing sudden and repeated attacks of intense fear.

- Feeling fearful of being out of control during a panic attack.

- Feeling fearful of physical sensations, such as a rapid heart rate or tingling in the arms and legs.

- Feeling fearful about when the next panic attack will strike.

How Mindfulness Can Help

Much of the anxiety we experience on a daily basis is triggered by fear of an imagined future. Developing mindfulness skills helps anchor us in the present moment. Mindfulness teaches us how to observe our thoughts, sensations, and emotions here and now, and can help us discern the difference between facts and feelings. As we've previously discussed, when we're in fight-or-flight mode, our higher brain goes offline. Remember, this is a survival instinct. If there is an imminent threat, we need to react first and think second. In the case of anxiety and panic, in which there is no real threat, the practice of mindfulness can bring the higher brain back online, which helps dampen the assault of the limbic response.

Avoiding the Avoidance Trap

A cognitive behavioral therapist explained it to me like this: Imagine your panic is a big, scary-looking dog that will chase you only if you run. While the dog might look and sound like Cujo, the reality is that the dog is really more like an anxious Chihuahua. Panic's bark is always louder than its bite. The moment you stop running, the dog stops chasing and, instead, cuddles up to you and begins to wag its tail.

The paradox of anxiety and panic is that the more we try to avoid them, the harder they pound on the door. If we simply open the door and invite them in, we begin to retrain our nervous system not to fear them.

Practice Becoming the Observer

Check in with yourself to begin. On a scale of one to ten (one being the lowest and ten being the highest), how would you rate your current level of anxiety?

Practice taking a few slow, deep, diaphragmatic breaths. Slowly and completely inhale and exhale through your nose. Feel your belly softly inflating like a balloon as you inhale and softly falling as you exhale. Begin to intentionally lengthen out your exhalations to a ratio of 2:1, making your out-breath twice as long as your in-breath. For example, inhale for a count of two, then exhale for a count of four. If this feels comfortable, gradually increase your inhalation to a count of four and exhalation to a count of eight. Breathe in this 2:1 ratio for 5 to 10 full cycles of breath. Extending your exhalations in this manner has a powerful calming physiological effect on your nervous system.

Now check back in. On a scale of one to ten, how would you rate your anxiety now? Perhaps nothing has changed, and that's okay. The act of simply observing is already helping to retrain your brain. Over time, you will come to realize that all anxiety does is go up and down. That's it! It might feel scary and life-threatening, but that's the lie of anxiety and panic. You are not in danger. It's just a false alarm.

It can be challenging to practice your mindfulness skills while in the throes of a full-blown panic attack, so arm yourself for success by practicing your skills during periods of relatively mild anxiety. Check in with yourself multiple times throughout the day. When you first wake up in the morning, rate your anxiety. When you're preparing your breakfast, where does your anxiety level sit? When you're stuck in traffic, check in with yourself and notice any sensations you might be experiencing. Give your anxiety a number. Begin to notice any patterns. Are there certain times of day or certain activities that trigger higher levels of anxiety? Are there certain times of day or certain activities that help ease your anxiety? Uncovering patterns will help you change them.

Getting acquainted with rather than avoiding your anxiety will fundamentally transform your relationship to it.

Breath and Mantra Meditation for Anxiety

This meditation has two phases—a mindful breathing practice to quickly calm your nervous system followed by a simple mantra meditation to quell anxiety and create a sense of safety and well-being in your body and mind.

Phase 1: 4–7–8 Breath

We covered this calming breathing technique in part II of this book and offer it again here as a powerful tool to help ease anxiety on the spot. Please refer to page 73 for instructions. The alternate nostril breathing practice on page 71 is also an effective breathing technique to soothe your nervous system when you are feeling stressed or anxious.

Phase 2: Mantra Meditation

- Find a comfortable seated position. Prop yourself up on a meditation cushion or folded blanket, or sit in a comfortable chair. You can also practice lying down. Draw your attention to all the points of contact of your body to whatever surface you are sitting or lying on. If you're in a chair, feel your feet firmly planted on the ground. Feel your butt supported by the seat of the chair. Feel your back supported.

- Next, begin to bring your attention to your breath. Take 5 slow, deep, and even diaphragmatic breaths through your nose. Feel your belly expand as you inhale and softly fall as you exhale.

- Once you feel grounded and anchored in your breath, begin to mentally repeat the affirmation: *I am safe.*

- Repeat *I am safe* silently to yourself for a few minutes. If you notice your mind start to wander, gently bring it back to the mantra. If you feel your body start to tense up or fill with unpleasant sensations, gently bring your attention back to your breath.

- Close your practice with a full, deep inhalation through your nose and an audible exhalation out through your mouth.

Meditation for Anger

Anger needs an outlet. We can think of anger as a teakettle. When the water comes to a boil, the steam and pressure need to be released through a hole in the spout.

Anger is not inherently bad. It is a normal human emotion that serves a healthy purpose. It helps us create boundaries and can be the catalyst for transformation and revolution. When we're sick and tired of being sick and tired, anger can spur us into action and activism. But anger becomes toxic when we hold on to it and let it fester in the dark.

I typically work with two types of people when it comes to anger—those who let their anger boil over and eventually explode onto the people around them, and those who repress their anger, deny its existence, and eventually implode on themselves. The former can show up as violence, which can lead to self-loathing and shame, while the latter may show up as depression.

The goal is to give our anger a healthy outlet to be felt and released so that we do not harm others or ourselves. This meditation for releasing anger is twofold: an active breathwork practice and a seated forgiveness practice.

If forgiveness seems like a stretch, don't force it. Allow it in on your own terms. Remember that anger is a mask for hurt. Forgiveness does not mean dropping our boundaries or giving someone who harmed us a free pass. It simply means we are no longer willing to carry the burden of our own pain.

Phase 1: Breath of Fire

We covered this stimulating breathing technique in part II of this book and offer it again here as a powerful tool to release anger and other deeply buried emotions. Please refer to page 78 for instructions and note the cautions and contraindications on page 79.

Phase 2: Forgiveness Meditation

- Find a comfortable position either seated or lying down. Close your eyes or keep them open, depending on what feels most comfortable to you.

- Begin to breathe in and out slowly through your nose. Take a few moments to anchor yourself in the sensation of your breath.

- Reflect on some of the ways you have been hurt or have hurt others. Acknowledge the hurt place inside you that guided your actions. Invite in forgiveness by repeating the following phrases silently to yourself:

    I practice forgiveness for the serenity of my spirit.
    For anyone I have intentionally or unintentionally harmed, please forgive me.
    For anyone who has intentionally or unintentionally harmed me, I forgive you.
    For the moments when I have intentionally or unintentionally harmed myself,
        I forgive myself.

- You can shorten the phrases to:
    Forgive me.
    I forgive you.
    I forgive myself.

- Observe and soften into whatever sensations, thoughts, and emotions arise. See yourself as a person who is deserving of forgiveness, compassion, and love. Close by offering yourself a moment of gratitude for practicing kindness and allowing forgiveness into your heart.

Meditation for Fear

Fear is our body's built-in defense mechanism that keeps us safe from harm. Fear was designed to protect us, but if we let it guide our thoughts, emotions, and actions, it can sabotage our relationships, career, health, and happiness. I used to think that being fearless was the goal. Surely none of the people I looked up to, like Oprah, Maya Angelou, or Brené Brown, felt fear. Then I watched an episode of *SuperSoul Sunday* and heard Brené Brown tell Oprah, "We're all afraid. We just have to get to the point where we understand it doesn't mean that we can't also be brave."

Throw out the concept of fearlessness. Remove it from your vocabulary and consciousness, because none of us is without fear; trying to eradicate fear from our lives will only set us up for failure. My goal is no longer to be fearless; my goal is to be courageous. One of the best definitions I've come across for courage is feeling fear and taking action anyway. Rather than eliminating fear and making it our foe, the meditation below will help you befriend fear so you can face it rather than run from it.

Befriending Fear Meditation

- Find a comfortable position either seated or lying down. Close your eyes or keep them open, depending on what feels most comfortable to you.

- Begin to breathe in and out slowly through your nose. Take a few moments to anchor yourself in the sensation of your breath.

- Bring to mind a situation in your life that has been a source of fear. If multiple scenarios arise, choose to work with the one that feels most relevant to your life right now.

- How does thinking about this situation make you feel? What thoughts and emotions come up? Scan your body. Where does this fear live? Notice any physical reactions or sensations, such as an accelerated heart rate, a rush of heat, or sweaty palms.

- Let go of the story or situation you visualized and simply stay with any feelings or sensations it left behind. Do your best to sit with what your fear really feels like for a few moments. Notice its weight, color, taste, shape, sensation, and location.

- The next step may sound a little out there, but bear with me. Give your fear a name. Yes, a proper name, like George or Diane. If possible, choose a neutral name—one that is not associated with anyone who triggers you. The name can be something totally silly, like Mrs. Skittles.

I know it sounds a bit ridiculous, but giving your fear a name instantly makes the fear itself less scary. It takes away some of its emotional charge. When your fear is named Mrs. Skittles, it's hard for it to have quite the same impact. Take a few moments to find a name that resonates with you.

- Thank your new fearful friend. Remember that, by evolutionary design, the function of fear is simply to protect you. My fear is named George. So I would say something along the lines of "Thank you, George, for showing up for me and protecting me. I know you are just trying to do your job. Thank you for all the times you looked out for me when I didn't know to look out for myself."

   Think of all the times fear has actually been a blessing in your life. Can you recall any times when fear actually served you? Were there any times when the alarm bells fear sounded helped you create boundaries or leave an unsafe situation or person? Genuinely thank your fear by name for doing its best job to protect you.

- There are two types of fear: fear that serves you and fear that keeps you stuck.

   Right now, let's concentrate on the latter and think of all the times fear has held you back. You will begin to create a healthy relationship with fear when you can discern the difference between real danger and false alarms.

- For any moments when your fear has held you back from saying, doing, creating, or achieving something in your life, invite your fear to stand down. Let your fear know by name that its services are no longer needed in that particular area. For example, "Thank you, George, for doing your job of protecting me, but your services are no longer needed. This is a job for my courage, not my fear."

- Now create a name for your courage. My courage is named Dory, after the little blue fish in Disney Pixar's animated film *Finding Nemo*. I know it's not exactly the name of a lionhearted warrior, but something always stuck with me about Dory's eternally encouraging mantra of "Just keep swimming!" Whenever fear stalls me to the point of inertia, I hear Dory's voice in my head: *Just keep swimming!* Because of this, I'm always able to move again.

   I think of my fear and my courage like my own personal football team; I can swap out the players and pick the best athlete for the next play. When you're swapping out your team, it is helpful to remember that fear and courage can feel almost identical. I once heard someone say that the physical effects of fear in our bodies (elevated heart rate, sweaty palms, faster breathing) are the exact same physiological effects of courage. So when you're walking into your boss's office at work to ask for a raise and you feel your heart in your chest, reframe your fear as your body stepping into an act of courage.

- Take a full, deep breath. On your next inhalation, call in your courage. With your next exhalation, release your fear. Continue breathing. Inhale to gather your courage. Exhale to set your fear free.

- Close your meditation with a few moments of affirmation, recited either silently or out loud:

    I am safe.
    I am supported.
    I am grounded.
    I am bold.
    I am brave.
    I am courageous.

- Take a moment to sit in silence. Bring your palms together at the center of your heart and offer yourself gratitude for meeting your fear with compassion.

Thunderbolt Mudra for Courage and Confidence

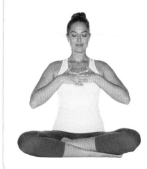

Mudras are hand gestures that can help shift our mental and emotional state. Thunderbolt mudra helps create self-confidence and courage. To do the mudra, loosely interlace your fingers. Keep your thumbs facing up and place your hands over your heart. Take a few deep breaths. You may choose to mentally recite the following mantra: *I am confident. I am courageous.* Or use an affirmation of your choice.

Meditation for Grief

Grief comes in many sizes, shapes, and forms. People usually pair grief with death, but grief can show up with a loss of any kind. We can grieve the loss of a marriage when it ends in divorce. We can grieve the absence of our children when they leave home for college. We can grieve the loss of a place we called home when we uproot. We can grieve the loss of a friendship, job, or the dream of a life we had planned. There is no right or wrong way to grieve. We can grieve in the arms of others. We can grieve in solitude. We can grieve through tears, laughter, meditation, movement, or prayer. The only rule is that we hold our hearts with the utmost care and allow ourselves the room to feel and the space to heal with no timelines or expectations.

I thought I would be an expert in navigating my grief when my mom died. After all, she was the person who showed me the ropes for coping with loss. As a funeral director and bereavement educator, my mom dedicated more than twenty-five years of her life to helping people move through grief.

Through this experience, I learned that nothing logical can truly prepare you for that type of loss. I remember my mom telling me that reality hits six weeks after the death of a loved one. Until then, you're either numb or preoccupied with the business of death: doctor bills, estate processing, communicating with family and loved ones. Then reality hits you with the force of a horse kicking you in the stomach. "You heal, but that business about getting over it? Nobody ever gets over it," my mother once said. "You learn to live with it. You learn to cope with the sadness, and eventually you learn to let joy back into your life. People say, 'You should feel this or that.' There is no *should* with feelings. They just exist."

She was right. For months I was numb. I wasn't there when she died and I didn't cry when I found out she was gone. In fact, I didn't skip a beat. I went to work the very next day and continued on with life as usual, despite the fact that everything had changed. When the emotions finally did come seven months later, they hit me over the head like a tidal wave, and I thought I would never be able to breathe again. But I did . . . and you will too.

Meditation to Release Grief

- Find a comfortable position either seated or lying down. Close your eyes or keep them open, depending on what feels most comfortable to you.

- Begin to breathe in and out slowly through your nose. Feel the sensation of your lungs inflating and deflating in your chest. Grief has a way of planting roots in our chest and winding around our heart. Focus your attention on any sensations in that area.

- Place one or both hands tenderly over your heart and set the intention to create a safe space of loving kindness for yourself. Breathe into the center of your heart and feel the support and comfort of your own loving touch.

- Bring to mind the loss you are experiencing. Breathe gently into whatever thoughts, images, memories, feelings, and sensations arrive. If tears come, let them flow. If anger comes, let it vent. If fear comes, embrace it with compassion. If sound comes, let it vibrate. Create room for your grief.

- To help your grief move through and out of you, inhale deeply through your nose and exhale slowly through your mouth, making an *sssssss* sound, like a hiss without the "h." It should sound similar to letting the air out of a tire. Sound vibration paired with breath is a powerful tool to help release emotion from our depths.

- Visualize golden light filling you as you inhale, and any grief leaving you as you exhale and make the *sssssss* sound. If tears come, let them flow; if no tears come, allow that to be your experience without any judgment. Continue for as many cycles of breath as needed until you feel complete.

- Take a moment to sit quietly and observe how you feel.

Meditation for Self-Worth and Unconditional Self-Love

You may have heard Groucho Marx's humorous and self-deprecating quote "I don't want to belong to any club that would have me as a member." These words never fail to make me laugh and want to cry at the same time. The sadness comes from that part in me that has never felt good enough. As long as I can remember, I've felt like an outsider. I was a shy, awkward, introverted kid who never felt smart enough, charismatic enough, funny enough, talented enough, beautiful enough, or cool enough. I carried this story of "not enough–ness" into adulthood, which led to self-sabotaging behaviors, toxic relationships, playing small in my career, a nonexistent social life, and an undercurrent of anxiety and depression.

In my workshops and teacher trainings, I always ask the group, "How many of you have ever felt not good enough?" Without fail, every single hand in the room goes up. Every time.

Beneath low self-esteem is a foundation of shame. Shame is a toxic emotion that slowly erodes our self-worth. It is the belief that we are inherently bad. And it's usually programmed into us before we even reach middle school. Shame keeps us locked in unconscious self-destructive patterns. In their book *Straight from the Heart*, authors Layne and Paul Cutright write, "A guilty mind expects punishment. Guilt will cause you to attract people and/or situations to validate your unresolved guilty thoughts about yourself."

While shame and guilt aren't exactly the same thing (guilt is usually defined as *doing* something we feel is bad versus believing that we *are* bad), they can both lead to self-sabotaging behavior when unhealed. To heal shame, we must first learn to embrace our shadow. Not a single person on this planet is without sin. We have all lied, cheated, manipulated, or hurt someone or ourselves somewhere along the way. It's part of being human. So be kind to yourself, dear human.

Offer yourself forgiveness. If your actions have caused suffering, find ways to make amends. In the Alcoholics Anonymous twelve-step program, step eight is making a list of all the people you have harmed and finding the willingness to make amends. Step nine is taking the action of making direct amends wherever possible, except when doing so would injure them or others. The people I know in recovery have all said these two steps have been the most impactful in cleansing themselves of shame. If the person you need to make amends with is yourself, practice the forgiveness meditation on page 201. Then proceed with the following meditation to help you invite in self-love.

Meditation for Generating Self-Worth and Unconditional Self-Love

- Find a comfortable position either seated or lying down. Close your eyes or keep them open, depending on what feels most comfortable to you.

- Begin to breathe in and out slowly through your nose. Feel your abdomen gently inflating as you inhale and gently falling as you exhale.

- Lovingly place one hand over your heart and the other hand on your belly. Shame likes to burrow into our gut. Breathe into your belly and welcome any sensations or emotions that arise.

- Mentally repeat the following affirmations:
    What I have *done* in the past does not define who I *am* in the present.
    I trust myself.
    I belong here.
    I am enough.
    I am worthy.
    I am capable.
    I am deserving of my own love and affection.
    I love and accept myself unconditionally.

- Take a moment to sit quietly and observe how you feel.

Mindfulness for Dissociation

Dissociation is a defense mechanism that kicks in when we've reached our threshold of mental and physical pain, as is the case with severe physical or emotional trauma.

Dissociation may show up as mild or extreme detachment, a separation of our memory or awareness from our present experience, or emotional or physical numbing. Brené Brown says, "We cannot selectively numb emotions; when we numb the painful emotions, we also numb the positive emotions."[1] When we've experienced pain, it's natural to want to avoid feeling, because we associate feeling with hurting. But numbing transports us away from the present moment. And the present moment is the only place where life happens. The work is to open ourselves up to feeling in small, safe doses and eventually expand our window of tolerance so we can safely experience larger sensations, thoughts, and emotions without getting overwhelmed or shutting down. Use the grounding mindfulness practice below to help you stay rooted in the present.

5–4–3–2–1 Grounding Practice

The 5–4–3–2–1 technique is a simple and powerful sensory awareness tool you can use any time you feel spaced out, anxious, or ungrounded. This exercise can be completed wherever you are right now.

- Name 5 things you see in your room or current environment. For example, a table or couch.
- Name 4 things you can feel, such as your feet on the floor or the texture of your shirt.
- Name 3 things you can hear, like the sound of your breath or traffic.
- Name 2 things you can smell. If there are no obvious scents around you, sniff your clothing or a nearby object.
- Name 1 thing you can taste. If you don't have any food or drink nearby, just notice the taste of your tongue or lips.
- Once you've completed the five steps, plant your feet firmly on the floor, breathe deeply in and out through your nose, and observe how you feel. I invite you to mentally repeat the following affirmations:

I am safe.	The earth supports me.
I am grounded.	My breath supports me.
I am balanced.	My body supports me.

Grounding Mudra and
Mantra Meditation for Dissociation

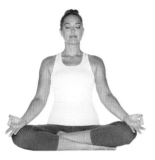

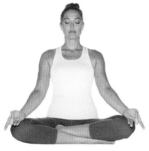

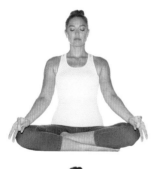

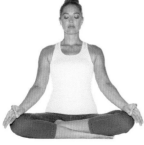

If you're feeling fragmented or disconnected from your body, use this grounding mudra and mantra meditation to anchor you back into your physical presence and cultivate peace of mind in the here and now. Start in a comfortable seated position with your hands resting faceup on your lap. Touch your index finger and thumb together on each hand. Next, release your index finger and bring your middle finger to touch your thumb. Release your middle finger and bring your ring finger to touch your thumb. Release your ring finger and bring your little finger to touch your thumb. Once each finger has connected with your thumb, start the sequence again from the top. To focus your mind, you may introduce the following mantra: *I feel to heal*. Mentally say each word as you touch each finger. For example, say "I" as you connect your index finger to thumb; "feel" as you connect your middle finger to thumb; "to" as you connect your ring finger to thumb; "heal" as you connect your little finger to thumb. Repeat the mantra in synchronization with the mudra as many times as needed to shift you into the present moment.

Meditation for Healing Sexual Trauma

There are few things more violating to our body, mind, and spirit than sexual trauma. The people I have worked with who have experienced sexual abuse describe feeling disconnected, detached, and even disgusted by their bodies. It is common to feel ashamed, numb, or even dirty in the aftermath of abuse, but it's important to remember you are not to blame. You did nothing wrong. Where you were, who you were with, what you were doing, what you were wearing, what you said or didn't say, or what you felt in that moment were not your fault. Sexual assault is *never* okay and it is *never* your fault. Release the weight of shame that is not yours to carry.

The journey of healing from sexual trauma is a journey of befriending your body, opening to your breath, and allowing yourself to feel again (pleasure included!) without any guilt or shame. Many healing modalities can help release the imprint of sexual trauma from our body and psyche, including breathwork, hypnosis, tension and trauma release exercises (TRE), eye movement desensitization and reprocessing (EMDR), sensorimotor psychotherapy, tantra, dance, yoga, meditation, and more. The key is finding what works for you. There is no right or wrong way to heal. I offer you the meditation practices and affirmations below to help you begin reclaiming your body, voice, power, and innate right to love and be loved.

Phase 1: Embracing Your Inner Child Meditation

If your trauma occurred when you were a child, I invite you to open up a loving conversation with your inner child so you can heal the wounds of your past together.

- Find a comfortable position either seated or lying down. Close your eyes or keep them open, depending on what feels most comfortable to you.

- Begin to breathe in and out slowly through your nose. Feel your abdomen gently inflating as you inhale and gently falling as you exhale.

- Tenderly place one or both hands over your heart as if you were caring for a small child, then take a few moments to visualize yourself as a small child. See yourself as you were when you were young. What age are you? What do you look like? What do you sound like? What are you wearing? What are your mannerisms?

- Begin to speak lovingly to your inner child. Perhaps even visualize cradling them in your arms as you speak. Tell your child how much you love them, and how sorry you are for everything they had to go through. Let your inner child know that nothing was their fault. They are not to blame. Acknowledge your inner child's strength and courage. Let your inner child know how proud you are of them for doing everything you had to in order to survive. Let your inner child know just how grateful you are to them and how resilient you have become. Tell your inner child how beautiful, radiant, whole, and perfect they are—then and today. Let your inner child know that they are now safe and free to finally be the carefree, joyful, playful child that they were always meant to be. Continue speaking to your inner child until you have said everything that needs to be said.

- Close by visualizing your current self lovingly embracing your child self. Allow your adult self and your child self to become one. See yourself as whole and fully integrated, deserving of love, kindness, and nurturing.

- Mentally repeat the following affirmations:

    I lovingly embrace and nurture my inner child.

    I am safe.

    I am whole.

    I am now free to live the life of joy, ease, purpose, and love that is my
        birthright.

    The Universe (or God or higher power) supports me in creating and fulfilling
        this life of joy and love.

Phase 2: Affirmations for Healing Sexual Trauma

If the inner child meditation didn't resonate with you or if your sexual trauma occurred later in life, I invite you to try the following affirmations instead:

- Find a comfortable position either seated or lying down. Close your eyes or keep them open, depending on what feels most comfortable to you.

- Begin to breathe in and out slowly through your nose. Feel your abdomen gently inflating as you inhale and gently falling as you exhale.

- Mentally repeat the following affirmations:

    I trust my body.

    My body is safe.

    It is safe for me to feel.

    I invite in feeling so I may begin healing.

    I lovingly embrace all parts of myself and my body.

    I claim my boundaries.

    I am worthy and deserving of love.

    I open the door to my heart.

- If some of the affirmations above don't resonate with you, feel free to create your own that feel more authentic. Remember, there is no wrong way to do this.
- Breathe into your belly and feel into your heart. Take a moment to sit quietly and observe how you feel.

After exploring the practices in this section, I invite you to consider the possibility of allowing forgiveness into your heart to additionally support your trauma healing. If you feel resistance or anger bubbling up at the mere thought of forgiving the person who harmed you, let that be okay too. Forgiveness is not a process to be rushed or approached disingenuously. Let go of the idea for now, and return to it only when you feel ready.

Forgiveness does not mean you condone, consent, absolve, or invite this person back into your life. Forgiveness doesn't ever need to be written or spoken out loud to this person. Forgiveness is not for them. Forgiveness is for you. Forgiveness doesn't give them any power; it helps you reclaim your own. If and when you feel ready for this step, refer to the forgiveness meditation on page 201, and as always, feel free to add your own affirmations and words that best honor your experience.

Mindfulness for Restful Sleep

Anyone who has struggled with insomnia knows how debilitating it can be. You've tried all the tricks in the book and nothing works. You're feeling more desperate by the minute. Anxiety about not being able to sleep creates a frustrating, self-fulfilling cycle of—you guessed it—the inability to sleep. Let go of sleep as your goal; instead, aim for total body relaxation. Tell yourself it's okay if you don't fall asleep right away or stay asleep, because deep relaxation can have almost as powerful healing and restorative effects on the body and mind as sleep.

I often practice yoga nidra (translated as "yogic sleep") to help me fall asleep when I can't shut off my racing thoughts. Yoga nidra is a deeply restorative form of yoga that involves little more than lying on your back and being guided methodically through every part of your body in order to induce a state of ultimate restfulness. A number of studies have confirmed the effectiveness of yoga nidra in treating PTSD, and more studies are emerging on yoga nidra as an intervention for chronic pain and treatment for sleep disorders. A 2014 study published in the *International Journal of Yoga Therapy* "showed significant decreases in negative thoughts of self-blame and depression" when yoga nidra was practiced twice a week for ten weeks at a VA medical center in Long Beach.[2] This study was specifically conducted with a group of women who had experienced rape and sexual trauma in the military.

In 2015, I had the opportunity to study and train with Richard Miller, clinical psychologist, researcher, and founder of the Integrative Restoration Institute and iRest yoga nidra. I caught a nasty cold the night before I had to travel and arrived at the training sleep-deprived and feeling terrible. I wasn't sure how I was going to make it through eight hours of training a day for five consecutive days. Fortunately, I had come to the right place! After just an hour of iRest yoga nidra, I felt as if my body had caught up on several hours of sleep.

It may sound too good to be true, but there's a proven scientific basis for why yoga nidra is so effective. It works like this: As we fall asleep, our brain waves shift from active, wakeful (and often stressful!) beta waves into the relaxed, slower state of alpha waves. Alpha waves produce a state of wakeful rest, which is a hallmark state of meditation. The transition from beta to alpha is considered a presleep stage. Stage 1 of sleep occurs when our brain transitions from alpha waves to theta waves, which are even slower in frequency than alpha waves. This stage is considered "light sleep," and it's common for people to report that they weren't really asleep if awoken during this stage.

Experienced meditation practitioners often reach a theta state during deep meditation, inducing a state of profound relaxation. In stage 2 of sleep, theta waves continue, body temperature decreases, and our heart rate begins to slow. Stage 3 is a transitional phase between light sleep and deep sleep where delta waves emerge. Stage 4 is our deepest sleep, where delta waves, which have the slowest frequency, predominate. Yoga nidra (and other deep forms of meditation) brings us to the threshold between alpha and theta, where our body "sleeps" while our mind is clear. So we emerge from a session feeling refreshed, alert, and well rested, even though we haven't slept.

The best way to practice yoga nidra is in a class with a trained teacher who can guide you through the process. The next best option is to download any number of meditation apps that offer guided sleep meditations. I recommend the Insight Timer app, which offers hundreds of guided meditations to choose from, including yoga nidra meditations specifically for sleep. Two of my bookmarked favorites on Insight Timer are the "Breathing into Sleep" meditation by teacher Bethany Auriel-Hagan and "Yoga Nidra for Sleep" by Jennifer Piercy. I can't tell you how they end, because I've never stayed awake long enough to finish either of them!

Apps aside, exercising during the day and creating a calming bedtime ritual at night will help your body release anxious energy so you can wind down to receive the rest you need. I recommend using the insomnia sequence, including progressive muscle relaxation, on page 152 as part of your nightly ritual. If you're still having trouble falling asleep, try these two calming breathing meditations.

Phase 1: Belly Breath for Deep Sleep

- Find a comfortable position lying down on your back. Gaze up at a point on the ceiling above and beyond eye level. This will make the muscles in your eyes have to work a little harder, which ultimately fatigues your eyes, making them heavy in preparation for sleep. As you stare at this point, count slowly backward from ten to one. Breathe deeply in and out through your nose, feeling your belly rise and fall as you count down. When you reach one, allow your eyes to gently close.

- Take 3 cycles of deep abdominal breath with your eyes closed, then open them again and stare at the same point on the ceiling. Repeat the count backward from ten to one. Repeat this cycle 2 more times.

  By the third round, your eyelids will crave being shut. Allow them to close gently and keep them closed (if it feels comfortable to you) as you move on to the next part of the breathing practice.

- Continue breathing in and out slowly through your nose. Feel your abdomen softly inflating like a balloon as you inhale and naturally falling as you exhale.

- Begin to mentally count the length of your inhalations and the length of your exhalations, with a focus of making your exhalations twice as long as your inhalations. For example, inhale for a count of 3, then exhale for a count of 6. Explore extending your breath a little longer, inhaling for a count of 4 and exhaling for a count of 8. If this feels too long or you find yourself running out of breath, go back to a ratio of 3:6 or try out 2:4.

  Stretching out your exhalations has the natural physiological effect of calming your body and brain. The added mental focus the counting provides helps silence the racing thoughts and mental chatter that often intrude when we're trying to sleep.

Phase 2: Left Nostril Breath

In the Kundalini yoga tradition, it is believed there are two energetic pathways that weave up our spine. The right channel is the *pingala nadi*, which begins below your root chakra (found at the base of your spine) and winds its way up to your right nostril. *Pingala* is associated with the sun and active, fiery, masculine energy. The left channel is the *ida nadi*. It also begins at your root chakra and ends in your left nostril. *Ida* governs the left side of the body and is associated with lunar, cooling, calming, feminine energy.

If that all sounds a little too woo-woo for you, you can just think of *pingala* as the equivalent of your sympathetic nervous system (activating, energizing, "sounding the alarm") and *ida* as your parasympathetic nervous system (calming, cooling, "rest and digest"). To move into sleep, we want to drop into our parasympathetic nervous system, which, according to Kundalini wisdom, can be accessed by breathing through your left nostril.

- Left nostril breathing is traditionally practiced seated with a tall spine. I recommend practicing it for between 3 and 11 minutes seated before tucking yourself into bed. (However, if you are already lying down, you can still practice on your back, making sure your spine is lengthened.) If this time frame seems oddly specific, that's because it is. Kundalini wisdom holds that it takes at least 3 minutes of breathing to have an effect on your circulation and blood chemistry; at 11 minutes, our pituitary gland and nerves start to learn and change.

- Close off your right nostril by placing your right thumb gently against it. Keep your left nostril open and take a full deep inhalation through your left side only. Exhale deeply out through your left nostril. Continue breathing in and out of your left nostril for 3 to 11 minutes.

- When you finish your breathing practice, release your right nostril and breathe normally through both nostrils.

Meditation for Chronic Pain

Living with chronic pain can rob you of life's vibrancy and joy. A close friend of mine suffered from chronic pain that started in her neck and wound its way down her spine. It hurt to turn her head, to sit, stand, and sleep; in other words, she was always in pain. She took painkillers, which made her feel foggy. She would often apologize for not being herself. On top of the pain, she struggled with anxiety. The pain fed the anxiety and the anxiety fed the pain.

Tired of living in a fog and desperately wanting a better solution, she reached out to me for help. I recommended a variety of natural supplements for inflammation to help manage the pain (I'll cover this in more detail in the section beginning on page 250); gentle stretches for her aching shoulders, back, and neck; and yup, you guessed it, meditation.

Dr. Danny Penman, author of *You Are Not Your Pain: Using Mindfulness to Relieve Pain, Reduce Stress, and Restore Well-Being—an Eight-Week Program*, says that pain comes in two forms: primary and secondary. "Primary pain arises from illness, injury, or damage to the body or nervous system. You could see it as the raw information sent by the body to the brain. Secondary pain is the mind's reaction to primary pain, but is often far more intense and long lasting. Crucially, it is controlled by an 'amplifier' in the brain that governs the overall intensity of suffering." Dr. Penman goes on to say that meditation "turns down the 'volume' control on pain" and can reduce chronic pain by 57 percent in beginning meditators and more than 90 percent in "accomplished" meditators.[3]

Meditation to Ease Chronic Pain

- Find a seated or lying position that feels comfortable and supportive. Close your eyes or keep them open, depending on what feels most comfortable to you.

- Allow your body to soften into the full support of the surface beneath you. Visualize yourself being cradled and lovingly held, releasing all physical effort.

- Begin to breathe in and out slowly through your nose. Feel your abdomen gently inflating as you inhale and gently falling as you exhale. Bring your attention to your nostrils. Notice the cool sensation of air as you inhale through your nostrils. Notice the slightly warmer sensation the breath takes on as it exits your nostrils. Stay with this gentle sensation of breath flowing in and out at the nostrils for a few moments.

- While continuing to breathe deeply, open your field of awareness to any strong, unpleasant, or painful sensations in your body. You may notice many sensations, but choose to focus on the one that feels the strongest and most palpable in this moment. Begin to explore all aspects of this sensation with gentle curiosity. Does this sensation have borders? Can you feel its edges? Note where it begins and where it ends. Does it travel to other places in your body or does it stay put? Does it have a shape, color, texture, or sound? What would this sensation say if it could speak? Does the sensation shift, change, diminish, or intensify just by virtue of you paying attention to it?

- Stay with your sensation as you begin to check back in with your breath. Focus on your exhalations. Visualize your exhalations as a source of healing energy and lovingly direct your healing breath toward your sensation. Feel your breath gently embracing your pain, cradling it as if it were comforting a child. Allow your breath to soften your pain, smoothing out its edges. Let your breath move directly into your pain with a whisper-soft touch, like a cloud caressing the sky. If any sensations become too intense, give yourself permission to back off.

- Continue lovingly sending your breath into your pain and notice any effects. With each exhalation, you may mentally say "soften," "release," or "let go." Continue breathing with or without the mental affirmation for a few more moments. Notice if your sensations are shape-shifting, fading, or backing off.

- Let go of your focus on the sensation and bring your attention back to the breath flowing in and out of your nostrils. Stay here for a few moments and observe how you feel without any judgment.

Energy Self-Massage to Ease Pain

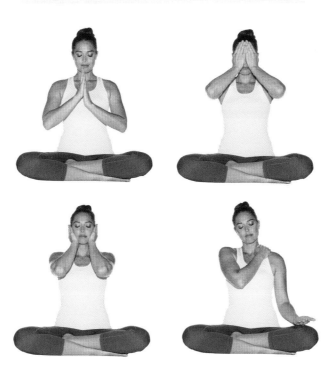

Our hands hold the power of self-healing. To access your own natural healing abilities, simply rub your palms together vigorously for approximately 30 seconds. Keep rubbing until you feel warmth starting to build between your hands. Gently cup your hands over your eyes and then your ears to help relieve fatigue, stress, and strain. Next, gently and lovingly place your hands over any other places on your body where you are experiencing tension, pain, or discomfort.

Mindfulness for Digestive Health

I have been guilty of scarfing down a bag of fast food in my car and shoveling fries into my face at a stoplight on more occasions than I would like to admit. These days, I've swapped out French fries for apple slices or a fresh fruit smoothie, but I still find myself eating on the go at least two or three times a week. I blame my busy schedule for rarely finding the time to actually sit down to enjoy a meal, but it occurred to me recently that I'm the one who sets my schedule.

Mindless eating is something we've all done. I'm sure you can relate to opening a bag of chips or a pint of your favorite ice cream, then plopping down on the couch in front of the TV. Twenty minutes later, you're holding an empty bag or cardboard container and nursing a stomachache and guilty conscience.

Mind*ful* eating is about changing your relationship to food by paying attention to what's on your plate and how it feels to your senses. It's tuning into your body's cues of hunger or satiety and noticing how your body responds. It's observing any thoughts, feelings, or emotions that arise surrounding your relationship with certain foods and taking the time to really ask if you are truly listening to your body. Research suggests that mindful eating can curb cravings, reduce stress-related eating, help lower blood sugar, improve cholesterol levels, and create an overall healthier relationship to food.

Mindful Eating

- Before each meal, ask yourself what you are really hungry for. The answer might be a cheeseburger or pizza. But inquire a little deeper. Are you hungry because your body needs the calories? Are you hungry for the social companionship that sharing a meal with friends can provide? Are you looking for a way to pass the time? Are you hungry for love or acceptance?

   Often we eat because we're bored, lonely, or stressed. When we ask ourselves what's behind our hunger, we may realize that the cheeseburger we are craving really isn't what we're hungry for at all. Release any judgment and ask these questions with simple curiosity.

- When you do sit down to eat, use all five senses throughout the experience. Notice the color, shape, texture, smell, consistency, flavor, taste, temperature, and sound of the food you are eating. Is it crunchy, chewy, flaky, sticky, hot, cold, bitter, sweet, savory, spicy, mild? Engage with all aspects of it. If it's a complex dish, can you distinguish each ingredient you taste on your palate? You may even visualize where these ingredients originally came from (such as turmeric from India).

- As you are eating, chew slowly and savor every bite. Digestion begins in your mouth. The better you chew your food and the smaller pieces you can break it into, the better you set your body up for healthy digestion and optimal absorption.

- As you continue eating, tune into your body's cues. Are you continuing to eat simply because you were taught to clean your plate? Or are you still eating because your body needs the fuel? Honor your body by nourishing it when it's depleted and stopping when you are full.

- Before, during, and after each meal, notice how you feel mentally, physically, and emotionally. Do you feel guilty or nurtured? Do you feel light, heavy, sluggish, tired, energetic, calm, anxious, irritable, or foggy? We'll explore all of this in much more depth in the next section, but for now, just start paying attention to how the food you consume makes you feel.

The Art of Mindfully Peeling an Orange

To practice mindful eating, here's a short and delicious exercise to try.

- Grab an orange. Hold it in both hands. Feel its weight and trace its shape. Feel the texture of the outer peel. Notice the color. Notice any spots, indentations, or markings. Hold it up to your nose and breathe in its scent.

- Begin to peel the orange slowly. Feel the peel underneath your fingernails. Notice the white part (known as the pith) between the skin and the fruit. What is its texture, taste, smell?

- Continue peeling until you reach the fruit. Slowly peel apart each piece. Notice the white "veins" in each slice. Notice the size and shape of each piece as you gently pull them apart.

- As you eat the orange, pay attention to the taste, texture, and sound it makes when you bite into it. Is it juicy, sweet, bitter, tangy? Notice the shape, texture, and color of any seeds. Feel the juice dripping down your fingers. Experience the orange with all your senses wide awake.

- When you're finished, take a moment to sit quietly and observe how you feel. What would it feel like to approach every meal with the same level of presence and sensory awareness?

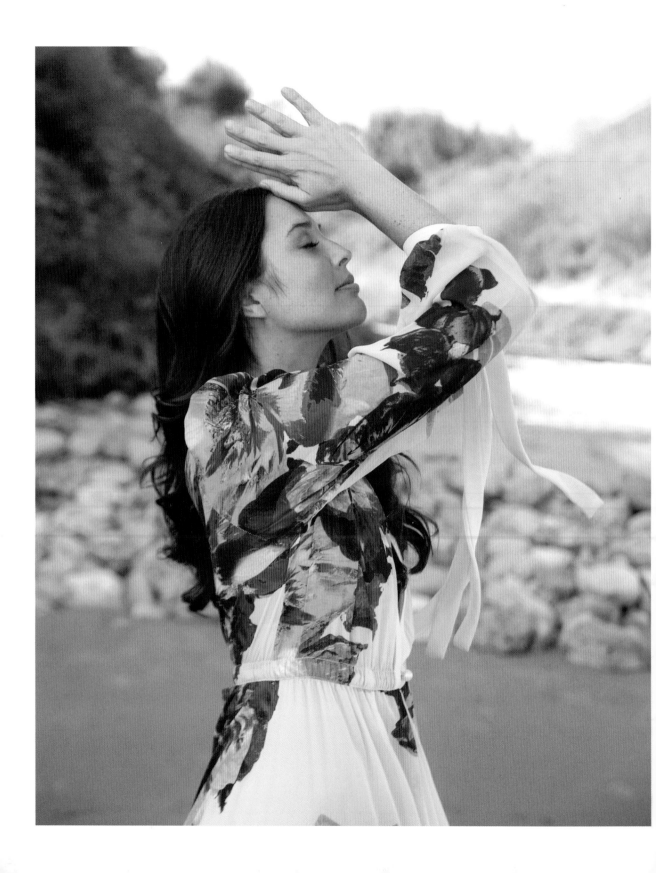

Part IV

Eat to Heal

Chapter 13

All Health Begins in the Gut

It is far more important to know what person the disease has than what disease the person has.
—Hippocrates

The landscape of nutrition can be incredibly confusing and filled with contradictions. Like politics and religion, food ranks among one of the most emotionally charged and hotly debated topics. More than once, I've witnessed doctors at health and wellness conferences bitterly clash over nutritional advice and information. I've heard stories of friendships and romantic partnerships ending over nutritional choices.

Food is often deeply rooted in our cultural, religious, and spiritual beliefs. It is so ingrained in our psychology that it can become a part of how we identify ourselves. We use labels to describe not just our food preferences, but who we are and what we stand for in life. When someone's label contradicts our own, it can trigger the deepest kind of indignation. For that reason alone, it's incredibly challenging to change someone else's view of food, let alone our own relationship to it.

So where to begin? I'll start by saying that no matter where you stand in the great food debate, the one universal truth is that what we eat profoundly affects our health—and not just on a physical level. Without question, our food choices greatly impact our mental health. Fortunately, nutritional therapy is being used more and more frequently in both treatment and prevention of some of the greatest mental health issues we face today, such as anxiety and depression. Turns out that Thomas Edison was right when he predicted, "The doctor of the future will give no medication, but will interest his patients in the care of the human frame, diet and in the cause and prevention of disease."

The second truth is there is no one-size-fits-all approach to food. What causes an inflammatory response in one person may have little to no effect on another. Some may do better on a diet that includes meat, while others may thrive on a vegetarian diet. Gluten may spell digestive disaster for one person yet be easily tolerated by another. Caffeine might greatly exacerbate someone's anxiety and wreak havoc on their adrenals, while it's fine in moderation for others. There are so many factors that play a role in determining how an individual reacts to food, including genetics, unique biochemistry, trauma and adverse childhood experiences (ACEs), medical history, use of antibiotics, how you were born (believe it or not, whether you were delivered vaginally or through C-section makes a big difference on your gut flora!), stress levels, lifestyle choices, drug and alcohol use—and the list goes on. The bottom line is that what works for others may not work for you, and no single book will be able to write a prescription for all individuals.

Precisely because of the individualized nature of healing, this book does not offer a specific diet plan. In fact, I really dislike the word *diet* altogether, as it is too often associated with restrictive eating and weight management. Navigating our way out of trauma is challenging enough; we certainly don't need to add on any guilt or shame about our size, weight, or appearance. If food is a struggle for you in any capacity, you are not alone and you won't find any judgment within these pages.

What you will find here is evidence-based information on how to help heal your gut and brain based on scientific studies and research from doctors, neuroscientists, and certified nutritionists who are setting the gold standard in their fields. You'll also find more than twenty-five exclusive mood-boosting, gut-healing recipes created in partnership with my dear friend Elise Museles, who is a brilliant chef, certified holistic health coach, and certified eating psychology coach. She is the author of *Whole Food Energy*, and her gut-healing recipes have been featured in the best-selling books *GutBliss* and *The Microbiome Solution*, by integrative gastroenterologist and microbiome expert Dr. Robynne Chutkan.

My hope is that the information and recipes that follow will open up a path of discovery for you to begin viewing food as one of your greatest allies on the road to greater physical health and mental well-being. This book is designed to meet you where you are today and to serve as a starting point for your journey. As your journey progresses, there may be certain areas where you need more guidance and support. I always recommend seeking out a certified nutritionist, naturopath, physician, or functional medicine doctor in your area to supervise any major dietary shifts and nutritional therapy. A qualified clinician can order a variety of blood, stool, and saliva tests to identify nutritional deficiencies, food allergies, and food sensitivities; screen for any harmful bacteria or parasites; measure cortisol levels; and prescribe the right dosages of nutritional supplements, including vitamins, minerals, glandulars, and amino acids.

But if you don't have the resources or access to a qualified nutrition professional, don't worry. Some of the simplest steps can create the most profound shifts. It is my great hope that the pages that follow will help you take those first steps toward achieving your greatest health and vitality.

My Journey with Food

My personal interest in nutrition started when my mom was diagnosed with stage IV pancreatic cancer. My mom's doctors told her chemotherapy could prolong her life by a few months but would do little to save her. With Western medicine telling us there was nothing they could do, my sister and I started researching holistic interventions that would, at the very least, give our mom some sense of control and empowerment in her fight. Through this, I started learning about the relationship between food and disease and the healing power of anti-inflammatory diets.

My own struggle with anxiety and panic attacks deepened my resolve to understand as much as I could, not only about food and physical disease but also the connection between food and mental health. I read every book I could get my hands on, sought out naturopaths and functional medicine doctors, took courses at the School of Applied Functional Medicine, and earned a plant-based nutrition certificate from Cornell University.

My own mental health journey and chronic digestive issues have made me a lifelong student of nutrition; however, I am not a doctor or dietician. Nonetheless, I could not fathom writing this book without including a section about what I consider to be the biggest missing link in helping people heal from trauma: food.

When I was going through my own dark night of the soul, I spent countless hours researching ways to help save myself from myself, yet couldn't find a single trauma healing resource that addressed trauma in all three places where it lives: the body, mind, and gut. It was an overwhelming and at times frustrating journey in which I was forced to put the pieces together myself. I want to save you that time.

Eating My Emotions

Being naturally tall and slender, I was able to get away with eating pretty much whatever I wanted most of my life while still giving off the impression of being "healthy." But if you could have peeked into my internal world during my formative years and most of my adulthood, my digestive tract would have painted a far more horrifying tale. I come from a large Hawaiian family—large in *every* sense of the word. For better or worse, food has always been what's brought us together. All of our holidays and family gatherings revolved around food—and lots of it. When there was a birth in the family, we ate. When there was a death in the family, we ate. When there was a wedding, a graduation, a football game, a celebration, or a tragedy, we ate. Food was my family's way of saying "I love you," and it was also a Band-Aid that we used to cover up our pain.

When I was a teenager, my grandfather was arrested for exposing himself to an underage boy at the beach. It was shocking news that created a lot of shame and embarrassment for my family. My parents were adamant about confronting my grandfather and staged an intervention at his home with a counselor present. I don't remember much of what was said that night, but I do remember sitting quietly in the corner crying, wanting it all to be a bad dream. When there was nothing left to say, my grandmother invited us all to eat as if nothing had happened. So we ate. When the meal was over, life went back to normal and we never spoke of it again.

In theory, our plate is the simplest place to make radical and lasting changes in our health and vitality. However, in practice, it is one of the most difficult, precisely because most of us have such a complicated, emotional relationship with food.

To be totally transparent, food is still the area where I struggle the most. While I have logged hours of research on the topic, worked with top naturopaths and functional medicine doctors, and dramatically overhauled my diet, I still have moments when I crave the sugary, processed "comfort food" of my past. Unsurprisingly, these cravings usually pop up during times of stress or emotional turmoil. Turns out there's a reason for this.

The Gut–Brain Connection

When I began suffering from panic attacks and crippling anxiety, I had no idea that the foods I was reaching for to help "take the edge off" were actually contributing to my anxiety and panic. Nor could I have ever imagined the possibility that, dating as far back as when I was in my mother's womb, my physical and mental health were already being shaped by my gut.

The gut is known as our "second brain" or enteric nervous system (ENS). It is made up of over 100 million neurons (more neurons than we have in our spinal cord!). The ENS governs our digestive system, but its work doesn't stop there. It influences our entire body through a network of neurotransmitters. And get this: it's our ENS, or our "gut-brain," that produces 95 percent of our body's serotonin! Yes, the same serotonin that psychiatrists once thought resided only in our actual brain actually *lives* in our gut! Our ENS is also responsible for the production of 50 percent of our body's dopamine, a critical neurotransmitter that is linked to our brain's pleasure and reward center as well as our ability to focus, learn, and retain information through memory. Inflammation in the gut can affect our body's ability to efficiently create these critical mood-balancing neurotransmitters.

Our gut and brain are in constant communication. Our gut sends signals to our brain not only about gut sensation, such as hunger, satiety, and nausea, but also about our well-being. Our brain responds back, thus generating gut reactions. These gut feelings of ours may seem fleeting, but they're not. Our brain keeps a virtual library of these feelings, which it accesses later on down the line when making decisions. This means that how we feel in our gut impacts not only what we eat but also our decisions and feelings about life in general.

We've all experienced the feeling of "butterflies" in our stomach when we are nervous or excited, or had a "gut feeling" about something that we couldn't shake. It turns out that gut feelings are real. According to Dr. Emeran Mayer, "Recent studies suggest that . . . the gut can influence our basic emotions, our pain sensitivity, and our social interactions, and even guide many of our decisions."[1] That's right—"gut instincts" and "trusting your gut" are much more than just colloquialisms. When our gut tells us something, it is the physiological result of anatomical functions between brain and gut and the signals that are passed back and forth between the two thanks to our bloodstream.

In his book, Dr. Mayer goes on to describe two fascinating studies on mice. In one study, transferring fecal pellets containing gut microbiota from an "extrovert" mouse to a "timid" mouse was enough to change the behavior of the latter mouse into a more "gregarious" creature that more closely resembled the behavior of the donor mouse. In the second study, transplanting stool from an obese mouse into a lean mouse turned the lean mouse into an eating machine.[2]

The implications of these and other emerging studies on the gut-brain connection could change the way we diagnose and treat physical and mental health issues. Imagine if part of the solution to a majority of our health woes might be as simple as changing what's on our plate.

Gut Health Begins Before We Do

New research indicates that our gut health starts in utero, before we're even born. For the past few decades, popular scientific belief has held that babies are born with a sterile gut and their first exposure to bacteria begins as the baby travels down the mother's vaginal canal, which colonizes the baby's gut with its first microbes. Babies pick up more microbes once they are out of the womb through skin-to-skin contact and breastfeeding and continue to add to their microbial garden throughout the first few years of life.

However, scientists have recently discovered small amounts of bacteria present in the amniotic fluid and placenta of the mother, as well as in the newborn's meconium (a scientific term for a baby's first poop!). This suggests that a baby's microbiome actually starts in the womb. One theory is that bacteria from the mother's mouth travel through the bloodstream and reach the baby in utero, through either the placenta or amniotic fluid. Another theory is that microbes find their way from the mother's vagina into the womb.

Maternal stress during pregnancy has long been linked to health issues for babies. Any physical and psychological stress your mother experienced during her pregnancy, as well as what she ate, helped set the stage for your future health.

Think back to your own birth story. Do you know what your biological mother's experience of pregnancy was like and what stressors may have been present? Were you delivered vaginally or born via C-section? Were you placed on antibiotics for any reason as an infant? All these things factor into shaping our microbiome.

In fact, you may experience symptoms of trauma from pain that is not actually yours but has been passed down through generations. With this in mind, I am absolutely fascinated by the work of Dr. Mayer. Through research, he has found that when a mother is stressed out during pregnancy, it literally changes her baby's brain and stress-response system. This is exacerbated by the mother's influence and interaction with her child post-birth. When a mother conveys the message to her child that the world is potentially dangerous, the child's gut feelings are biased in such a way as to be braced for exactly that. And it's not just that mother's child who bears the burden of this. According to Mayer, through the microbes in her vagina, a stressed-out or traumatized mother alters her infant's gut microbiome in such a way that key stress-response genes *that can last for several generations* are triggered.

This biological function is yet another example of a trait we have carried with us from the caveman days into modern times that no longer serves its intended function. When the world was less civilized, a child was well served by inheriting a strong fight-or-flight response and more careful, less outgoing and aggressive behaviors to better survive in a dangerous world. Today? Not so much.[3]

While there is a genetic predisposition to certain emotional aspects of our lives, we are also influenced by the events in our early lives. Mayer writes,

> For example, you may have inherited genes that predispose your fear or anger program to overreact to stressful situations. If you also experienced emotional trauma as a child, your body added chemical tags to these key stress-response genes. The net result is that as an adult, you will most likely experience exaggerated gut reactions to stress. This explains the common observation that two individuals exposed to the same stressful situation may show very different reactions to it: while one does not experience any noticeable gut reaction, the other one is incapacitated by nausea, stomach cramps, and diarrhea.[4]

The Gut and Immunity

The human body is made up of 30 to 50 trillion cells. Not a single one of these cells can function properly if our gastrointestinal system is in poor shape. A whopping 70 to 80 percent of our immune system resides in our gut. Aside from our skin, which is our body's largest organ, our gastrointestinal tract, or digestive system, is the main point of contact with the outside world. It's 25 to 30 feet in length, starting at our mouth and ending at our anus.

We ingest bacteria and microbes every single day. Some of these microorganisms are helpful and some are harmful. The gut has the incredibly important role of distinguishing between the two. What's wild is that the human cells in our body are actually outnumbered by foreign bacterial cells.

So how do we survive this onslaught of foreign invaders? Fortunately, the vast majority of bacteria in our bodies are beneficial. They serve as our gut's microbial partners by helping us digest our food and absorb nutrients; producing and secreting important enzymes, vitamins, beneficial fats, and amino acids; serving as a protective barrier to harmful toxins; and keeping our immune system in check by regulating inflammation. In fact, the entire length of our digestive tract is lined with a protective mucosal barrier inhabited by bacteria.

Clearly, we cannot function optimally without the help of our microbial friends. When we treat our microbes kindly, they repay us with health and vitality. Normal gut flora create the conditions for us to thrive. When our gut flora are compromised and our beneficial bacteria are damaged, the lining of our gut is weakened and we become more susceptible to invasion.

Gut Flora Foes

So what harms our friendly microbes? Let's take a look at some of the biggest stressors that can damage our gut flora and wreak havoc on our health.

Trauma

Trauma, and particularly childhood trauma, can have a major impact on our gut health. A recent study led by researchers at UCLA involving participants diagnosed with IBS versus a non-IBS control group indicated that childhood trauma can lead to lifelong changes in an individual's gut microbiome.[5]

In part I we touched on the fact that while we all experience trauma to varying degrees in our life, not everyone who experiences trauma will develop PTSD based on various risk and resiliency factors. Now, new research has indicated that there may be yet another factor to an individual's chances of developing PTSD: their gut microbiome. A new study by an international team of researchers out of Stellenbosch University in South Africa identified three different bacteria strains that appeared in significantly lower levels in individuals with PTSD. Lead researcher Stefanie Malan-Müller explains, "What makes this finding interesting is that individuals who experience childhood trauma are at a higher risk of developing PTSD later in life, and these changes in the gut microbiome possibly occurred early in life in response to childhood trauma."[6]

These three bacteria strains regulate our immune system. Not coincidentally, researchers have noticed that individuals suffering from PTSD have increased levels of inflammation and altered immune regulation. These two irregularities affect brain function and behavior. Although there is clearly a correlation between inflammation and immune regulation and PTSD, researchers are still trying to determine whether it's these factors that make us more susceptible to PTSD or if they are the consequence of PTSD. What we do know for sure is that the microbiome can be altered with prebiotics, probiotics, synbiotics (a combination of prebiotics and probiotics), and dietary intervention.[7]

Stress

Stress disrupts healthy digestion. As we've already discussed, digestion shuts off during the fight-or-flight response as blood gets diverted away from our gut and pumped into our extremities to help our muscles function at their peak for survival. Stress literally stops digestion in its tracks, inhibits absorption of vital nutrients, and can create uncomfortable symptoms such as heartburn, nausea, vomiting, diarrhea, and constipation. Whenever I take my dog to a new dog park, where she's met by a pack of unfamiliar dogs, she instantly gets diarrhea. It may seem like a silly example, but stress can literally make us (and our animals) sick.

My dog isn't the only example of this. Dr. Mayer cites studies done with adolescent rhesus monkeys that developed separation anxiety and diarrhea after leaving their mothers for the first time. He notes that many teenagers develop the same digestive symptoms as the young monkeys when they leave home for college.

While short-term stress has clear effects on our GI system, our gut flora usually bounce back quickly and return to normal levels of healthy bacteria after the stressful event has passed. Chronic stress, on the other hand, can lead to long-term damage for our digestive system. Short-term stress tasks the adrenal glands to produce more cortisol, which spikes our blood sugar temporarily to help generate more energy for an emergency response. When our cortisol levels get out of balance and stay out of balance, it can lead to food cravings, unhealthy fat storage, adrenal fatigue, hypoglycemia, diabetes, heart disease, depression, and anxiety.

Antibiotics

Antibiotics have one mission and one mission only: to destroy everything in sight. This is helpful and even lifesaving when it comes to eradicating a serious infection, but antibiotics these days are grossly overprescribed for even minor issues that are likely to resolve naturally on their own. The problem is that antibiotics lack the ability to discern between "good" and "bad" bacteria. As a result, they kill off beneficial bacteria in our gut, which leaves us susceptible to a host of GI issues. Studies have shown that long-term antibiotic use fundamentally alters our gut flora and can even make certain strains of bacteria resistant to the very same antibiotics, necessitating new, more powerful drugs. It can become a vicious cycle wherein our health and immunity are fighting a losing battle.

I made multiple trips to the emergency room for ear infections as a child, which were always solved with a prescription for antibiotics. Next came my GI issues. As early as I can remember, I have always had issues with severe bloating after eating. I also developed painful eczema as a teen, leading me to scratch my legs until they bled. I went on to develop debilitating allergies that were treated with multiple heavy-duty courses of drugs. Growing up, I never realized that these seemingly disparate issues could all be related. But as Hippocrates famously stated, "All disease begins in the gut."

Dr. Natasha Campbell-McBride, creator of the highly successful GAPS nutritional protocol and author of *Gut and Psychology Syndrome*, says that she has yet to meet a child with autism, ADHD/ADD, asthma, eczema, allergies, dyspraxia, or dyslexia "who has not got digestive abnormalities." In her book, she also notes that the majority of GAPS patients she sees have been exposed to numerous courses of antibiotics during their lives. "Given that many of these children had little chance to develop a healthy gut flora from the beginning, these courses of antibiotics have a devastating effect on their fragile gut ecology."[8]

Even if you haven't been exposed to antibiotics through your doctor, you've likely been exposed to them through your food. The meat and dairy industry is notorious for delivering antibiotics to animals whose meat, milk, and eggs end up at your local grocery store, and later in your digestive tract. And it's not just limited to meat and dairy; farmed fish are also given antibiotics.

Painkillers, Birth Control Pills, and Other Pharmaceuticals

Antibiotics are only one class of drugs that cause major damage to our gut. Other commonly used and prescribed drugs include painkillers such as aspirin, steroid creams, birth control pills, acid-reflux medications, statins (cholesterol-lowering drugs, like Lipitor), antidepressants, and antianxiety medications.

What these drugs have in common is that they stimulate the growth of bacteria that can lead to disease. They can also suppress the immune system and adversely impact gut flora. And worst of all, these drugs are often prescribed for long periods of time.

Drugs and Alcohol

Drugs and alcohol are often used as a means of coping with unresolved trauma, depression, and anxiety. Unfortunately, this strategy ends up creating a vicious cycle that only exacerbates these conditions. Alcohol is a depressant, which means that drinking too much can make us feel down and worsen any preexisting depression. It has also long been linked to anxiety disorders and PTSD. As if all of that isn't enough, doctors now know that alcohol abuse also creates severe damage to the gut, creates major nutritional deficiencies, and promotes the development of certain cancers.[9]

Diet

SAD is an acronym for the standard American diet, and it is indeed as sad as they come. The typical American diet is linked to obesity, heart disease, diabetes, and a host of other diseases that ultimately result in early death. Even if we are eating a fairly clean diet, there are so many ways we are sabotaging our own health and vitality through seemingly innocuous food choices. We'll talk about this in detail, but for a quick reference, you can check out the "Food Culprits" that may be undermining your health and your mood on page 234, as well as a list of common and accessible "Food Heroes" that can help heal your gut and boost your energy and your mood on page 242. But first let's take a look at the most common food sensitivities and allergies, how they may be affecting your health, and what you can do about it.

Food Sensitivities and Allergies

Food allergies can be very serious and potentially fatal, but the good news is that *true* food allergies are actually quite rare. In the case of a food allergy, our body produces antibodies (known as IgE) that trigger an immediate and aggressive inflammatory reaction. For example, peanut allergies can cause an immediate reaction of swelling, hives, difficulty breathing, and anaphylaxis.

Food sensitivities, on the other hand, are caused by a different type of antibody, known as IgG. Rather than experiencing an immediate inflammatory response, our body has a delayed reaction, which usually occurs anywhere between twenty-four and forty-eight hours after the consumption of a particular food. This delayed onset is the primary reason so many people have no clue they have a food sensitivity. Say you went out for pizza with friends. You ate, had a great time, and slept great that night. Two days later you wake up with a pounding headache. You may attribute it to stress or staying up too late, but chances are you're not going to associate it with the pizza you ate two days ago.

Most people associate food sensitivities with a stomachache or diarrhea, but the truth is that food sensitivities show up in a surprising number of ways, including eczema, acne, chronic headaches, fatigue, brain fog, depression, anxiety, heart palpitations, achy joints, sleep disturbances, nasal and sinus congestion, and more. While food allergies are estimated to affect approximately 4 percent of the U.S. population, food sensitivities are far more widespread, affecting millions of unsuspecting people. And often it's the foods we are most sensitive to that we crave the most. Eliminating a food your body is reactive to can radically transform your health and vitality.

Sensitivities occur when our immune system misidentifies something harmless as a threat. Our immune system can get overwhelmed and confused due to a variety of factors, including trauma, stress, lack of sleep, exposure to toxins, antibiotics, medications, poor dietary habits, nutritional deficiencies, and more. Remember that the majority of our immune system is housed in our gut. When our immune system is compromised, it can damage our gut lining, which serves the important function of protecting us from foreign invaders. Ultimately, this can lead to autoimmune diseases and a condition known as leaky gut. Once you have a leaky gut, you're highly susceptible to additional food sensitivities in the future.

Common Food Sensitivities

Here is a list of the most common food sensitivities. Note, however, that food sensitivities are highly individual and can vary from person to person.

- Citrus fruits
- Corn
- Dairy products (butter, cheese, milk, yogurt)
- Eggs
- Gluten (found in grains, including barley, Kamut, rye, spelt, triticale, and wheat)
- Nightshade vegetables (bell peppers, eggplant, potatoes, and tomatoes)
- Peanuts
- Refined sugars
- Shellfish
- Soy
- Yeast (baker's yeast, brewer's yeast, mold, vinegar, and wine)

Common Symptoms of Food Sensitivities

If you have any of the following symptoms, it may indicate a food sensitivity:

- Acne
- Anxiety
- Brain fog/inability to concentrate
- Canker sores
- Depression
- Eczema
- Fatigue/low energy
- GERD (gastroesophageal reflux disease)
- Headache

- Heart palpitations
- Joint pain/arthritis
- Mood swings
- Nausea
- Shortness of breath
- Sinus congestion or postnasal drip
- Stiff muscles or muscle pain
- Stomach pain
- Weight gain/inability to lose weight

If You Have a Food Sensitivity

The best way to determine if you have a food sensitivity is to perform an elimination test. Here's how:

- If you think you may be sensitive to one of the foods listed on the previous page, eliminate it from your diet completely for 4 weeks. If you don't know which food you may be sensitive to, consider eliminating *all* of the foods on the list (I know—it's a hefty order). Cutting down the offending foods to just once a week won't work, nor will having just a little nibble or bite here and there. Our immune system will inevitably find out and react.

- Keep a food journal during the 4-week elimination period, tracking how you feel physically, mentally, and emotionally.

- After 4 weeks, reintroduce one food group at a time. Eat the food daily for at least 3 days and track any symptoms. Compare how you felt during the elimination period to how you feel during the reintroduction.

- If your symptoms return during the reintroduction period, that particular food is highly likely to be a trigger and should be eliminated from your diet. You can retest again after a few months to see if the food still causes sensitivity.

Chapter 14

Food Heroes and Zeros

The food you eat can be either the safest and most powerful
form of medicine or the slowest form of poison.
—Ann Wigmore

What's on our fork can make or break our health. Identifying the foods that support your mental and physical health and those that worsen it puts the power of healing in your own hands. Below you'll find a list of common foods that may be secretly sabotaging your health and well-being. You'll also learn which foods you should be incorporating to keep your brain and your body in tip-top shape.

Common Food Culprits

Here are the most common food culprits that can negatively impact our mood, drain our energy, and exacerbate—and in some cases even *cause*—mental health issues and symptoms that mimic depression. As you read through the list, notice which common culprits have a strong presence in your life, pay attention to any cravings and symptoms described, and compare them with any symptoms you may be experiencing. Eliminating or cutting back on these foods can do wonders for your health.

Sugar and Refined Carbohydrates

It's common knowledge that excessive consumption of sugar from processed foods like candy, cake, cookies, and other sweets can lead to weight gain, obesity, and diabetes. But sugar is also linked to a variety of mood and mental health issues, including depression and anxiety. Studies have shown that it can even affect our cognitive abilities, including learning and memory.

Sugar is highly addictive, with some public health officials going so far as to call it "the most dangerous drug of the times." Research has shown that excessive sugar consumption can increase dopamine levels in our brain in a way similar to drugs such as tobacco, cocaine, and morphine.[1] With prolonged consumption, our dopamine levels actually decrease over time, creating a cycle similar to substance abuse, wherein we need increasingly higher dosages of sugar to satisfy the pleasure centers in our brain in order to stave off low moods. It's a vicious trap of cravings, crashes, anxiety, and mood swings, which can lead to feelings of shame, guilt, and depression.

Consuming refined sugar can swing our blood sugar levels wildly out of control. When our blood sugar rises, our insulin levels respond by rising as well. After the initial spike, there is an inevitable crash in blood sugar. When your blood sugar falls, your body craves more sugar to pick you back up, and the cycle continues.

Sugar crashes can lead to irritability, mood swings, anxiety, fatigue, foggy thinking, and headaches. Blood sugar swings also tax the adrenal glands, which respond by producing more cortisol. As you may recall, when our adrenal glands are burdened with a long-term overproduction of cortisol, they can tire out and actually end up underproducing cortisol, which can lead to adrenal fatigue and exacerbate anxiety or depression. Refined sugar also depletes our body of vital nutrients such as B vitamins and minerals such as zinc, manganese, magnesium, and calcium, many of which help to stabilize our mood.

If sugar addiction is something you struggle with, know that it's not your fault and you are not alone. Many people beat themselves up for lacking willpower or the self-discipline to conquer their sugar cravings and fall into self-loathing every time they reach for something sweet. Take a moment and offer yourself a huge dose of kindness and compassion. You are not weak. You are not a failure. Sugar changes your brain chemistry, which quite literally renders willpower useless. And it is insidiously hidden in some of the most common foods, including those marketed as "healthy." You can find it lurking in cereals, packaged oatmeal, packaged bread, yogurt, canned and instant soups, salad dressings, bottled sauces, "healthy" snack bars (including granola bars and protein bars), ketchup, and many more foods.

Getting your sugar consumption under control is a top priority to take back your health and balance your mood. As a first line of defense, try eliminating all sugar for thirty days. If you just can't kick the habit, I recommend seeking out a naturopath or physician who can test and address any neurotransmitter imbalances, candida overgrowth, or adrenal issues that might be at play. Addressing these imbalances can radically shift your health by curbing your cravings and ultimately improving your mood.

Dr. Kelly Brogan, who specializes in treating depression through nutritional interventions, writes in her book *A Mind of Your Own: The Truth About Depression and How Women Can Heal Their Bodies and Reclaim Their Lives* that "the secret to ending your depression could very well be in stopping the highs and lows (the sugar roller coaster) that are taking place in your bloodstream and, by implication, your brain." She goes on to write that balancing blood sugar chaos can also potentially spare you from panic disorder, generalized anxiety, symptoms associated with ADHD diagnoses, and bipolar disorder, as well as staving off the need for potentially detrimental medications.[2]

CONSIDER ELIMINATING THE FOLLOWING SOURCES OF PROCESSED SUGAR:

- Bread
- Breakfast cereals
- Candy, cakes, cookies, pies
- Fruit juice
- Ice cream
- Pasta
- Soda and diet soda
- Sports drinks
- Sweetened yogurts

Sugar by Any Other Name . . .

. . . well, it may still be as sweet, but it's also just as bad for you. Read your labels carefully! Avoid all artificial sweeteners like aspartame, saccharin, and sucralose, and be on the lookout for these commonly added sugars with sneaky names:

- Beet sugar
- Corn syrup
- Dextrose
- Evaporated cane juice
- Fructose
- Fruit juice concentrate
- Glucose
- High-fructose corn syrup
- Invert sugar
- Lactose
- Malt sugar
- Maltose
- Molasses
- Sucrose
- Syrup

Tips to Curb Your Sugar Cravings

I know, I know. Knowing you should cut out sugar is one thing, but actually *doing* it is an entirely different matter. But here's the thing: food manufacturers know that too. Put the power back in your own hands. Here are some of my favorite tips for kicking that sugar habit—or at least cutting it down.

- *Consume enough protein, especially at breakfast.* Incorporating protein into your breakfast will help control your blood sugar levels as you start your day. Quality sources of protein include eggs, wild fish, organic meats, and poultry. If you don't eat meat or eggs or prefer to drink your breakfast rather than eat it, add a scoop of your favorite plant-based protein powder to a green smoothie. You can cut down on the sugar content by replacing banana with avocado or steamed and frozen cauliflower.

- *Incorporate healthy fats into your diet.* Our brain is almost 60 percent fat and functions best when fueled with healthy fats. When you swap out sugar as a primary fuel source for healthy fats such as avocado, coconut, nuts, and nut butters, you can get off the blood sugar roller coaster. Healthy fats also satiate your appetite and keep you feeling full longer, so you're less likely to reach for a sugary snack.
- *Drink water infused with fresh fruit.* Add slices of lemon, lime, orange, or cucumber to make your water feel more like a treat.
- *Ditch artificial sweeteners.* This doesn't mean you have to sacrifice taste. Try replacing them with spices like cinnamon or licorice, which can help satisfy sweet cravings.

Dairy

I used to live for cheese. I had a serious love affair with that beautiful gooey gold, but I never considered the possibility that it was contributing to so many of my health and digestive woes. My naturopath suggested I eliminate dairy for a few weeks to see if it would help clear up some of my allergies and pesky eczema. In less than a month, my allergies virtually disappeared and my skin issues cleared. I no longer started off each morning with my attractive sinus-clearing ritual of shooting globs of mucus out of my nose and coughing up little balls of phlegm into my sink before brushing my teeth. Gross, I know!

While the dairy industry refutes any connection between milk products and increased mucus production and research into the topic admittedly hasn't been conclusive, many naturopaths, functional medicine doctors, and holistic health practitioners recommend that clients eliminate dairy products from their diets, to great effect. Dr. Andrew Weil, a pioneer in the field of integrative medicine and director of the Arizona Center for Integrative Medicine at the University of Arizona, encourages eliminating dairy products to relieve allergy symptoms, including asthma and eczema.[3]

Allergies aside, it's estimated that approximately 75 percent of the world's population is lactose intolerant. Lactose is a type of sugar found in milk. Those who are lactose intolerant lack the enzyme lactase, which is needed to digest lactose. Symptoms include stomach pain, bloating, diarrhea, and gas.

When I reach for cheese now, I choose nondairy plant-based options such as almond or cashew cheese (I like the brands Kite Hill and Daiya), but I admit that the sight and smell of a cheese pizza still makes my head turn and my mouth water. I know I'm not alone in this. As Dr. Kelly Brogan notes in her book *A Mind of Your Own*, dairy (and wheat) actually include morphine-like exorphins, which cause our opiate receptors to perk up.[4]

And while we're speaking of the brain, recent studies associate casein, a protein found in dairy products, with schizophrenia, depression, and autism. I would say this makes a compelling case for trying a casein-free diet by eliminating dairy. Yes!.

One final note on dairy: remember that what works for some may not work for all. If you eliminate dairy from your diet to little or no result, dairy might not be an issue for you, and you can safely incorporate it back into your diet. *Dr Neal Barnard*

CONSIDER ELIMINATING THE FOLLOWING DAIRY SOURCES:

- Baked goods such as cake, cookies, muffins, and scones, which usually contain milk as an ingredient
- Butter
- Cheese (including all cheese from cow's and goat's milk, cottage cheese, and cream cheese)
- Cream/half-and-half (be on alert for dairy in creamy salad dressings, cream sauces, and cream soups)
- Custard
- Ice cream
- Milk and buttermilk
- Processed foods containing whey protein or casein, which is usually found in protein powders and protein bars
- Sour cream and crème fraîche
- Yogurt

Substitutions for Dairy

Replace your cravings for milk, butter, and yogurt with dairy-free alternatives such as nut milk (almond, rice, hemp, cashew, or coconut milk), coconut yogurt, and nut butters.

Gluten

Gluten is a protein found in wheat, rye, and barley. It derives its name from its glue-like consistency, which holds flour together and helps dough keep its shape. Similar to casein, gluten can have an opioid-like effect on the brain, triggering addictive cravings and accompanying crashes that keep us reaching for the bread basket.

Dr. David Perlmutter, author of *Grain Brain: The Surprising Truth About Wheat, Carbs, and Sugar—Your Brain's Silent Killers*, calls gluten "a modern poison."[5] Gluten impedes the absorption of nutrients and can't be easily digested, which can ultimately result in the deterioration of our small intestine lining.

While many may be alerted to their body's negative reaction to gluten through symptoms such as abdominal pain, nausea, diarrhea, and constipation, even worse, others don't experience obvious signs of gastrointestinal distress while other parts of their body, such as their nervous system, are under silent assault.

While celiac disease (a serious autoimmune disorder that causes damage to the small

Only True alem For R 2%)!

intestine and is triggered by eating gluten) affects only about 1 percent of the American population, gluten sensitivity affects far more people, most of whom don't have any clue it's an issue. Dr. Marios Hadjivassiliou, professor and researcher at the Royal Hallamshire Hospital in England, claims that gluten sensitivity can be a primarily neurological disease. Operating under that theory, he tests for gluten sensitivity in all patients who come to him with mysterious neurological complaints. Dr. Perlmutter summarizes Dr. Hadjivassiliou's findings: "People with gluten sensitivity can have issues with brain function without having any gastrointestinal problems whatsoever."[6]

And it doesn't stop here. Gluten can adversely impact us in a whole host of very serious ways, including depression, seizures, headaches, multiple sclerosis/demyelination, anxiety, symptoms associated with ADHD diagnoses, ataxia (loss of control of bodily movements), and nerve damage.[7]

As Trudy Scott, nutritionist and author of *The Antianxiety Food Solution*, writes, "I've seen so many clients experience dramatic mood improvements when they avoid gluten, so I always recommend that my clients with anxiety and other mood problems go gluten free. Doing so may completely resolve symptoms of anxiety, especially among people who aren't benefiting from antianxiety medications."[8]

CONSIDER ELIMINATING THE FOLLOWING GLUTEN SOURCES:

- Barley
- Bulgur
- Durum wheat
- Farina
- Graham flour
- Kamut
- Kashi
- Matzo meal
- Rye
- Semolina
- Spelt
- Triticale
- Wheat

Goad For Mac & Us

AVOID "HIDDEN" GLUTEN IN THE FOLLOWING FOODS:

- Baked goods such as cookies, cakes, pastries, pies
- Baking soda and baking powder
- Beer and wine coolers
- Bread
- Bread crumbs (and breaded foods like fried foods)
- Candy
- Cereal
- Crackers and chips
- Croutons
- Imitation meat or seafood
- Pasta
- Salad dressing
- Sausage
- Seitan
- Soups and gravy
- Soy sauce
- Stuffing
- Tabbouli
- Teriyaki sauce
- Tortillas

Substitutions for Gluten

Swap out gluten products for these gluten-free alternatives: rice, amaranth, arrowroot, millet, buckwheat, teff, nut flours, ground flaxseed, quinoa, sweet potatoes, and oats (make sure they are labeled "gluten free").

Caffeine

Many people can't imagine life without their daily cup or three of coffee. If you need caffeine to get you through the day, it may be time to rethink your relationship with it. Caffeine is a stimulant drug, albeit a legal one. And like any drug, it can have side effects. When I suggest to my clients that their caffeine habit could very well be exacerbating their anxiety, irritability, insomnia, and fatigue, I'm usually met with strong protests. The loudest protestors often later concede that giving up their morning cup was the best decision they ever made because it significantly reduced their anxiety and panic.

If you're still clinging to your coffee cup, perhaps it will help to know that there's a mountain of research to back up the link between caffeine and anxiety, which can be particularly problematic if you're predisposed to panic disorders and social anxiety.[9] For instance, heavy caffeine use may lead to increased use of antianxiety medications.[10] It can cause lactate buildup, which contributes to anxiety and panic attacks. Caffeine can also stimulate panic-attack-like symptoms, such as heart palpitations and tremors.[11, 12] A small but notable 1989 study followed six patients with anxiety disorders who regularly consumed 1½ to 3½ cups of coffee per day. Cutting out caffeine improved their symptoms within a week, where pharmaceuticals and psychotherapy had previously had no effect. They remained improved for at least a six-month follow-up period by only abstaining from caffeine![13]

If anxiety, panic attacks, chronic fatigue, and insomnia aren't issues for you, then eliminating all caffeine may not be necessary. Again, the key is to understand your own unique needs and make the changes that support you as an individual.

Weaning Off Caffeine

If you do decide to remove caffeine from your diet, be aware that quitting coffee cold turkey can create withdrawal symptoms, so it's best to wean yourself off slowly. I've found success with the following strategy:

- Start slowly introducing decaf into your cup. Brew three-fourths regular coffee to one-fourth decaffeinated coffee for a week. Then switch to half regular coffee and half decaf for week two. For week three, switch to one-fourth regular coffee and three-fourths decaf. From there, you can completely eliminate regular coffee all together.

- If you drink multiple cups of coffee a day, you can also experiment with simply cutting down to just one cup a day, then half a cup.
- You can also try swapping out coffee for green tea and, eventually, swapping out green tea for hot water with lemon.
- Drink plenty of filtered water throughout the elimination process.
- Consider supplementation during the elimination process. Trudy Scott, a certified nutritionist and author of *The Antianxiety Food Solution*, has found great success managing withdrawal symptoms like headaches and fatigue in her patients by having them take the over-the-counter supplement tyrosine. Check with your certified nutritionist, naturopath, or doctor to see if tyrosine may be a fit for you.

  Dr. Mark Hyman, director of the Cleveland Clinic's Center for Functional Medicine, recommends taking 1,000 milligrams of vitamin C with breakfast and dinner. Vitamin C can help ease withdrawal symptoms while supporting your adrenal glands. A magnesium supplement can also help, especially if you're experiencing irritability or difficulty sleeping. Dr. Hyman suggests a combination of 500 milligrams calcium citrate and 250 milligrams magnesium citrate before bed.[14]

Alcohol

We briefly discussed alcohol and the way it affects the gut, but will touch here on why eliminating alcohol is imperative for those who suffer from anxiety. According to Dr. Joseph Pizzorno and Dr. Michael Murray, authors of *Textbook of Natural Medicine*, alcohol causes nutritional deficiencies, depletes nutrients that are important for preventing anxiety, and can result in reactions similar to food sensitivities, all of which heighten anxiety.[15] It can lead to lower levels of serotonin and has been linked to anger and even violence.[16] It has also been linked to anxiety, depression, and sleep problems.

Alcohol also lends itself to a vicious cycle. It causes blood sugar levels to drop up to twelve hours after consumption, which leaves people craving sugar and more alcohol—both of which make matters worse. Low blood sugar can result in anxiety, dizziness, headache, and fatigue.[17]

Alcohol Recovery

Recovering from alcohol addiction can take many forms and will look different for each individual. The best approach is a multifaceted one that includes multiple avenues of support. This might include therapy to address any underlying trauma, support groups like Alcoholics Anonymous or other religious or spiritual organizations, exercise, mindfulness, and nutritional therapy.

To help reduce your dependency on alcohol, it can be helpful to understand when you use it and why. Do you use alcohol as a stimulant for energy? Does it help pick you up? Or does it calm you down? Do you use it as a sleep aid? A muscle relaxant or a painkiller? According to Trudy Scott, identifying how you use alcohol can help you identify solutions to balance your brain chemistry, improve your mood and alleviate symptoms like anxiety.[18] Her book, *The Antianxiety Food Solution,* along with Julia Ross's book *The Mood Cure,* are both great resources to dive deeper into the topic of nutritional therapy and amino acid supplementation as a means to improve your mental health and emotional well-being.

Food Heroes

We've discussed common food culprits that can sabotage our physical and mental well-being—and now it's time to discover foods that support our mental health, stabilize our moods, and create energy and vitality!

Healthy Fats

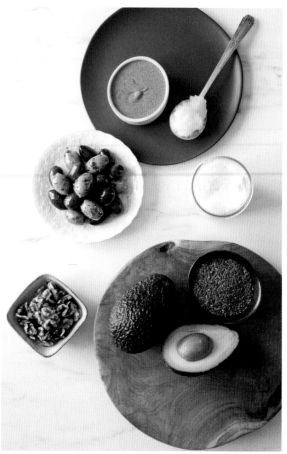

Fat has been unfairly demonized over the last few decades. Saturated fat, in particular, started getting a bad rap in the 1950s, when it was hypothesized in what has become known as the lipid hypothesis that dietary fat increased cholesterol and heart disease. The American Heart Association jumped on board the anti-fat train and began discouraging the consumption of butter, eggs, meat, and other foods high in saturated fat.

And thus the low-fat craze was born. Big food brands seized the opportunity to repackage and market unhealthy foods as new healthy "low-fat" options like low-fat cookies, muffins, frozen yogurt, breakfast cereals, salad dressings, and more. What they didn't tell consumers, however, is that when they cut the fat, they added sugar, effectively making these "low-fat" treats less healthy than ever before.

More than half a century later, doctors and researchers are finally clearing up the fat myth. Astonishingly, our brain is actually made up of more than 60 percent fat. "Fat—not carbohydrate—is the preferred fuel of human metabolism and has been for all of human evolution," says Dr. Perlmutter in *Grain Brain*.[19]

Good Fat vs. Bad Fat

There's a popular meme about two cartoon avocados. One of the avocados is running away in tears while the other avocado chases after his friend, exclaiming, "I said you're the *good* kind of fat!" Navigating the landscape of "good fat" versus "bad fat" can be confusing. Let me help simplify it. Fats are categorized into two main groups: saturated and unsaturated.

In the saturated group, we have foods like meat, eggs, cheese, butter, and coconut oil. Saturated fats have historically been classified as "bad" fats, but emerging research is changing that. We now know that in fact saturated fats are essential for our good health.

Consider this: breastfed babies are literally raised on saturated fats, which constitute 54 percent of the fat in breast milk. This isn't surprising, because each and every cell in our body requires saturated fats; they are responsible for 50 percent of our cell membrane. Saturated fats are vital to the proper functioning of our lungs, heart, bones, liver, and immune system. Our bones require saturated fats, as does our liver. Saturated fats also help our immune system destroy germs and ward off tumors.[20]

Now, with that in mind, it's also important to understand that not all saturated fats are created equal. Processed and canned meats that contain nasty additives and artificial preservatives should be avoided, including hot dogs, ham, Spam, sausages, corned beef, packaged deli meats, and beef jerky. Grain-fed beef should also be avoided. Grain-fed cows are moved to crowded feedlots with the purpose of fattening them up quickly on a diet based mostly of corn and soy. They are often given hormones to promote faster growth and antibiotics due to unsanitary living conditions. What an animal eats determines the quality of its meat and actually changes the composition of the meat. Grain-fed beef lacks the healthy omega-3s that are found in grass-fed beef. Whenever possible, choose grass-finished over grass-fed and grass-fed over grain-fed. What's the difference? While the term *grass-fed* may conjure up images of happy cows grazing on green pastures, "grass-fed" cows aren't required to have a strictly grass diet to earn the label on beef packaging. Many grass-fed cows are transferred to grain feedlots before going to slaughter. *Grass-finished*, on the other hand, refers to cattle that were raised from start to finish on a grass and forage diet. Factory-farmed meat and dairy should also be avoided. Not only are factory-farmed animals given antibiotics and artificial growth hormones, they are also subjected to cruelty and raised under inhumane conditions.

There's also another group of saturated fats that should be avoided at all costs: artificial trans fats. The majority of trans fats consumed today are synthetically produced and can be identified on food labels as "partially hydrogenated oil." Trans fats are found in margarine, partially hydrogenated vegetable oils, and a host of other processed foods, including frozen pizza, cookies, crackers, doughnuts, chips, and fried foods.

The unsaturated group is divided into monounsaturated and polyunsaturated fats. Monounsaturated fats include avocados, nuts, olives, and olive oil, all of which are "good" sources of fat. By now, most of us know that olive oil is known for its health benefits—but did you know that it was also shown to help reduce anxiety in a recent animal study?[21]

Polyunsaturated fats include omega-3 fatty acids found in fatty fish (salmon, trout, catfish, mackerel), as well as plant-based sources like walnuts and flaxseeds, which are also considered "good" sources of fat. Joseph Pizzorno, a prominent naturopathic physician, points to flaxseed oil in particular as being helpful for patients with agoraphobia. Aside from that biggie, flaxseed oil also helps with things like dry skin, dandruff, brittle fingernails, and nerve disorders.[22]

Making Sense of Omegas

You may have heard the health world buzzing about the benefits of omega-3 fats, while warning about overconsumption of omega-6 fats. But most of us don't know what the difference is. Both are essential fatty acids that our body doesn't naturally produce; therefore we need to get them from our food sources.

Omega-3s are the superheroes of brain health. They have been shown to fight depression and anxiety, reduce symptoms of ADHD in children, balance mood swings, reduce the occurrence of relapses in people with schizophrenia and bipolar disorder, reduce the risk of age-related mental decline and Alzheimer's disease, and reduce inflammation.

While omega-3 fatty acids have been shown to decrease inflammation, omega-6 fatty acids are known for *increasing* inflammation. However, omega-6 fats in their unprocessed form (such as nuts and seeds) aren't all bad. When consumed in moderation, they have their own benefits for brain and immune function.

The problem is not the existence of omega-6s, but the ratio of omega-3s to omega-6s in the standard American diet. Anthropological research indicates that human beings evolved consuming omega-6 and omega-3 fats in a ratio of roughly 1:1.[23] Western diets today have a disproportionately high consumption of omega-6 to omega-3 fats, with a ratio ranging from 15:1 to 17:1. This imbalance has been linked to a host of negative effects on our health, including cardiovascular disease, cancer, and inflammatory and autoimmune diseases.[24] Omega-6s are found in high quantities in processed vegetable oils, including canola, corn, cottonseed, safflower, soybean, and sunflower oil.

Fats to Include	Fats to Avoid

HEALTHY OILS:
• Avocado
• Coconut
• Flaxseed (don't use for cooking, as flaxseed oil is unstable when heated; drizzle it onto salads cold)
• Macadamia
• Olive
• Pumpkin seed
• Walnut
• Fish   *No Oils:*
       Dr. Esselstn
        Dr. Klaper
	OILS:
	• Canola
	• Corn
	• Cottonseed
	• Peanut
	• Safflower
	• Sunflower
	• Soybean
	• "Vegetable"

BUTTER: • Ghee (clarified butter) *None*	**BUTTER SUBSTITUTES:** • Margarine • Shortening
MEAT, FISH, AND EGGS: • Grass-fed beef • Organic, pasture-raised poultry • Organic, pasture-raised eggs • Wild fish *Avoid*	**MEAT, FISH, AND EGGS:** • Grain-fed beef • Factory-farmed poultry • Conventional eggs • Farmed fish
NUT MILKS AND NUT BUTTERS: • Almond • Cashew • Coconut • Hemp	**DAIRY:** • Cow's milk
NUTS AND SEEDS: • Almonds • Brazil nuts • Cashews • Chia seeds • Flaxseed • Sunflower seeds • Pumpkin seeds • Walnuts	
FRUITS: • Avocados • Olives	

Cholesterol—Friend or Foe?

Like saturated fat, cholesterol has also been vilified over the past fifty years. But emerging research shows that it's not completely deserving of its bad reputation. Did you know our brain needs cholesterol to develop and function properly? In fact, 25 percent of the cholesterol in our bodies is found in our brains. So when our cholesterol levels get too low, our brain doesn't function optimally.

Too little cholesterol can result in a host of neurological problems, ranging from depression to dementia. A 1998 study showed that deceased Alzheimer's patients had a significantly low level of cholesterol in their cerebrospinal fluid.[25]

On a more day-to-day level, a study published by Boston University in 2005 showed that there is a relationship between cholesterol levels and cognitive performance. It negatively impacted skills like attention, abstract reasoning, and word fluency.[26]

Before you start dreaming of bacon and butter for every meal, know that *none* of the research suggests that anyone should eat a diet comprised primarily of butter, meat, and eggs. In his Brain Maker diet, Dr. David Perlmutter recommends that fibrous fruits and vegetables that grow aboveground should make up the majority of your plate, with protein as a side dish, rather than the main dish.

Protein

Protein is vital for physical and mental health. It contains amino acids, which affect the neurotransmitters that impact our mood. When I was experiencing panic attacks and adrenal fatigue, eliminating sugar and carbs as my main source of fuel and replacing them with protein and healthy fats made a world of difference in helping to balance my mood, diminish my anxiety, and prevent energy crashes.

Proteins are commonly referred to as the "building blocks of life." They provide essential fuel for our cells and play a role in almost every function of our body. Proteins are found in both plant and animal sources; however, they contain different amino acid profiles. Animal sources of protein include meat, poultry, eggs, and fish. Plant sources of protein include legumes, nuts, seeds, hemp, and soy. Unfortunately, the standard American diet is loaded with low-quality protein, and many people consume far more than is nutritionally needed by the body. When choosing animal sources of protein, select humanely raised, organically and grass-fed meat.

On the other end of the spectrum, vegetarians and vegans often consume too few "complete" proteins (which contain more essential amino acids than "incomplete" proteins). There are many excellent plant-based sources of protein, but to obtain adequate proportions of essential amino acids, vegetarians often need to combine proteins to form complete amino acid profiles. Eating too little protein and incomplete proteins can impact neurotransmitter function and affect mood and mental health.

Many vegetarians and vegans choose a plant-based lifestyle not just for greater health but for deeply held spiritual and ethical reasons. The desire not to harm animals is an admirable trait and one that scientists agree can help the planet on a large environmental scale. I have personally gone back and forth between being vegetarian and, at times, completely vegan, but have recently shied away from labels that feel too restrictive. My current diet is primarily plant-based, with an emphasis on fruits, veggies, and healthy plant-based sources of fat, but I do supplement with fish oil and incorporate sparing amounts of humanely raised, organic, grass-fed animal protein when my body calls for it. Bottom line: listen to your own body and make choices that honor yourself.

Quality Animal Protein Sources	Quality Plant Protein Sources
• Organic, grass-fed, humanely and pasture-raised meats free of antibiotics and hormones (beef, pork, lamb, poultry)	• Legumes (lentils, beans, chickpeas)
• Wild, sustainably caught fish (salmon, sardines, anchovies)	• Nuts (raw almonds, walnuts, cashews, Brazil nuts, and more)
• Organic, pasture-raised eggs	• Seeds (hemp, flax, chia, pumpkin, sunflower)
• Bone broths (chicken and beef)	• Organic, fermented, or sprouted soy (tempeh, tofu, edamame) (Soy is a common food allergen and non-organic sources should be avoided.)
• Organic hydrolyzed collagen (may be mixed into smoothies or beverages)	• Gluten-free grains (Quinoa is technically a seed but is usually eaten in meals like a grain.)

Proteins to Avoid
• Commercially (or "conventionally") raised meat and eggs
• Whey protein
• Soy protein isolates (This type of soy product has been artificially processed and linked to allergies, thyroid problems, and more.)

Vegetables and Fruits

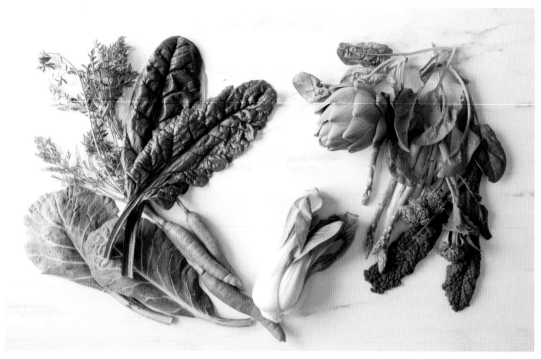

In a confusing and often contentious landscape of nutritional information, there's one thing all of the experts agree on: eat your veggies! Vegetables should be an essential part of your diet, as they provide a diverse array of necessary nutrients, including vitamins, minerals, fiber, and antioxidants, and are known to help reduce the risk of chronic diseases.

There are a few groups of vegetables in particular that should be a staple in any "good mood" diet.

Cruciferous Vegetables

Cruciferous vegetables are a good source of nutrients, minerals, and fiber. They also feature sulfur-containing compounds called glucosinolates, which have been studied for their potential cancer-fighting benefits. In one study, concentrated amounts of the glucosinolate glucoraphanin were found to improve autistic behaviors.[27] It should be noted that some studies have found a link between high levels of cruciferous vegetables and thyroid dysfunction, but the risk is generally thought to be very low for the majority of the population.

Cruciferous vegetables include:

- Arugula
- Bok choy
- Broccoli
- Brussels sprouts

- Cabbage
- Cauliflower
- Collard greens
- Kale

- Mustard greens
- Radishes
- Turnips
- Watercress

Sea Vegetables (Seaweed)

Sea vegetables are nutritional powerhouses and among the richest sources of minerals, including iodine, iron, magnesium, calcium, and phosphorus. Their exceptionally high mineral content supports thyroid and nervous system function. Calcium and magnesium help support muscles, and magnesium in particular is a powerful natural muscle relaxer and can also help improve sleep. Sea vegetables also contain vitamins, proteins, lipids, and amino acids. They can be used in soups, as toppings for salads or main dishes, as snacks, or as healthy gluten-free alternatives to wraps.

They include:

- Arame
- Dulse

- Kelp
- Kombu

- Nori
- Wakame

Root Vegetables

In Ayurveda, an ancient mind-body healing system developed thousands of years ago by sages in India, root vegetables are revered for their emotionally grounding properties. They are thought to be healing and balancing during times of stress and anxiety. Root vegetables contain essential vitamins and minerals, including vitamin A, which has been linked to healthy brain function.

Root vegetables include:

- Carrots
- Parsnips
- Squash
- Sweet potatoes

- Turnips
- Yams
- Yucca

Fruits

Fruits are an important part of a whole foods diet, and like vegetables, they are packed with essential vitamins, minerals, fiber, and antioxidants. They are also known to help reduce the risk of chronic diseases like heart disease and cancer. If blood sugar crashes are an issue for you, fruits should be consumed in moderation.

Low-sugar fruits include:

- Avocados
- Berries
- Lemons
- Limes
- Pumpkin

High-sugar fruits include:

- Apricots
- Bananas
- Cherries
- Figs
- Grapes
- Mangoes
- Melons
- Pineapples
- Plums

Herbs and Spices

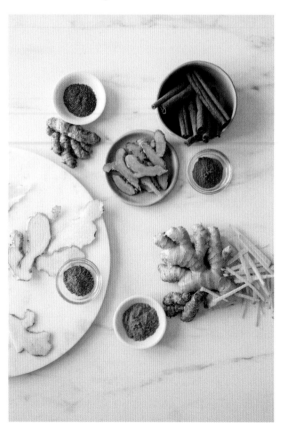

Herbs and spices are a wonderful source of nutrients that have many benefits for physical and mental health. Following are three superstar spices that will make powerful additions to your gut-healing and mood-boosting toolbox.

Turmeric

Turmeric is a golden spice that has long been touted for its disease-preventing, anti-inflammatory, and medicinal properties. Numerous studies have shown its effectiveness at helping the body fight inflammation, even rivaling the power of some anti-inflammatory drugs. According to a study published by James A. Duke in the October 2007 issue of *Alternative & Complementary Therapy*, turmeric outperformed many pharmaceuticals against several chronic, debilitating diseases, with virtually no negative side effects.[28]

Curcumin, the active compound in turmeric, has also been linked to improving brain health and helping to lower the risk of brain diseases like Alzheimer's.

Turmeric can be found at most local grocery stores in its powdered form as a spice or as a supplement and is sold as a whole root at many specialty groceries. It can be used in a variety of dishes and beverages to spice up any dish with healing properties.

Try Healing Turmeric Latte recipe on page 260 to help ease inflammation, reduce pain, and nourish you from the inside out.

Ginger

Ginger stands out as one of the most medicinally healing foods on earth. It is effective at relieving nausea and is used as a seasickness remedy and a natural antinausea remedy for chemotherapy patients and patients recovering from surgery. It has also been studied for its effectiveness in relieving nausea associated with morning sickness in pregnant women.

As a powerful anti-inflammatory, ginger is also a natural reliever of muscle and joint pain, and studies have shown it to be as effective as ibuprofen for menstrual pain. Like its cousin turmeric, ginger may also improve brain function and help lower the risk of Alzheimer's disease. It also aids with digestion and can soothe stomach pain and gas.

Saffron

Saffron is a vibrant, aromatic spice renowned for its flavor and medicinal properties. One of its most notable and exciting healing benefits is its link to treating anxiety and depression. In one study involving the treatment of mild to moderate depression, saffron was found to be similar in efficacy to the drug imipramine.[29] It was also more recently found to positively impact anxiety, with minimal side effects.[30]

Probiotics

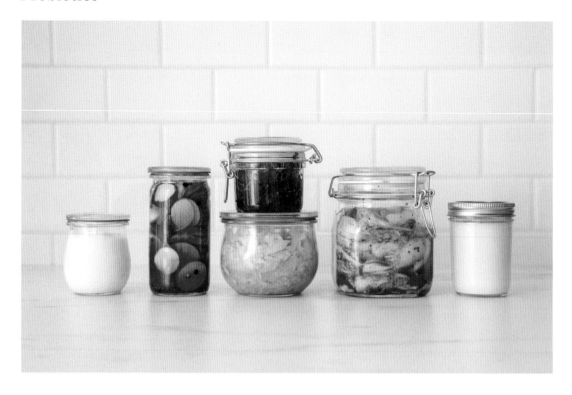

What's all the hype about probiotics? Probiotics are beneficial live bacteria that help improve immune function, reduce inflammation, aid digestion and nutrient absorption, prevent infections, and protect our gut from harmful bacteria. Probiotics can also help reestablish healthy bacteria balance after a course of antibiotics (which destroys both good and bad bacteria). They are also being increasingly studied for their role in improving mood and in reducing anxiety, stress, and depression.

We receive probiotics by eating fermented foods. Because of this, fermented foods are a staple in my household, as they should be for anyone who wants to improve their digestive health and mood. Fermented foods are hailed for their probiotic power, and when consumed regularly, they help keep our gut flora flourishing. You can easily make fermented foods at home. In fact, you'll find flavorful gut-friendly recipes for homemade coconut yogurt, kimchi, pickled radishes, and miso soup in the recipe section that starts on page 260.

Fermented food sources of probiotics include:

- Kefir
- Kimchi
- Miso
- Pickles
- Sauerkraut
- Yogurt

Prebiotics

You may be familiar with probiotics, but what are prebiotics? In *Nutrition Essentials for Mental Health*, author Leslie Korn explains it like this: "Prebiotics set the stage in the colonic 'garden' so probiotics or microbiota can flourish and not allow the harmful bacteria to propagate, much like healthy soil allows seeds to develop into fruit and be resistant to the effects of 'pests.'"[31]

Prebiotics include:

- Asparagus
- Bananas
- Beans
- Chia seeds
- Chicory root
- Dandelion
- Garlic
- Jerusalem artichokes
- Leeks
- Onions (both raw and cooked)

Mood-Boosting Vitamins and Supplements

While whole foods are optimal sources of essential nutrients and vitamins, in many cases it can be of great benefit to bring in reinforcements in the form of supplements to help improve mood, reduce anxiety, and increase energy. I always recommend seeking out a qualified nutritional therapist or doctor to work with when starting a supplementation program. They can prescribe accurate and individualized dosages that are beyond the scope of this book. They can also order blood and saliva tests to help identify specific nutrients you may be lacking, as well as identify any contraindications and potential drug interactions with any current medication you may be taking.

When taking supplements, make sure you check with your nutritional therapist or doctor and always read the label so that you know how and when to take a supplement. This is important because some supplements are best taken with food, while others work best on an empty stomach.

The list below is by no means exhaustive. There are a wide variety of vitamins, minerals, essential fatty acids, amino acids, enzymes, and glandulars that can help support a variety of physical and mental health issues.

Zinc

When I interviewed my friend Dr. Robin Berzin, a physician and the founder and CEO of Parsley Health, about her top five go-to supplements for brain health, zinc was at the head of her list. She shared that there is a strong correlation between zinc deficiency and depressive disorders, impaired memory, and mood disorders. She says, "For those individuals with depression who are not responsive to medication, zinc supplementation can be effective."

B Vitamins

B vitamins are critical for regulating mood and nervous system function. There are eight B vitamins—B_1, B_2, B_3, B_4, B_5, B_6, B_7, B_9, and B_{12}. You can find a B-complex at any local grocery store or pharmacy that includes all eight of these B vitamins. Or you can supplement with individual B vitamins as necessary.

Vegans and vegetarians are encouraged to supplement with B_{12}, as it's found only in animal sources, not plant sources. B_{12} deficiencies can lead to depression, paranoia, memory loss, and nerve damage, which is often accompanied by numbness or tingling. When I was struggling with panic disorder, supplementing with B_{12} was an essential component of getting my anxiety and panic under control. Because I was a vegetarian at that time, my diet had no sources of B_{12}, which left me more susceptible to anxiety and depression. When my vegetarian and vegan students who struggle with anxiety or panic begin supplementing with B_{12}, many of them experience a dramatic relief from symptoms. You can also get regular B_{12} shots from a naturopath or functional medicine practitioner.

Vitamin D

Vitamin D is a fat-soluble vitamin that occurs naturally in only a few food sources. The two main food sources of vitamin D are fatty fish (like salmon) and eggs. We also naturally produce vitamin D when exposed to sunlight, but it can be challenging to get enough vitamin D through diet and sun exposure alone, leaving many deficient.

Vitamin D helps regulate the absorption of calcium and phosphorus, and boosts our immune system. It also plays a role in balancing our mood. In one study, researchers found that vitamin D deficiency was linked to anxiety and depression in fibromyalgia patients.[32] It has also been used to improve symptoms of seasonal affective disorder, like depression and anxiety.

No: Dr. Popper

Quick Tip:
Avoid the Winter Blues

If you live in a part of the world with limited sun exposure, take a vitamin D supplement and consider buying a light box to help relieve depression and SAD (seasonal affective disorder).

Magnesium

Ah, calm. That's what magnesium provides us with. It helps relieve anxiety, fear, nervousness, restlessness, and irritability by going straight for the nervous system. It also protects the heart and arteries, which helps quell anxiety and panic attacks. Studies have shown that even small amounts of magnesium make a big difference, so this is a case of a little going a long way.

If you struggle with anxiety or insomnia, wind down your evening with a soothing Epsom salt bath. Epsom salts are a form of magnesium that is easily absorbed through your skin while you soak in the tub.

You can also make your own sleep concoction by simply mixing water with Natural Calm, a magnesium supplement that, when added to water, transforms into a fruity antistress drink. It's available online and at most health food stores, as well as big retailers like Walmart and Target.

Fish Oil

Fish oils support cognitive function, including learning and memory, help improve depression, and can help relieve symptoms of PTSD. They are also powerful anti-inflammatories.

No Oils: Fish w/Mercury et al

Probiotics

We already discussed the power of probiotics, which can be acquired through diet in the form of fermented foods. However, many people don't get adequate levels through diet alone, in which case a probiotic supplement is recommended. The most popular strain is acidophilus.

However, to get the most benefit, it is generally recommended that you take a probiotic that includes a diverse variety of strains with a large number of bacteria. In her book *Gut and Psychology Syndrome*, Dr. Natasha Campbell-McBride recommends a probiotic with at least 8 billion bacterial cells per gram.

Also note that different strains offer different benefits. For example, some probiotics are more effective in relieving constipation, while others help stop diarrhea. It's always a good idea to work with a qualified clinician to help you choose the right probiotics for you.

Turmeric

We've already spoken at length about this anti-inflammatory wonder spice. You can cook with it (turmeric is traditionally used in curry dishes), juice it, boil it (for turmeric tea), or take it in supplement form. However, it's important to know that in order for turmeric to best be absorbed by our bodies, it should be consumed with fats or oils, as well as black pepper or piperine (a compound of black pepper), which helps increase its bioavailability. When choosing it in supplement form, read the label to find a brand that contains black pepper extract or piperine.

Chapter 15

Feel-Good Recipes for Optimum Gut and Brain Health

Everyone has a doctor in him or her, we just have to help it in its work. The natural healing force within each one of us is the greatest force in getting well. Our food should be our medicine. Our medicine should be our food.
—Hippocrates

When I first started exploring the world of healthier eating, I bought a bunch of "healthy" cookbooks and spent a fortune on fancy hard-to-find, hard-to-pronounce ingredients like *ashwagandha*—which, to be fair, is actually quite an incredible adaptogenic herb (meaning that it helps us adapt to stress). But I digress. My excitement and motivation quickly fizzled as I took my first bite of what was supposed to be a "mouthwatering" gluten-free, dairy-free, plant-based sunflower seed pizza (which took me almost two hours to make!), only to discover that my tantalizing creation tasted like a piece of soggy cardboard. Disappointment set in, and Domino's pizza was at my door fifteen minutes later.

I want to spare you from similar disappointment. In the coming pages, you'll find more than twenty-five easy-to-follow, gut-healing, mood-boosting recipes, carefully crafted in partnership with my dear friend, certified eating psychology coach Elise Museles. The recipes were designed to be time-saving and budget friendly, using everyday ingredients. Best of all, they truly are mouthwatering!

While many of the recipes can be whipped up in thirty minutes or less, there are a few recipes that require a little more patience (such as homemade kimchi). If the thought of fermenting your own food in jars doesn't delight your inner chef, skip it and go for the store-bought version. There is no shame in taking time-saving shortcuts! The intention is to integrate these gut-healing foods into your life in an accessible and sustainable way.

May these recipes tantalize your taste buds, lift your mood, energize you from the inside out, and inspire you to take your health into your own hands.

Shopping Tips

Here are a few shopping tips to help you navigate the grocery store like a seasoned pro.

- Buy organic whenever possible.
- Buy local and seasonal foods whenever possible.
- If consuming animal protein, opt for grass-finished meat, pasture-raised poultry and eggs, and wild fish. No: FUHRMAN
- Swap out dairy for any of the following plant-based milks: ✓

Almond	Oat
Cashew	Pea
Coconut	Rice
Flax	Soy (choose organic only)
Hazelnut	Tigernut
Hemp	

- Limit your time in the inner aisles of the grocery store and do most of your shopping around the perimeter, where most whole foods, fresh fruits, and veggies are found.
- Buy in bulk to save money.
- Buy frozen berries to save money and retain antioxidant value (frozen berries are picked and preserved at their peak of freshness).
- Check out your local ethnic food markets for less expensive herbs, spices, roots, and fermented foods.

Smoothies, Drinks, and Bowls

Note that yields throughout this chapter may vary depending on the size of components used, such as bananas and coconuts.

Healing Turmeric Latte

Go for the gold! This warm and soothing drink is made with turmeric, a close relative of ginger and one of the most potent anti-inflammatory spices. Curcumin, the healing compound in turmeric, gives the spice its vibrant yellow color, not to mention a host of health benefits for both body and brain. Add this latte to your morning routine in place of coffee or as a nourishing way to wind down at the end of a busy day.

Makes one 8-ounce latte

1 cup unsweetened almond or coconut milk
1 tablespoon grated fresh turmeric root (or 1 teaspoon ground)
1 tablespoon grated fresh ginger (or ¾ to 1 teaspoon ground)
1 teaspoon ground cinnamon, plus extra for garnish
2 teaspoons coconut oil
Splash of pure vanilla extract
Pinch of freshly ground black pepper
Raw honey or natural sweetener of choice to taste

1. Gently warm the almond milk in a small saucepan without bringing to a boil. Add the turmeric, ginger, cinnamon, coconut oil, and vanilla and gently heat until the coconut oil is melted and the drink is at your preferred temperature. Pour the warm mixture into a blender and add a pinch of pepper and your sweetener of choice. Blend for 30 seconds to 1 minute, until well combined.

2. Pour the latte into a mug and top it with more cinnamon as desired. Sip and savor this healing drink!

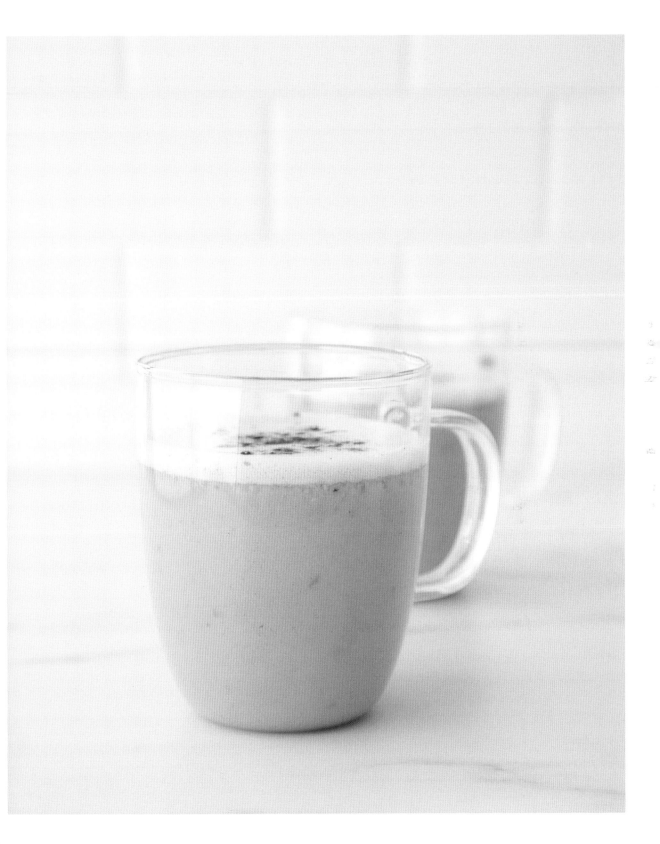

AB&J Smoothie

Create the flavors of this popular childhood sandwich with a healthy twist! This creamy smoothie is loaded with antioxidants, omega-3 fatty acids, and a hefty dose of plant-based protein. Just fill up the blender with these nutrient-dense and blood-sugar-stabilizing ingredients whenever you need a burst of energy that will keep you going all morning (or afternoon) long.

Makes one 16-ounce smoothie

1 cup plant-based milk, such as almond milk, or more as needed

1 serving vanilla plant-based protein powder (I like VeganSmart, available at Whole Foods, your local health food store, CVS, and Amazon)

½ cup steamed and frozen cauliflower florets

½ cup frozen raspberries

½ cup frozen strawberries

2 tablespoons almond butter

2 teaspoons flax meal (ground flaxseeds)

¼ teaspoon ground cinnamon

Pinch of sea salt

1 fresh strawberry (optional), for garnish

Almonds, sliced (optional), for garnish

Put the plant-based milk and protein powder in a high-speed blender and blend until smooth. Add the cauliflower, raspberries, strawberries, almond butter, flax meal, cinnamon, and salt and blend until the smoothie is thick and creamy. Adjust the liquid to your desired consistency. Garnish with strawberries and sliced almonds, if desired.

> *Blending Basics:* Not all blenders are created equal; there are high-speed (or high-performance) blenders and regular blenders. High-speed blenders are designed for maximum efficiency and make blending harder ingredients like nuts, frozen fruits and veggies, and fibrous greens a breeze. Many high-speed blenders can also be used to make nut milks, nut butters, spreads, and even soup! The downside is that most come with a hefty price tag, but if you plan on doing a lot of blending, they are a worthwhile investment. Regular blenders are less powerful, but much more affordable and can generally get the job done with a little more patience and planning. If using a regular blender, add ingredients in order from hardest to softest and blend in stages rather than all at once. You can also soften harder ingredients, such as nuts, by soaking them in water first to make them easier to blend.

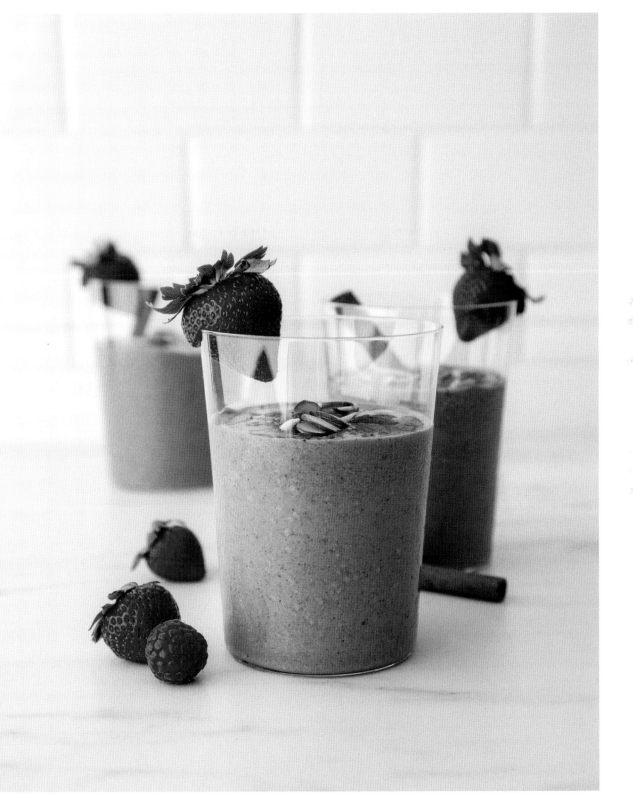

Grounding Pumpkin Chai Spice Smoothie

Pumpkin is a fall favorite, and no wonder: it has an energetic quality that is grounding and stabilizing. Pumpkin is rich in beta-carotene and helps balance blood sugar and support insulin regulation. The anti-inflammatory spices in this recipe, including the blood-sugar-stabilizing cinnamon, blend together to create a healing smoothie that will keep you even and steady with every flavorful sip.

Makes one 16-ounce smoothie

1 cup unsweetened almond or coconut milk,
   or more as needed
½ cup unsweetened pumpkin puree
¾ cup steamed and frozen cauliflower florets
1 frozen sliced banana
1 tablespoon almond butter
½ teaspoon pure vanilla extract

½ teaspoon ground cinnamon,
   plus a pinch for garnish
Pinch of ground cloves
Pinch of ground cardamom
½-inch piece of fresh ginger
Pinch of sea salt

1. Combine the almond milk, pumpkin, cauliflower, banana, almond butter, vanilla, cinnamon, cloves, cardamom, ginger, and salt in a high-speed blender and blend until smooth and creamy. Adjust the liquid to your desired consistency.

2. Top with a sprinkle of cinnamon and serve immediately.

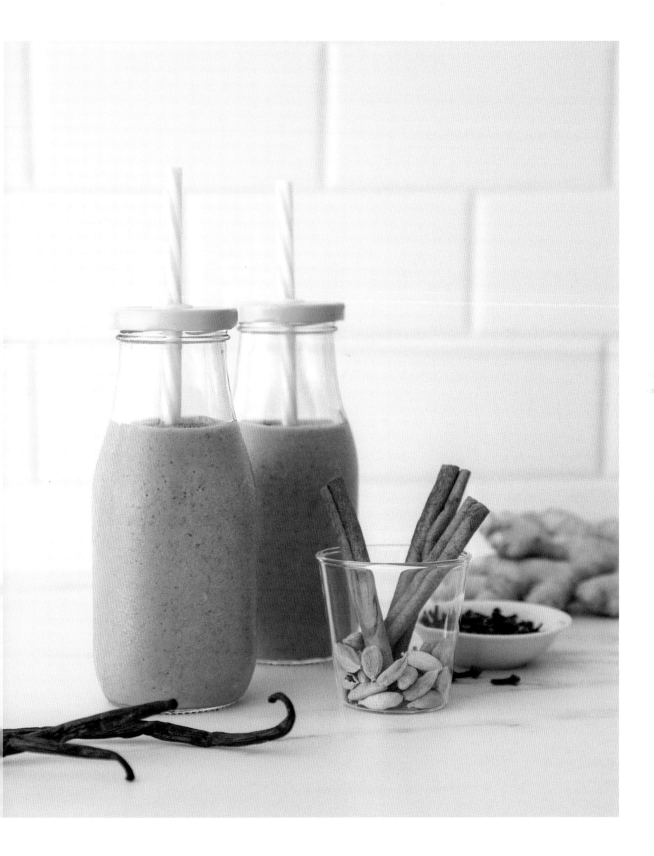

Tropical Green Smoothie

Savor the taste of the tropics with a refreshing green blend that is cleansing, healing, detoxifying, and hydrating. With pineapple for easy digestion and cilantro to support detoxification, this smoothie is just as delicious as it is nutritious.

Makes one 16-ounce smoothie

1 cup unsweetened coconut milk
1 cup spinach
1¼ cups frozen pineapple chunks
½ avocado
Juice from half an orange

2 tablespoons chopped fresh cilantro
1 tablespoon hemp seeds, plus more for garnish if desired
Pinch of sea salt

1. Combine the coconut milk and spinach in a high-speed blender and blend until smooth. Add the pineapple, avocado, orange juice, cilantro, hemp seeds, and salt and blend again until combined, adjusting the liquid to your desired consistency.

2. For an extra kick of omega-fatty acids, sprinkle hemp seeds on top to garnish. If desired, place fresh pineapple chunks on a skewer and insert into the smoothie for a tropical twist.

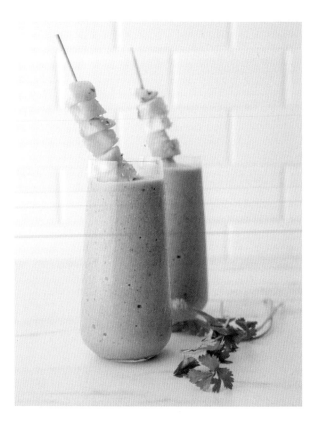

Uplifting Chocolate Oatmeal Smoothie

This smoothie may taste like sinful cookie dough, but it is packed with calming magnesium and good-for-you carbohydrates. Toss some raw cacao into the mix for a phytonutrient-filled creation that also happens to be mood-boosting and energizing, too!

Makes one 14-ounce smoothie

1 cup plant-based milk, or more as needed
¼ cup old-fashioned rolled oats (gluten-free if necessary)
1 tablespoon cashew butter (or the nut butter of your choice)
1 frozen sliced banana
½ cup steamed and frozen diced zucchini
1 to 1½ tablespoons cacao powder or cocoa powder
½ teaspoon ground cinnamon
1 Medjool date, pitted
Pinch of sea salt
1 tablespoon cacao nibs (optional)

1. Put the plant-based milk and oats in a high-speed blender and blend until smooth. Add the cashew butter, banana, zucchini, cacao powder, cinnamon, date, and salt and blend until well combined. Adjust the liquid to your desired consistency.

2. Mix in the cacao nibs, if using, and pulse 3 or 4 times until they are incorporated.

Berry Matcha Smoothie Bowl

Thicker than the traditional smoothie, this berry and green combination is served in a bowl and topped off with the nutritional boost of your choice. While all the ingredients in this bowl are loaded with antioxidants, the spinach and blueberries contain calming nutrients and the matcha provides a burst of steady energy from L-theanine. However, even if you are in a pinch and don't have matcha on hand, this smoothie bowl is still delicious and nourishing.

Makes one 12-ounce bowl

½ to 1 cup almond milk, or more as needed
1 cup spinach
¼ avocado
1 teaspoon matcha (green tea) powder
1 Medjool date, pitted
1 cup frozen blueberries
1 serving vanilla plant-based protein
   powder (I like VeganSmart, available at
   Whole Foods, your local health food store,
   CVS, and Amazon)

Pinch of sea salt
Toppings of your choice (I like fresh berries,
   sliced bananas, nuts, seeds, shredded
   coconut, bee pollen, and granola)

1. Combine the almond milk, starting with less and adding more as necessary (this bowl should be thick!), and spinach in a high-speed blender and blend until smooth. Add the avocado, matcha powder, date, blueberries, protein powder, and salt and blend until smooth and creamy. If necessary, adjust the liquid to your desired consistency, but make sure it is thick enough that the toppings don't sink.

2. Pour the mixture into a bowl and top with the nutritional boosts of your choice.

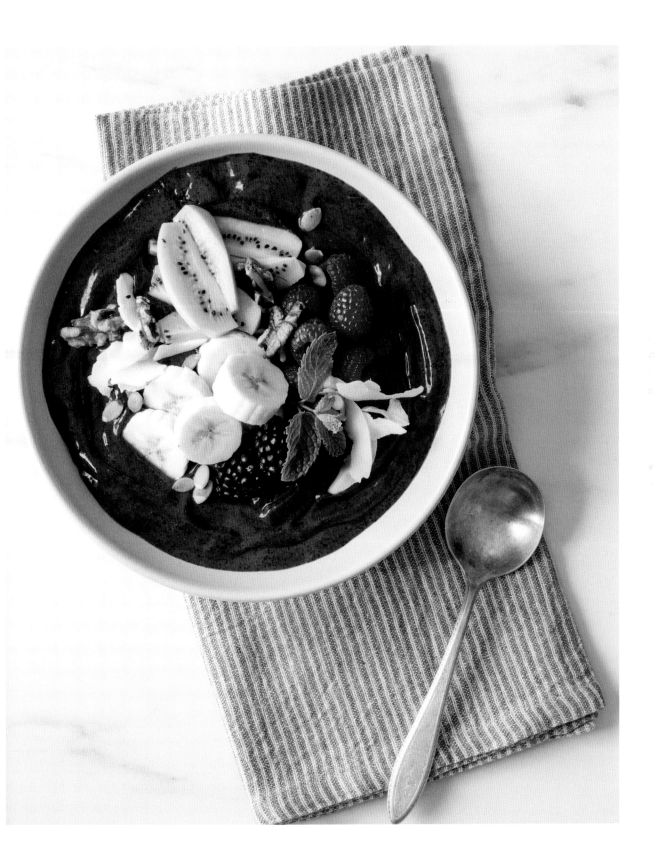

Breakfast

Happy Belly Yogurt

There's nothing more satisfying than replacing a store-bought item with a homemade version. This DIY coconut yogurt is easy to make and filled with beneficial bacteria to keep your gut healthy and your mind happy! Coconut meat is also a healthy source of plant-based fat for brain fuel and is high in manganese, a trace mineral that helps metabolize fat and protein, stabilize blood sugar levels, and support our nervous system. Add this probiotic-rich yogurt into smoothies, overnight oats, or chia seed pudding, or just eat it on its own!

Makes 2 to 3 servings

2 young Thai coconuts (available at natural food stores or Asian supermarkets)
2 teaspoons freshly squeezed lemon juice
½ teaspoon probiotic powder (approximately
   2 capsules, opened)

Optional flavorings to blend into the yogurt after it has fermented

Berries	Mango
Peaches	Pure vanilla extract
Papaya	Lemon zest

1. Open the coconuts and scrape out the meat. Reserve the coconut water in a separate bowl.

2. In a blender, combine the coconut meat, ⅓ cup of the coconut water, and the lemon juice and blend until smooth. Adjust the liquid as necessary. Spoon the mixture into a nonmetal bowl (this is important, as the live cultures in the probiotic react when in direct contact with metal). Use a wooden spoon to mix in the probiotic powder until well incorporated.

3. Pour the mixture into one or two glass jars and cover them tightly with a lid. Place the jars on the counter and let them ferment for 24 hours.

4. Mix the yogurt well in the jars. If you prefer a creamier texture, pour the mixture into a blender and blend on medium speed until the desired consistency is reached. If you have blended the yogurt, return it to the jars and store them in the refrigerator with the lids tightly shut for up to 5 days.

5. To serve, stir in or top with the fruit and flavorings of your choice or enjoy your yogurt plain and simple!

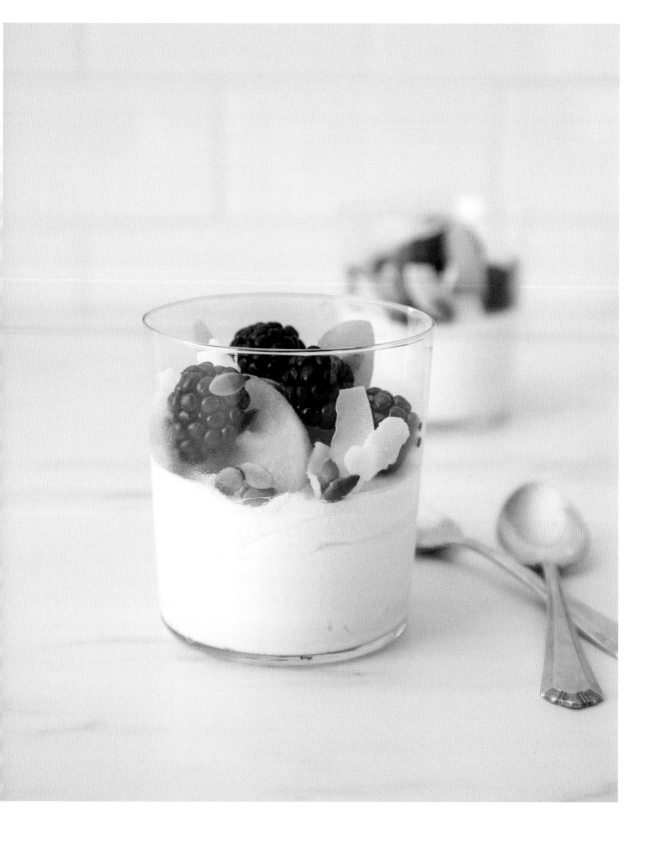

Savory Kimchi Oatmeal Bowl

Who says oatmeal needs to be sweet? Prepare the oats as you traditionally would, but instead of adding berries and sweeteners, toss in some nutrient-dense greens and gut-healing probiotic-rich kimchi, top with a brain-boosting egg, and finish with omega-rich seeds. And a bonus: some people find that starting the day off on a saltier note can be more grounding and stabilizing.

Makes 1 bowl

1 cup water (or ½ cup water and ½ cup
   vegetable broth for more flavor)
Sea salt
½ cup rolled oats (gluten-free if necessary)
3 teaspoons olive oil
2 cups spinach
Pinch of crushed red pepper flakes
Freshly ground black pepper to taste

1 egg
½ cup kimchi, store-bought or homemade
   (page 274; note that the kimchi should
   ferment for 3 to 4 days before use)
Sliced avocado
1 tablespoon hemp seeds
Hot sauce (optional)

1. Bring the water and a pinch of salt to a boil in a small or medium saucepan over high heat, then add the oats. Turn the heat down to a simmer and let the oats simmer uncovered for 3 to 5 minutes. When the oats have cooked to your taste, remove from the heat and set them aside in the pot.

2. In a medium saucepan, heat 2 teaspoons of the oil. Add the spinach and a pinch each of red pepper flakes, sea salt, and pepper and sauté for 2 to 3 minutes, until the spinach is slightly wilted. Place the oats in a bowl and top with the spinach.

3. In the same saucepan, heat the remaining 1 teaspoon oil and add the egg. Cook for 2 to 3 minutes over medium-high heat, until the egg is golden around the edges and cooked to your liking. Place the egg in the bowl with the oats and spinach. Sprinkle with salt and pepper to taste.

4. Add the kimchi to the bowl and top the bowl with a few slices of avocado and the hemp seeds. Season with sea salt and pepper to taste and add a hot sauce drizzle if you like.

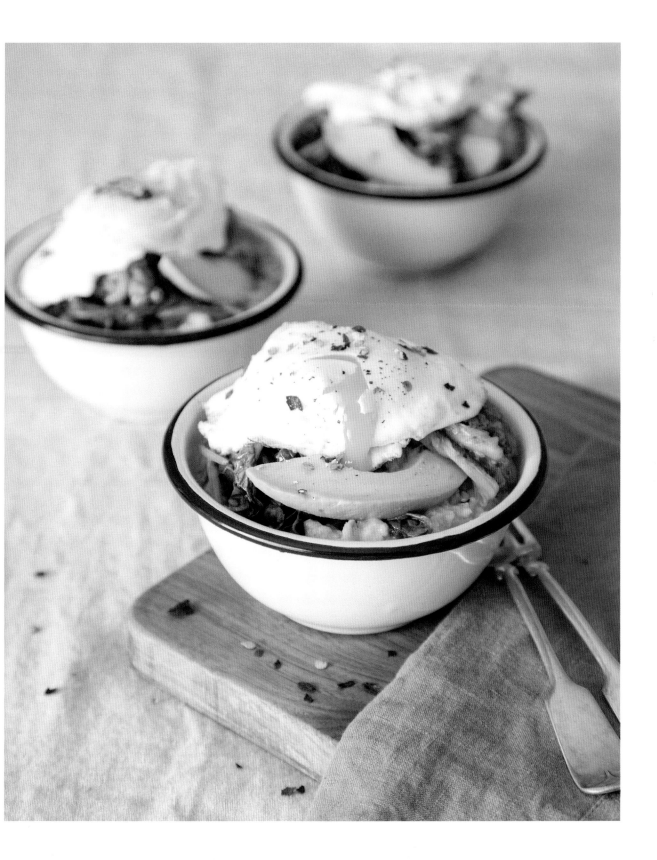

Kimchi

Fermented foods contain gut-healing probiotics that can help balance the body's pH, regulate immunity, and control inflammation. Try making your own version. It's easy!

Makes approximately 6 cups

1 head Napa cabbage or green cabbage, cut into 1-inch strips
6 cups warm water (filtered if possible)
¼ cup sea salt (for soaking)
3 green onions, thinly sliced (green parts only)
6 red radishes, grated
1 apple, cored and pureed in a blender or food processor

2 carrots, peeled and thinly sliced
2 large garlic cloves, minced
1 teaspoon grated fresh ginger
2 tablespoons Korean chile pepper flakes or paste (gochugaru, available in Asian supermarkets and online)

1. Put the cabbage in a large bowl.

2. In a separate bowl, combine 2 cups of the warm water with the salt and stir until the salt dissolves. Add the remaining 4 cups warm water to the mixture and stir until mixed well. Pour the liquid over the cabbage and make sure the cabbage is submerged. Cover the bowl with a plate or lid to speed the fermenting process. Let the cabbage soak for 5 hours, or until the cabbage has wilted. Reserve ¼ cup of the liquid, then drain and rinse the cabbage.

3. In the large mixing bowl, combine all the remaining ingredients with the cabbage and mix until well incorporated. Add the reserved soaking liquid to the mixture.

4. Divide the mixture among clean glass jars (such as canning jars) and press down to make sure that the brine covers the vegetables. Place the jars in a warm, sunny spot on the counter. Let the mixture sit for 3 to 4 days, checking daily to see if it is ready and sampling to make sure it is properly fermented.

5. Store the kimchi in a tightly sealed jar in the refrigerator for up to 2 months.

Apple Pie Overnight Oats

Spend just a few minutes before bed putting all the ingredients for this delicious oat breakfast together in a jar, then sleep in and wake up to a nutrient-dense and energizing breakfast that magically prepared itself while you were sleeping! Oats increase healthy gut bacteria, improve blood sugar control, and are a good source of magnesium—a calming mineral that can help ease anxiety. You also get the benefit of fiber-rich apples and blood-sugar-stabilizing cinnamon.

Makes 1 cup

½ cup rolled oats

1 tablespoon flaxseeds

½ cup plant-based milk, or more as needed

1 tablespoon almond butter
  (or other nut butter)

½ apple, cored and grated, plus apple slices
  for garnish

½ teaspoon ground cinnamon, plus a pinch
  for garnish

Splash of pure vanilla extract

Pinch of sea salt

Maple syrup, raw honey, or other natural
  sweetener (optional)

Sliced almonds, for garnish

1. Put the oats, flaxseeds, plant-based milk, almond butter, apple, cinnamon, vanilla, and salt in a glass container and stir until well combined. Cover and refrigerate the oats overnight or for at least 4 hours.

2. When you're ready to serve, remove the oats from the refrigerator and stir. Add extra plant-based milk as desired for a thinner consistency.

3. Eat the oats straight out of the jar or heat them up in a saucepan until warmed through if you prefer your oats hot. Sweeten if you like. Top with additional cinnamon, apple slices, and almonds.

Blueberry Cobbler Overnight Oats

This recipe offers all of the same ease and nutritional benefits as the Apple Pie Overnight Oats (page 275), but with antioxidant-rich blueberries. Blueberries are packed with calming nutrients and vitamins, which are beneficial for easing anxiety, as well as boosting brain health.

Makes 1 cup

½ cup rolled oats (gluten-free if necessary)
½ banana, mashed
1 tablespoon flaxseeds
½ cup plant-based milk, or more as needed
1 tablespoon almond butter
   (or other nut butter)
½ cup blueberries, plus more for garnish

½ teaspoon ground cinnamon,
   plus a sprinkle to garnish
Splash of pure vanilla extract
Pinch of sea salt
Maple syrup, raw honey, or other natural
   sweetener (optional)
Sliced almonds

1. Put the oats, banana, flaxseeds, plant-based milk, almond butter, blueberries, cinnamon, vanilla, and salt in a glass container and stir until well combined. Cover and refrigerate overnight or for at least 4 hours.

2. When you're ready to serve, remove from the refrigerator and stir. Add extra plant-based milk as desired for a thinner consistency.

3. Eat the oats straight out of the jar or heat them in a saucepan until warmed through, as desired. Sweeten if you like. Top with additional cinnamon, fresh blueberries, and almonds.

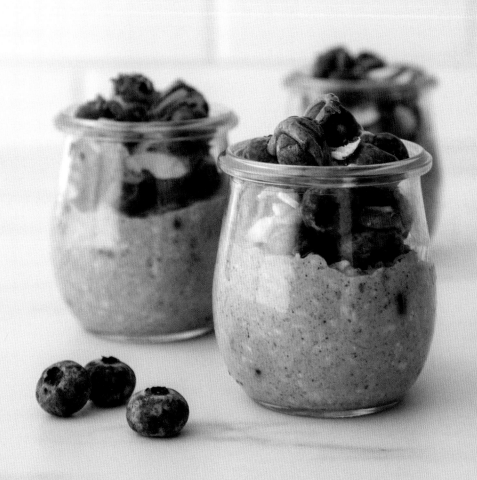

Brain Power Mini-Frittatas

Add a serving of protein (and veggies!) to your morning meal with the ease and convenience of frittata cups. This version offers all the same protein, vitamins, and minerals as a traditional frittata—including the brain-boosting choline found in eggs—but is made using muffin tins for easy, on-the-go individual servings. You'll also get an extra boost from turmeric, one of the most potent anti-inflammatory spices. Turmeric not only supports your brain but can also be used for alleviating depression.

Makes 12 frittata muffins

1 tablespoon olive oil, plus extra to grease
   the muffin tins
½ cup thinly sliced spinach
¼ cup finely diced onion
½ cup grated zucchini
12 large eggs

Splash of unsweetened almond or
   coconut milk
Sea salt and freshly ground black pepper
   to taste
1 teaspoon ground turmeric

1. Preheat the oven to 350°F. Grease a muffin tin with oil.

2. Heat the 1 tablespoon oil in a medium saucepan. Add the spinach, onion, and zucchini and sauté for 2 to 3 minutes, until the vegetables are slightly tender. Remove from the heat and set the veggies aside to cool.

3. In a large bowl, whisk the eggs and add the almond milk. Season with salt, pepper, and turmeric.

4. Add the vegetables to the egg mixture and mix until incorporated. Divide the mixture among the muffin tin wells, filling each almost to the top.

5. Bake for 22 to 25 minutes, until the frittatas are golden around the edges. Eat immediately or store them in the refrigerator for 3 days or in the freezer for up to 2 months.

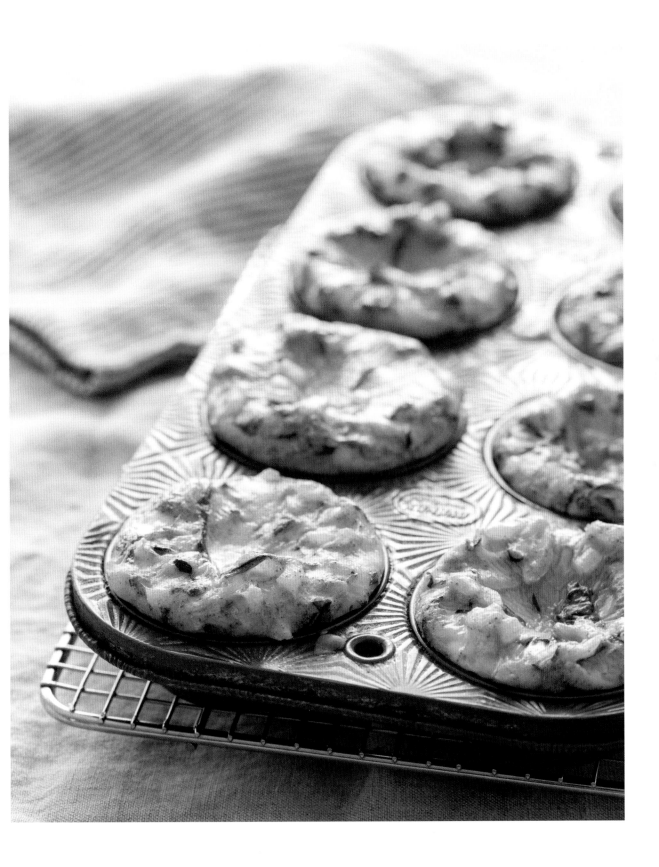

Chocolate Almond Flour Pancakes
with Cacao Nibs

Healthy never tasted so good! Toss some raw cacao into these grain-free gems for a scrumptious breakfast loaded with phytonutrients and mood-boosting properties. Almond flour is a rich source of healthy fats and can help keep your blood sugar steady and your body satisfied all morning long.

Makes 12 pancakes

3 large eggs NO. CHIA SEEDS

2 tablespoons maple syrup, plus more for
  serving

1 tablespoon almond milk

½ teaspoon pure vanilla extract

1½ cups almond flour (preferably blanched
  flour, for best texture)

¼ to ½ teaspoon sea salt

¼ teaspoon baking soda

1 tablespoon cacao powder or cocoa powder

½ teaspoon ground cinnamon

1 tablespoon coconut oil, plus more
  as needed

Fresh berries and/or sliced banana

1. Whisk the eggs in a large bowl. Add the maple syrup, almond milk, and vanilla and mix until smooth.

2. In a medium bowl, mix the almond flour, salt, baking soda, cacao powder, and cinnamon. Add the dry mixture to the wet mixture and stir to combine thoroughly but do not overmix.

3. Melt the coconut oil in a large skillet over medium-low heat. Drop approximately 2 tablespoons of batter onto the skillet for each pancake, leaving enough space in between pancakes to flip them. Cook the pancakes on one side until small bubbles form, then flip them to the other side. Repeat with the remaining batter and add fresh oil when necessary.

4. Serve with a drizzle of maple syrup and berries and/or bananas.

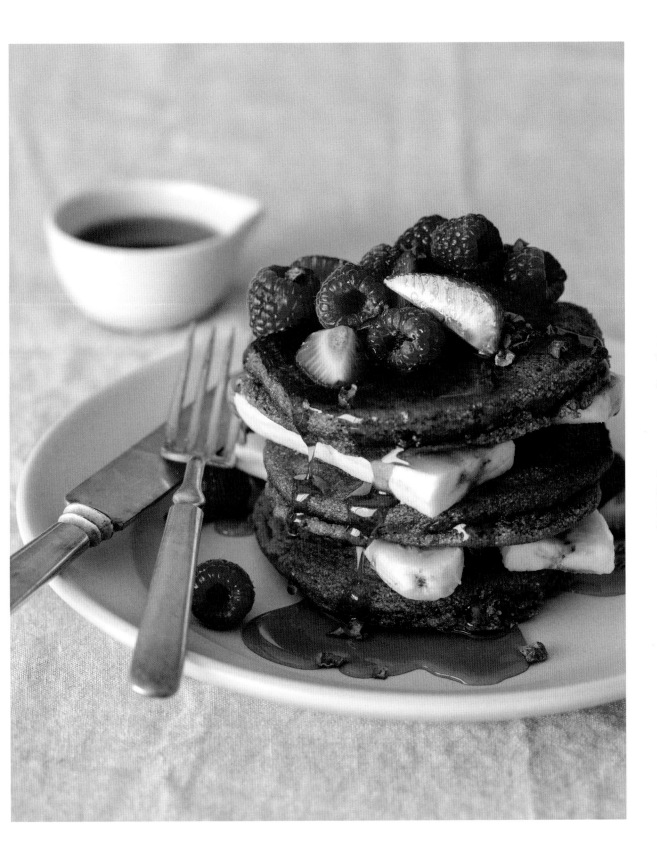

Beet, Orange, and Walnut Salad in Butter Lettuce Cups with a Lemony Shallot Vinaigrette

A simple but elegant salad that is a nutritional powerhouse with minimal ingredients. Walnuts are rich in omega fatty acids and support brain health, while beets are energizing and loaded with iron and B vitamins. You'll also get an extra dose of immune-boosting vitamin C from the orange and the lemon juice in the vinaigrette!

Makes 2 meal-size salads or 4 appetizer salads

Salad

2 medium to large beets

Drizzle of extra-virgin olive oil

2 fennel bulbs, trimmed, quartered, and thinly sliced

1 large navel orange, peeled and sliced into rounds

¼ cup walnuts

3 tablespoons fresh mint leaves

1 large head of butter lettuce

Lemony Shallot Vinaigrette

¼ cup freshly squeezed lemon juice

2 teaspoons Dijon mustard

2 teaspoons pure maple syrup

1 tablespoon chopped fresh parsley

2 teaspoons minced shallot

¼ to ½ teaspoon sea salt

¼ teaspoon freshly ground black pepper

¼ cup olive oil

1. Make the salad: To roast the beets, preheat the oven to 400°F. Line a baking sheet with parchment paper.

2. Cut off the top of the beets and scrub their roots clean. Place the beets on the baking sheet and drizzle them with a touch of oil. Roast until the beets are tender and can be easily pierced with a knife or fork, 45 to 55 minutes. Let the beets cool to room temperature, then peel and cut the beets into 1½-inch cubes.

3. In a medium bowl, combine the beets, fennel, orange, walnuts, and mint.

4. Make the vinaigrette: In a separate bowl, whisk the lemon juice, mustard, maple syrup, parsley, shallot, salt, and pepper. Slowly drizzle in the oil and whisk again until emulsified.

5. Arrange the lettuce leaves on individual plates. Drizzle the dressing over the vegetable mixture, toss to combine, and place the mixture on top of the lettuce. Season with salt and pepper as desired. Serve immediately.

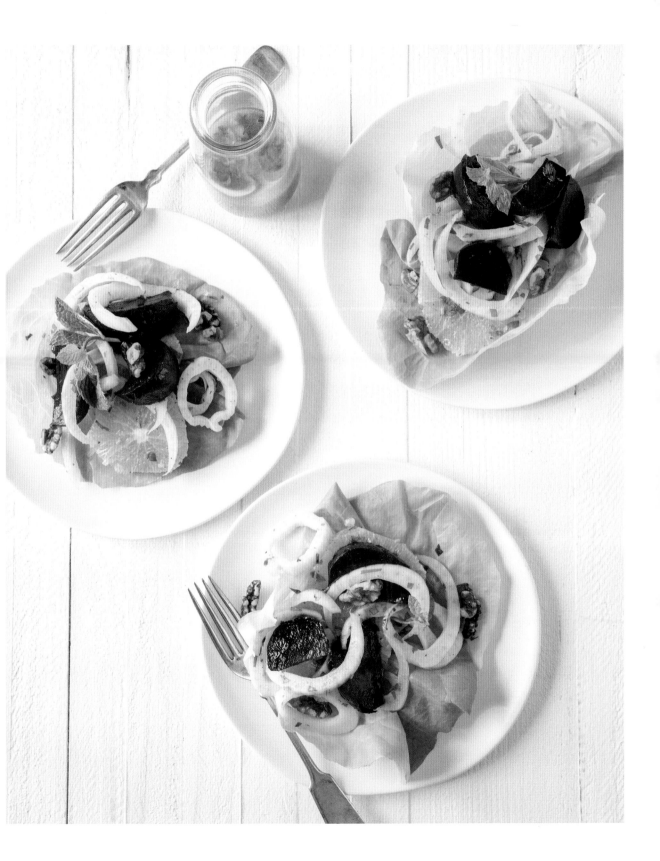

Rainbow Salad with Grilled Chicken and Apple Cider Vinaigrette

One of the simplest ways to take the stress out of healthy eating is to count colors, not calories or carbs! Focus on filling your plate with all the hues of the rainbow to fill your body with an array of nutrients. Each color contains its own set of healing properties and health benefits, and this salad has them all! Add the grilled chicken to balance the meal with protein or choose a plant-based protein for a vegetarian option. Top off this vibrant dish with a vinaigrette made with apple cider vinegar, which supports healthy digestion and cleanses your system. Eating clean never looked (or felt!) so good.

Makes 4 meal-size salads

Chicken (see Note)

2 tablespoons olive oil ~~No~~

2 tablespoons freshly squeezed lemon juice

½ teaspoon paprika

1 garlic clove, minced

¾ teaspoon sea salt

Freshly ground black pepper

1 pound boneless skinless chicken breasts ~~No~~

Apple cider vinaigrette

1 garlic clove, minced

¼ cup apple cider vinegar

3 teaspoons raw honey
  (or pure maple syrup)

2 teaspoons Dijon mustard

¼ to ½ teaspoon sea salt

Freshly ground black pepper to taste

¼ cup extra-virgin olive oil

Pinch of crushed red pepper flakes
  (optional)

Salad

6 cups leafy greens (such as kale, romaine, arugula, spinach, or mixed greens)

1 cup strawberries, tops removed

2 carrots, peeled and cut into ¼-inch rounds

1 cup 1-inch-cubed pineapple

2 cups thinly sliced purple cabbage

1 cucumber, cut into ¼-inch rounds

1 large avocado, pitted, peeled, and cut into 1-inch dice

¼ cup thinly sliced radishes

½ cup microgreens

¼ cup sunflower seeds

Optional nutritional boosts

Hemp seeds, flaxseeds, pumpkin seeds, pine nuts, sliced almonds, pecans, dried cranberries, goji berries, pomegranate seeds

1. Make the chicken: In a medium bowl, combine the oil, lemon juice, paprika, garlic, salt, and pepper. Set the chicken in the marinade, coat both sides, and let the chicken marinate at room temperature for 15 to 20 minutes.

2. Preheat a grill to high heat (or set a grill pan over high heat). Grill the chicken until it is cooked through with an internal temperature of 165°F, 7 to 8 minutes per side. Set the chicken aside to cool, then slice it into strips. (The chicken can be prepared the day before and refrigerated.)

3. Make the apple cider vinaigrette: In a medium bowl, combine the garlic, vinegar, honey, mustard, salt, and pepper. Slowly drizzle in the oil and whisk until the dressing is emulsified. Season with salt and black pepper or crushed red pepper flakes to taste.

4. Make the salad: Toss the greens, strawberries, carrots, pineapple, cabbage, cucumber, avocado, radishes, and microgreens in a large salad bowl. Place the sliced chicken on top of the salad. Toss the salad with enough dressing to coat. Store the remaining vinaigrette in a tightly sealed container in the refrigerator for up to 5 days.

5. Sprinkle the salad with sunflower seeds and add the nutritional boosts of your choice. Enjoy eating every hue of the rainbow!

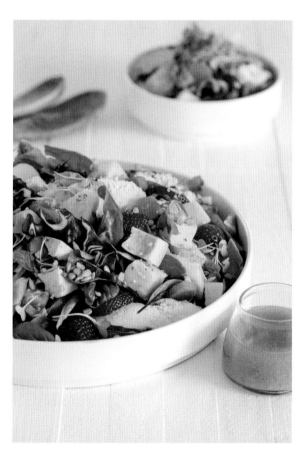

Note: Use any chicken or the protein of your choice. The leftovers can be tossed into other salads or meals throughout the week for a quick and nourishing source of added protein.

Kale and Quinoa Salad with Carrot-Ginger Dressing

Whip up this Asian-inspired salad in a matter of minutes. Kale is often called the king of greens because it's such a nutritional powerhouse. Plant-based quinoa contains all of the essential amino acids and is a protein, not a grain or carb. The sprinkle of hemp seeds and drizzle of carrot ginger dressing are the icing on this nutritional cake. Just wait until you see how this mood-boosting salad floods your body with both nutrients and flavor!

Makes 4 meal-size salads

Dressing

3 medium carrots, peeled and
  roughly chopped
1-inch piece of fresh ginger, peeled
¼ small white onion, roughly chopped
3 tablespoons rice vinegar
1 tablespoon maple syrup
1 tablespoon unrefined toasted
  sesame oil
1 tablespoon tamari or coconut aminos
3 tablespoons olive oil
¼ teaspoon sea salt, or to taste
Crushed red pepper flakes (optional)

Salad

1 cup cooked quinoa
1 bunch lacinato kale or curly kale,
  thinly sliced and massaged with olive oil
4 cups sliced Napa cabbage or Savoy
  cabbage
2 carrots, peeled and grated
1 cucumber, peeled and cut into ¼-inch
  rounds
2 green onions, thinly sliced
1 large pear, cored and cut into ¼-inch slices
2 tablespoons hemp seeds

1. Make the dressing: Put the carrots in a food processor or high-speed blender and pulse until they are almost smooth. Add the ginger, onion, vinegar, maple syrup, sesame oil, and tamari and pulse again. Pour in the olive oil and 1 tablespoon water and process until the dressing has a smooth and creamy texture. Add more olive oil to reach the desired consistency. (Any remaining dressing will keep in a tightly sealed container in the refrigerator for up to 5 days.)

2. Make the salad: Combine the quinoa, kale, cabbage, carrots, cucumber, green onions, and pear in a large bowl. Drizzle the dressing over the salad and toss to lightly coat. Sprinkle the hemp seeds over the top and serve.

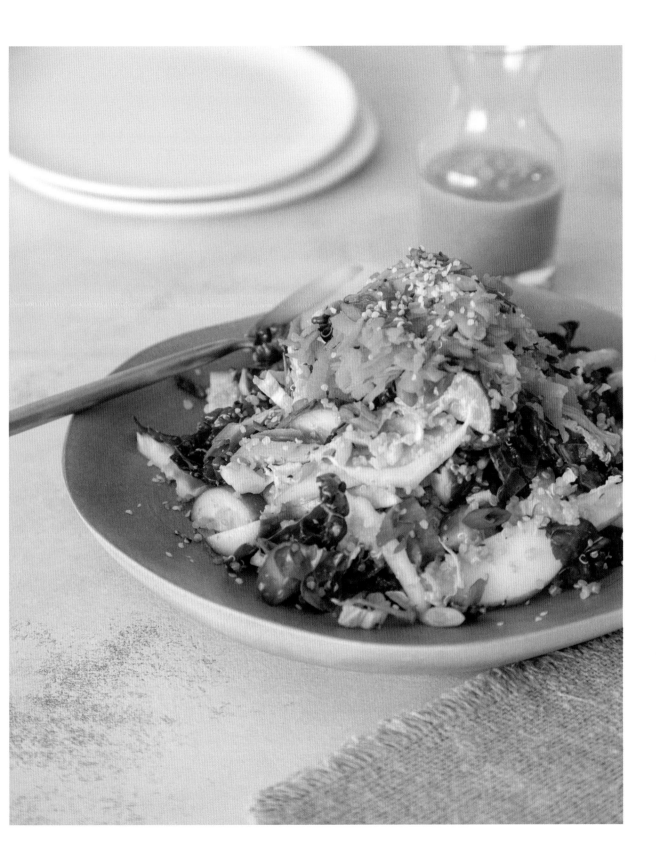

Red Lentil Soup

Nothing nourishes your body and soul like a warm bowl of soup. Filled with cumin, garlic, turmeric, veggies, plant-based protein, lemon, and greens, this dish brings comfort food to a whole new healing level. Lentils are a rich source of choline and vitamins B₁ and B₅, all of which support mental well-being. The garlic and onion are high-prebiotic foods that add a gut-healing element to this fiber-filled, plant-powered meal. As if all of that isn't enough, the addition of spinach and lemon take it up a notch in nutrition and flavor.

Makes 6 to 8 servings

2 tablespoons olive oil

1 yellow onion, finely chopped

2 garlic cloves, minced

1 teaspoon ground cumin

1 teaspoon ground turmeric

1 teaspoon dried oregano

2 large carrots, peeled and cut into
  ¼-inch rounds

2 large celery stalks, finely chopped

1½ cups chopped tomatoes, including juices
  (if good fresh tomatoes aren't in season,
  use one 15-ounce BPA-free can
  or carton of diced tomatoes)

4 cups low-sodium organic vegetable broth,
  or more as needed

1 cup uncooked red lentils, rinsed

½ to 1 teaspoon sea salt, or more to taste

Freshly ground black pepper to taste

2 tablespoons chopped fresh parsley

3 cups spinach

1½ tablespoons freshly squeezed lemon juice
  (or juice of ½ large lemon)

1. In a large stockpot, heat the oil over medium-high heat. Add the onion and sauté until almost translucent, 5 to 6 minutes. Add the garlic, cumin, turmeric, oregano, carrots, and celery and cook, stirring continuously, for 7 to 8 minutes, until the vegetables begin to soften. Add the tomatoes and cook for 1 minute, then mix until well combined.

2. Add the broth, lentils, ½ to 1 teaspoon salt, and a generous amount of pepper. Bring the mixture to a boil, then turn the heat to medium-low. Cover the pot and let the soup simmer until the lentils are softened, 35 to 40 minutes. Add water or extra broth for a thinner consistency or if the liquid evaporates too quickly. Stir in the parsley, spinach, and lemon juice and season the soup with salt and pepper to taste.

3. Ladle the soup into bowls and serve warm. Store any remaining soup in a tightly sealed container in the refrigerator for up to 5 days, or up to 3 months in the freezer. Enjoy!

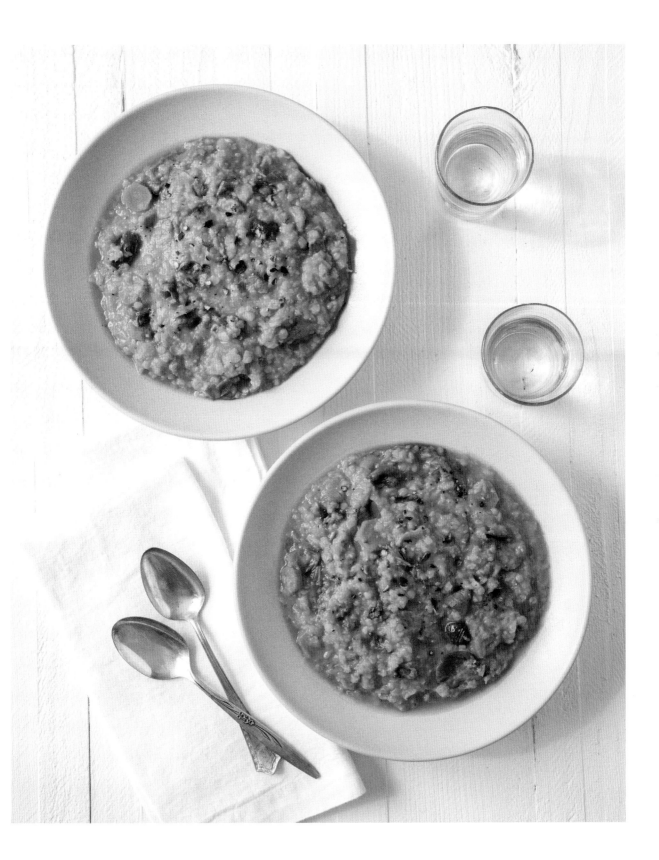

Go with Your Gut Miso Soup

Miso soup is a gut-healing superstar! It also happens to be easy to make and a light addition to any meal. Shiitake mushrooms are known for their anti-inflammatory properties and ability to improve immune function. Seaweed has an especially high mineral content, including magnesium, iron, iodine, calcium, phosphorus, and sodium, which helps to support nervous system function, mental well-being, and muscle relaxation. Top this light dish with greens for an additional nutritional boost!

Makes 2 to 4 servings

4 cups water or vegetable stock
½ cup thinly sliced green onions, plus more for garnish
½ cup shiitake mushrooms, quartered (or any mushrooms)
1 cup chopped spinach (or any leafy greens)
1 sheet nori seaweed, sliced into thin strips
¼ cup miso paste
Sea salt and freshly ground black pepper to taste

1. Bring the water to a low boil in a medium saucepan over medium heat. Lower the heat to a simmer, add the green onions and mushrooms, and cook for 2 minutes, until heated through. Add the spinach and seaweed and cook for 1 minute, or until wilted, taking care not to let the soup boil again.

2. Remove from the heat and ladle about ½ cup into a bowl. Add the miso paste to the bowl and stir until dissolved. Return the mixture to the soup and stir to combine. Season with additional salt and pepper.

3. Ladle the soup into bowls and garnish with more green onion. This soup is best served immediately but will last in the refrigerator for up to 3 days.

Bone Broth *No!*

Health experts are raving about bone broth, and for good reason! It is recommended by leading doctors as a superfood that can help alleviate anxiety and depression as part of a gut-healing protocol. Bone broth can be easily integrated into your lifestyle and enjoyed on its own as a warming beverage or used to add nutrients to soups, rice, quinoa, or vegetable dishes. It is a simple, but lengthy process. Plan on starting in the morning and letting it simmer on the stove all day. Make sure the bones are from grass-fed or organic chickens. Also, be sure not to skip the apple cider vinegar step, as it helps break down the minerals and enhance the nutritional profile of the bone broth.

Makes 4 to 6 quarts broth

2 to 3 pounds chicken bones
   (from a butcher or a roasted chicken)
2 tablespoons apple cider vinegar
Enough filtered water to cover the chicken
   bones, plus 4 quarts filtered water
1 onion, quartered
1 leek, trimmed, rinsed, and roughly
   chopped
2 carrots, roughly chopped

3 celery stalks
1-inch piece of fresh ginger, peeled
1-inch piece of fresh turmeric root, peeled
2 garlic cloves
¼ cup fresh parsley (and/or other herbs
   of your choice, such as rosemary and
   oregano)
1 teaspoon sea salt, or more to taste
Freshly ground black pepper to taste

1. Rinse all the bones thoroughly. Put the bones and vinegar in a large stockpot and add enough filtered water to cover the bones. Let sit for 1 hour to allow the vinegar to leach minerals from the bones.

2. After 1 hour, add the onion, leek, carrots, celery, ginger, turmeric, and 4 quarts filtered water and bring to a hard boil over high heat. Skim any scum that rises to the top of the pot. Turn the heat to low, cover, and simmer for at least 12 hours and up to 18, checking periodically to remove the impurities on top of the broth.

3. About 30 minutes before the end of cooking, add the garlic, parsley, and any other fresh herbs you would like to include.

4. Remove from the heat and let the broth cool. Remove the bones and strain the broth. Refrigerate the cooled broth for at least 2 hours (and up to overnight), until the fat congeals on top. Remove the fat with a skimmer and discard it. Season with salt and pepper.

5. Store the broth in a tightly sealed container in the refrigerator for up to 5 days or in the freezer for up to 4 months.

Happiness Kebabs

Salmon is among the richest dietary sources of vitamin B_{12}, which has been studied for its effects on relieving depression and impacting mood. It's also high in choline, a vitamin that improves brain metabolism and memory. Aside from all of these healing benefits, the kebabs are delicious, colorful, and crowd pleasers, too!

Makes 8 kebabs

Salmon and marinade

2 tablespoons olive oil No

1 garlic clove, finely minced

2 tablespoons tamari

2 tablespoons rice vinegar

¼ teaspoon dry mustard

Crushed red pepper flakes

1 tablespoon honey

1 tablespoon sesame oil

1 pound salmon fillet, cut into 1-inch cubes No

3 tablespoons sesame seeds, plus more
  for garnish

Kebabs

1 zucchini, cut into ½-inch-thick rounds

1 yellow squash, cut into ½-inch-thick
  rounds

Extra-virgin olive oil No

Sea salt and freshly ground black pepper
  to taste

1 green onion, sliced

Special equipment: 8 bamboo skewers

1. Marinate the salmon: In a medium bowl, combine the olive oil, garlic, tamari, vinegar, mustard, red pepper flakes, honey, and sesame oil and stir well. Add the salmon and stir to coat it with the marinade. Marinate the salmon in the refrigerator for 1 hour, then add the sesame seeds and stir to coat the cubes.

2. Meanwhile, soak the skewers in water for 45 minutes. Preheat the grill to medium-high heat.

3. Make the kebabs: Place the marinated salmon, zucchini, and squash on the skewers, alternating the ingredients. Drizzle the skewers with oil and sprinkle with salt and pepper as desired. Use tongs to place the skewers on the grill and cook for 3 to 4 minutes per side, until the salmon and vegetables are cooked through but not overdone. Place the kebabs on a plate or platter to rest a few minutes before serving.

4. Sprinkle the kebabs with sesame seeds and green onion to serve.

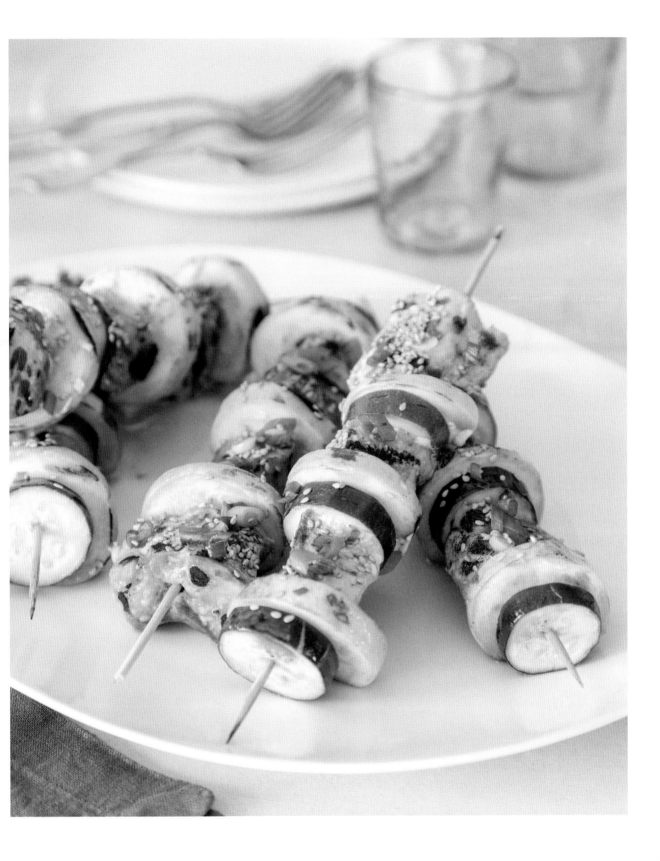

Stress-Free Sheet Pan Dinner

Take the stress (and mess!) out of midweek dinners with this one-pan meal that is roasted and served on a single baking sheet! This is one of my go-to dinners when I need to get some quick sustenance at the end of a long day. The Moroccan anti-inflammatory spices included in this dish are healing, while the chicken contains tryptophan, which can help you relax and settle in after a long day. Toss in some veggies for fiber and added nutrients. And one more bonus: you can store any remaining leftovers in the refrigerator and toss them into a salad or reheat them to get two meals for the price of one.

Makes 4 servings

Moroccan spiced chicken

1 tablespoon extra-virgin olive oil
¼ teaspoon paprika
¼ teaspoon ground cumin
¼ teaspoon ground coriander
¼ teaspoon ground turmeric
½ teaspoon sea salt
Pinch of cayenne pepper
1 pound boneless skinless   No
   chicken breasts

Vegetables

1 lemon, half thinly sliced
1 large sweet potato, peeled and cut into
   ½- to 1-inch cubes (about 2 cups)
1 zucchini, sliced into ¼-inch rounds
1½ cups cauliflower florets
1 cup cherry or grape tomatoes
1 tablespoon extra-virgin olive oil   No
½ teaspoon sea salt
¼ teaspoon freshly black ground pepper
1 garlic clove, finely chopped
¼ cup chopped fresh cilantro

1. Preheat the oven to 450°F.

2. Line a rimmed baking sheet with parchment paper.

3. Make the Moroccan spiced chicken: In a large bowl, whisk the oil, paprika, cumin, coriander, turmeric, salt, and cayenne. Add the chicken and stir to coat. Set aside.

4. Arrange the sliced lemon, sweet potato, zucchini, cauliflower, and tomatoes on a large parchment-lined sheet pan. (It may be necessary to use a second pan.) Drizzle with oil and season with the salt and pepper. Sprinkle the garlic over the vegetables.

5. Lay the chicken breasts among the vegetables in a single layer. Bake for 20 to 25 minutes, then stir and flip the chicken breasts over. Bake for 10 minutes more, until the vegetables and chicken are browned around the edges and the chicken reaches an internal temperature of 165°F. Sprinkle the cilantro and squeeze the other half lemon over the pan.

6. Serve warm on the baking sheet for easy cleanup!

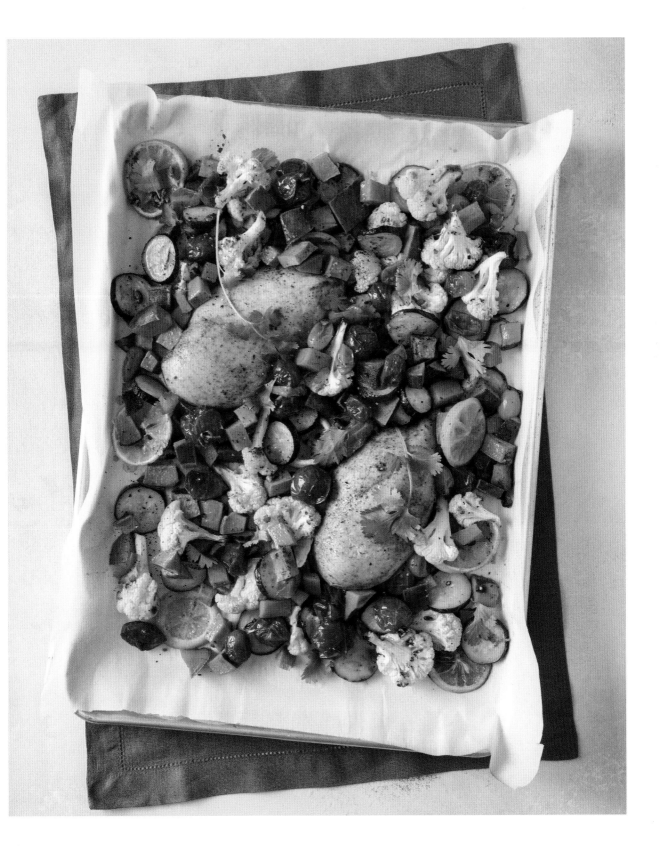

Turkey Meatballs N⌀

Try this modern version of the classic dish. Replace the beef with turkey to garner a hefty dose of vitamin B6, a necessary nutrient for maintenance of the nervous and immune systems, then whip up a batch of homemade marinara sauce and combine them on top of twirl-worthy zucchini noodles for an extra serving of veggies and fiber. Now that's what I call a healthy twist! If you're short on time, feel free to use store-bought marinara sauce in place of the homemade version in this recipe—just be sure it is low in added sugars.

Makes 4 servings

Turkey meatballs

1 pound ground turkey breast
1 egg, beaten
1 teaspoon dried oregano
½ teaspoon dried basil
1 tablespoon tomato paste
¼ cup chopped fresh parsley
¾ teaspoon sea salt
¼ cup flax meal (ground flaxseeds)
½ cup grated onion
1 garlic clove, minced

Tomato sauce

2 tablespoons olive oil
2 garlic cloves, minced

½ teaspoon crushed red pepper flakes
    (optional)
2 pounds tomatoes, quartered
    (fresh tomatoes or organic tomatoes in
    glass jars or BPA-free cans)
2 to 3 tablespoons tomato paste
    (or more for a thicker sauce)
½ teaspoon sea salt, or more to taste
1 tablespoon thinly sliced fresh basil, plus
    more for garnish if you'd like
Fresh flat-leaf parsley leaves (optional)

Zucchini pasta

4 large zucchini
Drizzle of extra-virgin olive oil

1. Make the turkey meatballs: Preheat the oven to 400°F. Line a baking sheet with parchment paper.

2. In a large bowl, combine the turkey, egg, oregano, basil, tomato paste, parsley, salt, and flax meal. Mix well by hand or with a wooden spoon. Add the onion and garlic and mix until well combined, but do not overmix.

3. Form 1½-inch balls and place them on the prepared baking sheet. Bake for 16 to 18 minutes, until the meatballs are browned on the outside and the center is no longer pink.

4. While the meatballs are cooking, make the tomato sauce: Heat the oil in a medium saucepan over medium heat. Add the garlic and the red pepper flakes, if using, and sauté for about 1 minute, until the garlic is browned around the edges. Add the tomatoes, tomato paste, and salt, cover the pan, lower the heat to a simmer, and cook for 18 to 20 minutes, until the sauce begins to thicken. Adjust the seasonings to taste. For a thinner sauce, puree half of the mixture with an immersion blender or regular blender. Pour the sauce back into the pan and add the basil and cooked meatballs to simmer for 3 to 4 minutes.

5. Make the zucchini pasta: Use a julienne peeler or knife to make long, thin zucchini slices. If you own a Spiralizer, that's the least labor-intensive way to make the noodles. While the meatballs are simmering, drizzle oil in a skillet and heat the noodles over medium-low heat for 2 to 3 minutes, until heated through.

6. Transfer the pasta to a bowl and top it with the meatballs and tomato sauce. Garnish with red pepper flakes and basil or parsley.

7. Store any remaining sauce in a tightly sealed container in the refrigerator for 5 days or in the freezer for up to 3 months.

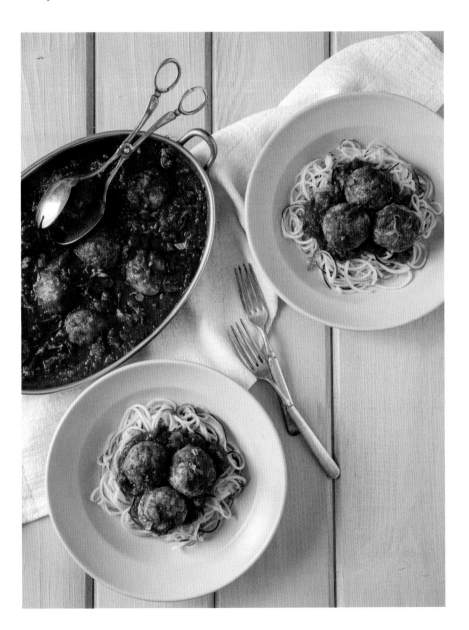

Colorful Curry and Shrimp Stew

This bright dish has it all: healing anti-inflammatory spices, grounding root vegetables, hearty greens, plant-based protein, and brain-boosting nutrients thanks to the shellfish. Just looking at the array of colors included on this plate is enough to make you smile even before you experience the warmth and satisfaction of eating this meal. Serve over quinoa flavored with a squeeze of lime for some added flavor and zest!

Makes 4 to 6 servings

1 tablespoon coconut or olive oil
1 small yellow onion, finely diced
1 to 2 tablespoons Thai red curry paste (according to taste, as some pastes are spicier than others)
1 tablespoon grated fresh ginger
1 to 2 garlic cloves, minced
1 tablespoon grated fresh turmeric root, or 1 teaspoon dried turmeric
2 teaspoons sea salt
Pinch of cayenne pepper
2 carrots, peeled and cut into ¼-inch rounds
2 celery stalks, cut into ¼-inch slices
2 cups cauliflower or broccoli florets
1 sweet potato, peeled and cut into ½-inch cubes

¼ cup chopped fresh cilantro, plus more for garnish if you'd like
One 14-ounce can full-fat unsweetened coconut milk
1 to 2 cups vegetable broth (as needed), store-bought or homemade
1 pound large shrimp, peeled, deveined, and tails removed
1 bunch of curly kale, stalks removed, leaves loosely sliced
Juice of 1 lime, plus more for garnish
Sea salt and freshly ground black pepper to taste
Crushed red pepper flakes

1. In a large Dutch oven or heavy-bottomed stockpot, heat the oil over medium-high heat, add the onion, and sauté until soft. Add the curry paste, ginger, garlic, turmeric, salt, and cayenne and cook for 1 minute. Add the carrots, celery, cauliflower, and sweet potato and cook for 5 minutes, until softened slightly. Add the cilantro, coconut milk, and just enough broth to cover the vegetables) and bring to a boil. Lower the heat to a simmer, cover, and cook for 20 to 25 minutes, until all the vegetables can be pierced with a fork.

2. Add the shrimp, cover the pot, and cook for 2 to 3 minutes, until the shrimp are pink and cooked through. Turn off the heat and add the kale, mixing with a spoon to distribute it evenly. Squeeze in the lime juice and season with salt, pepper, and red pepper flakes to taste.

3. Serve the curry hot and garnish with a squeeze of lime, some cilantro, and red pepper flakes.

Rise Bowl with Tahini Sauce

Rise up! The power of health is in your hands with this bowl. You can boost your energy, alleviate anxiety, regulate your mood, and heal from the inside out. Note that this recipe will need a bit of planning, as you will need to give the radishes between three and four hours to pickle before serving. If you are running short on time, kimchi, sauerkraut, or any other pickled vegetable you might have on hand can be used in place of the radishes.

Each ingredient in this signature bowl is carefully selected to nourish body and mind. The beneficial probiotics carried in fermented vegetables are a vital part of any gut-healing protocol. Squash is a rich source of vitamin A, which boosts immunity. Shiitake mushrooms are loaded with vitamin B_5 to support neurotransmitters, balance blood sugar, and protect against emotional stress and anxiety. Avocados feed your brain, and the tahini sauce pulls it all together with healthy fats to keep you happy and satisfied.

Makes 2 bowls

Pickled radishes

1 bunch of radishes, thinly sliced
1 garlic clove
1 heaping teaspoon black peppercorns
½ teaspoon crushed red pepper flakes
⅔ cup raw apple cider vinegar
2 tablespoons raw honey
1 teaspoon sea salt

Roasted butternut squash

1 small to medium butternut squash
1 tablespoon extra-virgin olive oil
Sea salt and freshly ground black pepper
  to taste

Tahini sauce

3 tablespoons tahini
2 tablespoons freshly squeezed lemon juice
1 garlic clove, minced
½ teaspoon grated fresh ginger
1 tablespoon apple cider vinegar
1 tablespoon pure maple syrup
2 tablespoons extra-virgin olive oil
½ teaspoon sea salt

Rise bowl

1 tablespoon extra-virgin olive oil
1 bunch of curly kale, stems removed,
  leaves thinly sliced
1 cup shiitake mushrooms
Sea salt and freshly ground black pepper
  to taste
1 to 2 cups cooked quinoa
½ cup dried wakame (available at most
  natural foods stores, Asian supermarkets,
  and online), soaked in water for 4 to
  5 minutes
½ to 1 avocado, pitted, peeled, and thinly
  sliced
¼ cup sliced almonds, toasted (see note on
  the next page)

1. Make the pickled radishes: Put the radishes in a pint-size heatproof glass jar and add the garlic, peppercorns, and red pepper flakes. Be sure there's enough room in the jar for the liquid.

2. In a small saucepan, combine the vinegar, honey, salt, and ⅔ cup water. Bring the liquid to a boil for 2 minutes, then remove from the heat. Stir until the honey is dissolved. When the liquid has slightly cooled, pour it into the jar over the radish mixture. Cover the jar and refrigerate for 3 to 4 hours, until you are ready to serve. The pickled radishes will keep in the refrigerator for up to 2 weeks.

3. Make the roasted butternut squash: Preheat the oven to 400°F. Line a baking sheet with parchment paper. Peel the squash, then halve it lengthwise. Using a spoon, scoop out and discard the seeds. Dice the squash into bite-size cubes (about 1 inch). Put the cubes in a large bowl and coat them evenly with the oil, salt, and pepper. Spread them in a single layer on the baking sheet. Roast, tossing the squash cubes occasionally, for about 30 minutes, or until just tender and golden brown around the edges.

4. Make the tahini sauce: In a medium bowl, combine the tahini, lemon juice, garlic, ginger, vinegar, maple syrup, oil, and salt. Whisk, adding 1 tablespoon water at a time until you have achieved a creamy consistency that can be drizzled over the bowl.

5. Make the rise bowl: Heat a medium or large sauté pan over medium-high heat and add the oil. Stir in the kale and mushrooms and sauté for 2 to 3 minutes, until the mushrooms begin to soften and the greens slightly wilt. Remove from the heat. Sprinkle the vegetables with sea salt and pepper to taste.

6. To assemble the bowls, divide the quinoa, kale-mushroom mixture, and butternut squash evenly between the bowls. Place the pickled radishes and wakame on top of the greens, then add the avocado and almonds. Drizzle the bowls with the tahini dressing. Season with salt and pepper to taste, serve warm, and enjoy!

Note: To toast the almonds, preheat the oven to 350°F. Place the almonds in a single layer on a baking sheet or toaster oven tray. Bake for 3 to 4 minutes, until the almonds are golden brown around the edges. Make sure to check the almonds every minute, as ovens vary and nuts can burn quickly.

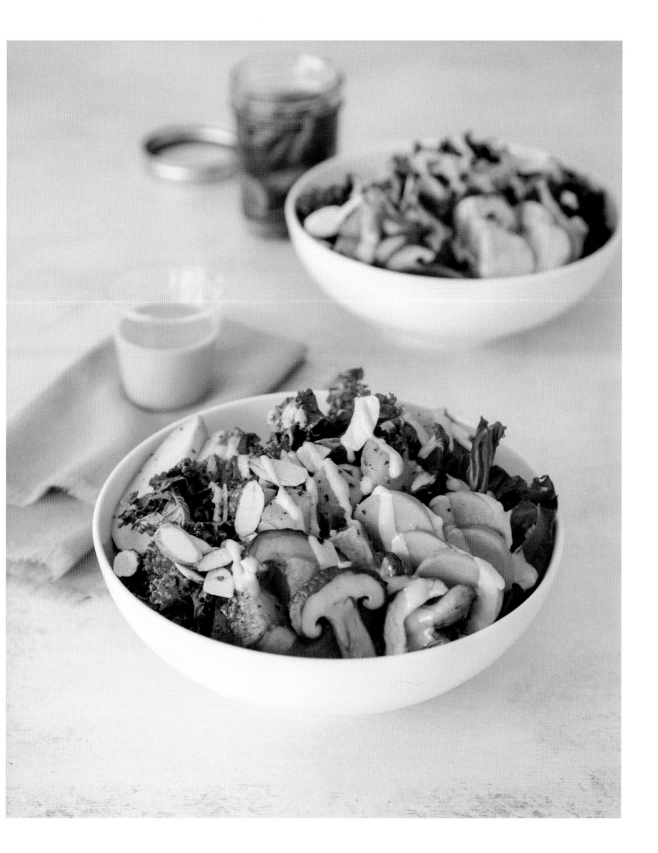

Chocolate Almond Nice Cream

This easy-to-make nice cream is dairy free and refined sugar free and uses potassium-rich bananas as the base. Add a dose of healthy fats from the almond butter, a serving of antioxidant-rich cacao, and a dose of gut-healing probiotics for a recipe that is mood-boosting and satisfies your sweet tooth, too!

Makes 2 bowls of nice cream

3 sliced and frozen bananas

1 to 2 tablespoons plant-based milk
 (as needed for blending)

2 tablespoons almond butter

2 tablespoons cacao powder or
 cocoa powder

1 tablespoon cacao nibs (optional)

½ teaspoon probiotic powder
 (or 2 capsules, opened)

1. Place the bananas in a food processor, adding just enough plant-based milk to blend. Process the mixture, which will maintain a chunky texture, then become creamy and smooth. If necessary, scrape down the sides of the processor midway through. When the mixture is smooth, add the almond butter and cacao powder. Process again until all the ingredients are well incorporated. If you'd like to add an extra kick of crunchy chocolate, pulse in the cacao nibs.

2. Pour the mixture into a bowl and stir in the probiotic powder (be sure to add the probiotics after you've processed the nice cream, since contact with the metal blade of the blender can weaken its effectiveness).

3. Grab some spoons and dig in! Nice cream is best when eaten immediately.

Lemon Coconut Bliss Balls

These tasty, sweet yet tangy treats are made for snacking! With healthy fats from the coconut and cashews plus a dose of plant-based protein, vitamin C–rich bliss balls will help keep your blood sugar stable and your sweet tooth satisfied. Make sure to prepare a batch at the beginning of the week to have a healthy snack or dessert available when that sweet tooth strikes!

Makes twenty 1-inch balls

1 cup cashews or almonds

1 cup pitted Medjool dates

½ cup unsweetened shredded coconut, plus more for coating the balls

½ teaspoon pure vanilla extract

3 tablespoons freshly squeezed lemon juice

Pinch of sea salt

2 teaspoons lemon zest

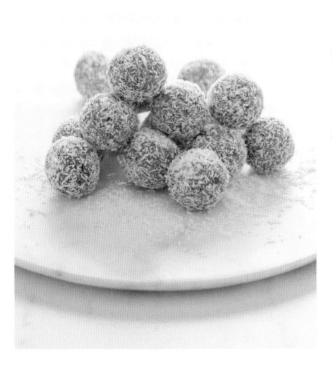

1. Put the nuts in a food processor and blend until they are finely chopped but not completely smooth. Add the dates, coconut, vanilla, lemon juice, and salt and process until the mixture is well combined. Add the lemon zest and pulse a few times, until all the ingredients are incorporated.

2. Using a small spoon, scoop out the mixture and use your hands to roll it into 1-inch balls. Roll each bliss ball in shredded coconut.

3. Refrigerate the bliss balls for at least 1 hour before serving. Store any remaining bliss balls in an airtight glass container in the freezer for up to 1 month.

Strawberries and Cream Chia Pudding

The tiny chia seed produces big benefits. Aside from being a nutritional powerhouse filled with an easily digestible form of protein that is a rich source of iron, magnesium, calcium, and phosphorus, chia seeds also contain essential omega-3 fatty acids. Whip up this easy and satisfying pudding and then take it to the next level by tossing in strawberries for an extra serving of immune-boosting nutrients. If strawberries aren't your jam or you feel like mixing it up, feel free to experiment with other fruits, such as peaches, raspberries, blackberries, or blueberries. If you like, go over the top by adding a swirl of Happy Belly Yogurt (page 270) for a dose of gut-healing TLC!

Makes 2 servings

1 cup unsweetened coconut milk
  (or other nut milk)
½ teaspoon pure vanilla extract
1½ tablespoons maple syrup
¾ cup strawberries, plus more sliced
  strawberries for garnish

Pinch of sea salt
½ teaspoon lemon zest (optional),
  plus more for garnish
¼ cup chia seeds
Unsweetened shredded coconut (optional),
  for garnish

1. Put the coconut milk, vanilla, maple syrup, strawberries, and salt in a blender and blend until smooth. Mix in the lemon zest, if using, and pulse until well combined. Put the chia seeds in a bowl or mason jar. Pour the blended mixture over the chia seeds and mix well. Stir every few minutes for about 10 minutes, then place the pudding in the refrigerator for at least 1 hour to set.

2. To serve, divide the pudding between two cups or bowls and top with sliced strawberries, shredded coconut, and more lemon zest, if using.

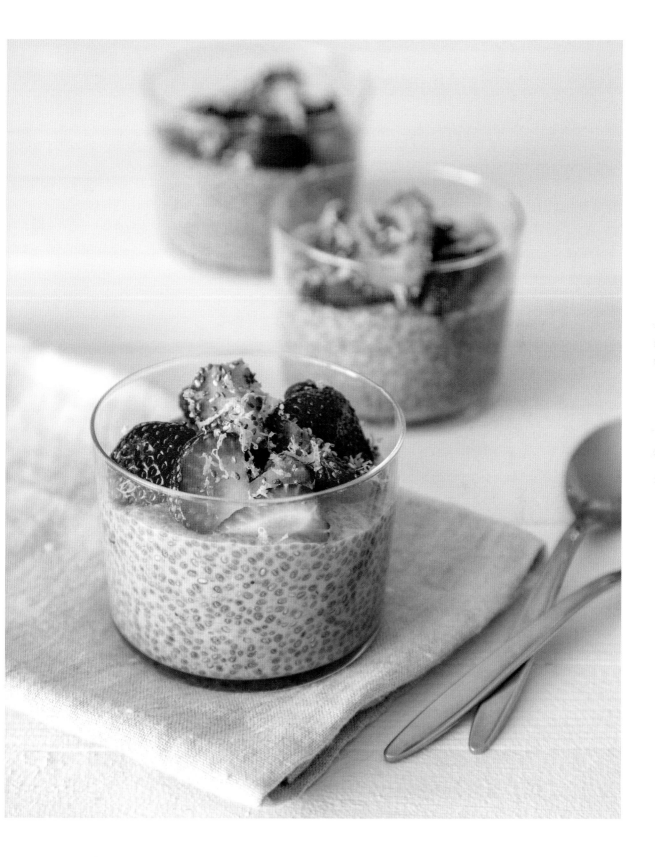

Mood-Boosting Chocolate Avocado Pudding

This rich and decadent chocolate pudding is not only quick and easy to make, but it's also loaded with mood- and brain-boosting ingredients to keep your mind and body happy. The avocado whips into such a creamy and satisfying dessert that nobody will even know it's hidden beneath the chocolate!

Makes 2 to 3 servings

2 large ripe avocados, pitted and peeled
3 tablespoons cacao powder or cocoa powder
¼ cup maple syrup
½ teaspoon pure vanilla extract
1 tablespoon almond butter
Pinch of sea salt
2 tablespoons coconut or almond milk

Optional toppings

Raspberries
Chocolate shavings
Shredded coconut

1. Combine the avocados, cacao powder, maple syrup, vanilla, almond butter, salt, and coconut milk in a blender and blend until smooth, scraping down the sides as necessary.

2. Divide the pudding between two or three bowls and top it with raspberries, chocolate shavings, shredded coconut, or any other nutritional boosts that sound tasty to you. Avocado pudding is best when eaten immediately.

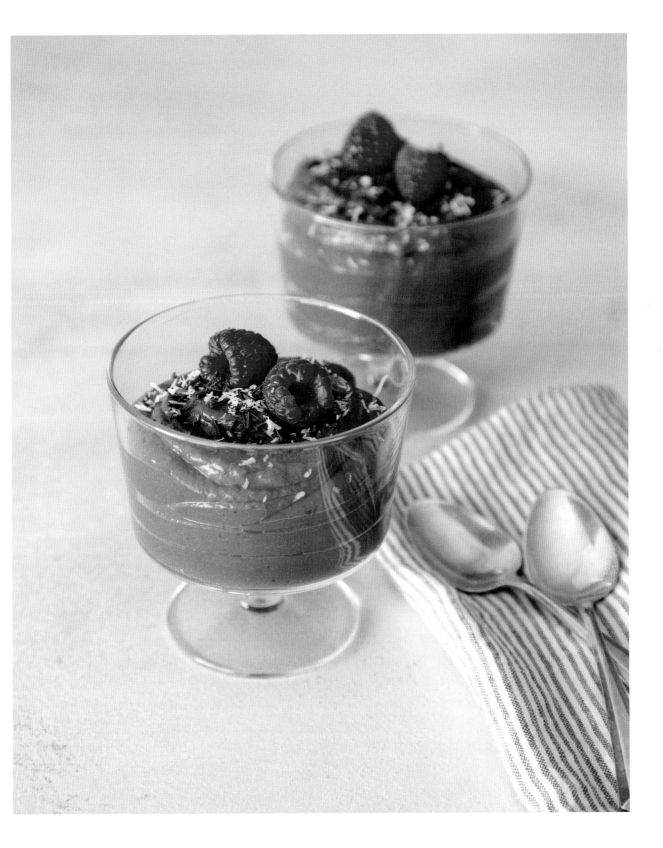

Sweet Potato Toasts with Toppings

These sweet potato treats are better than sliced bread! Satisfy that craving for toast by using sweet potatoes rather than processed grains as your base. Root veggies grow underneath the ground, where not only are they the anchor and foundation of a plant, but they also soak in enormous amounts of minerals. Serve this easy-to-make "toast" just as you would serve traditional toast and top it with your favorite brain- and mood-boosting toppings, such as avocado, a poached or fried egg, microgreens, tahini, fresh berries, hemp seeds, a nut butter, bananas, or strawberries for a nutrient-dense snack that can work as a breakfast, too!

Makes about 5 slices

1 large sweet potato, scrubbed
   (peel if desired, but it's not necessary)
Toppings of choice (I like almond butter and
   berries for a sweeter version or avocado
   and an egg for a savory twist)
Pinch of sea salt

1. Cut the sweet potato lengthwise into ¼-inch slices. Toast it in a toaster (you will probably need two cycles) or in a toaster oven for about 10 minutes, until the potato has cooked through and is golden brown around the edges. Add the toppings of your choice and sprinkle with a pinch of sea salt. Get creative!

2. Store any unused "toast" in an airtight container in the refrigerator for up to 3 days and reheat before serving.

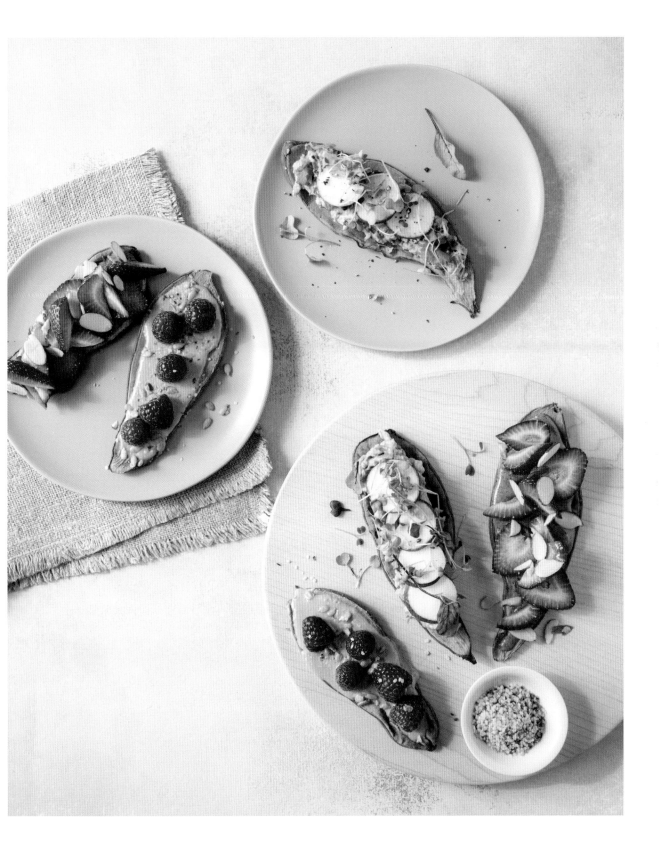

Superfood Trail Mix

Trail mix makes an easy on-the-go snack that helps stabilize mood and blood sugar in between meals. Nuts are a brain-boosting source of healthy fats, and the goji berries and cacao nibs are known as superfoods because they are nutrient powerhouses that pack large doses of antioxidants, polyphenols, vitamins, and minerals. Pack up a mason jar and store it in your desk, make individual serving packets to throw in your bag, or take this it along on your next travel adventure.

Makes six ½-cup servings

¾ cup walnuts
¾ cup pumpkin seeds
½ cup sunflower seeds
¼ cup Brazil nuts
2 tablespoons cacao nibs
¼ cup goji berries
½ cup coconut flakes

1. Combine and mix all the ingredients in a large bowl.

2. Store the trail mix in a glass jar or divide it into individual servings for an easy grab-and-go option.

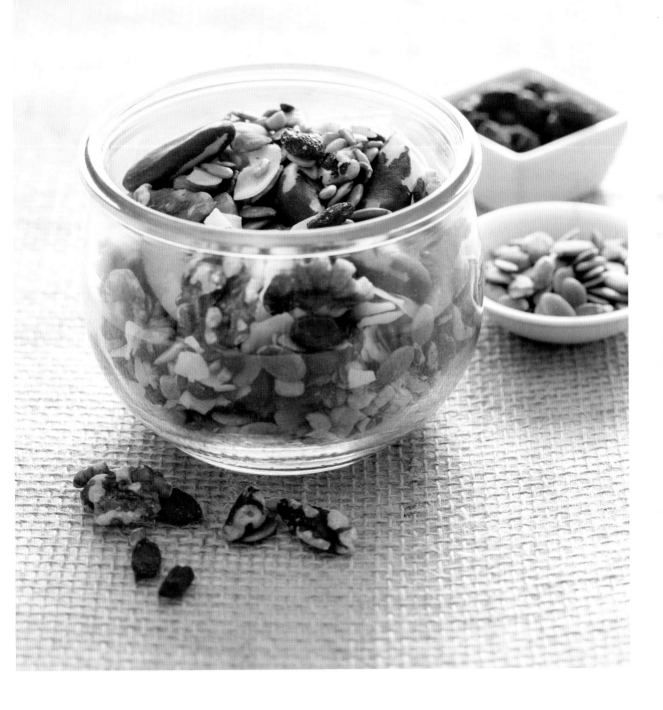

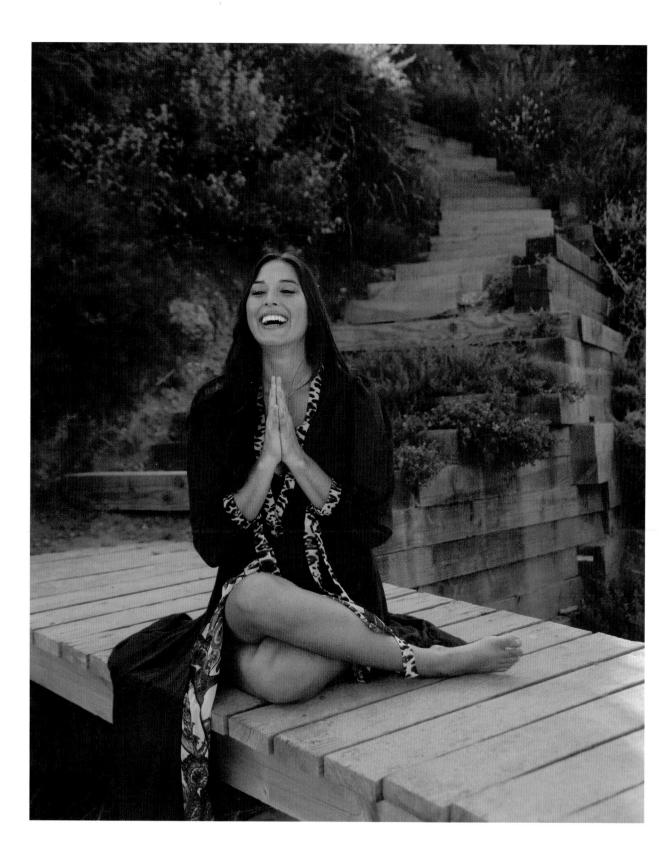

Acknowledgments

I never fully understood the meaning of "it takes a village" until I embarked on this journey of birthing a book. I must first thank my incredible literary agent, Coleen O'Shea, who is singlehandedly responsible for making this book happen. Your patience, support, guidance, and belief in me were unwavering. Thank you from the bottom of my heart for all that you are and all that you do.

To my wildly talented editor, Nikki Van Noy, "thank you" doesn't even begin to express the depth of my gratitude. It is no mistake that the universe brought us together. Thank you from the bottom of my heart for being my biggest champion and keeping me sane throughout this process. This book is as much yours as it is mine. I truly could not have done it without you. You have a friend in me for life.

Deepest gratitude to my wonderful editor at William Morrow, Cassie Jones, and the entire publishing family at HarperCollins. Working with such an all-star team has been a dream come true. Thank you for taking a chance on an unknown author and giving me a platform to share my voice, passion, and purpose.

Heartfelt thanks to Elise Museles, my rockstar recipe developer. You are a powerhouse! I am in awe of your energy and talent. You truly went above and beyond, and I am eternally grateful for your huge contribution to this book.

To my manager, Amy Stanton, and the entire team at Stanton & Co., especially Denege Prudhomme, Kara Froula, and Sadie Ruben, thank you for all the support throughout the years and for being my biggest advocates.

To my most cherished friend, Robert Sturman. I can think of no greater honor than having you step in front of the camera to grace the pages of this book with me. You have shown up for me during my darkest hours, held my heart in your hands, and restored my faith in humanity on more occasions than I can count.

To my soul sister Kate Berlin, I must have done something right in this lifetime to be able to walk this path with you by my side. Thank you for your courage to show up so authentically in life and for inspiring me to do the same.

To the fiercely resilient, wildly talented, and beautifully empowered women who lent their courageous voices and personal stories to this book, including Sheri Poe, Susan Alden, Jenny Burke Mathews, Tori Palatas, Kristin, and Nancy Shappell—thank you, thank you, thank you. Your words are the heart of this book. And to all those who supported me and championed this book through their gracious praise, testimonials, interviews, contributions, and moral support, including Rachel Brathen, Kimberly Snyder, Dr. Robin Berzin, Dezryelle Arcieri, Jennifer Pastiloff, Annalise Oberts—I bow deeply to you in love and gratitude.

To my stellar creative team, including my talented lifestyle and movement photographer, Collin Stark; hair and makeup artist Jessica Stark; food photographer Christina Peters; food stylist Nicole Kruzick; prop stylist Aneta Florczyk; and assistant Yuuki Yamagiwa—thank you for all your tireless help behind the scenes. Your support in bringing this book to life was invaluable. I am eternally grateful.

To Adam Brewer, thank you for your unconditional love. Your kindness is my compass. I couldn't have asked for a better partner or a more incredible father for our son. I love you.

To my dad, Ken Ordenstein, and sisters, Cherie Akina and Milika'a Vierra—thank you for loving me through all my learning curves. You helped shape me into the woman that I am today. I inherited my strength, courage, and resiliency from all of you. Mom used to always jokingly say that our family put the "fun" in *dysfunctional*, but there's no other family I would have chosen to be born into. To my mom, Anne Sage—I inherited my love of books from you. I wish you were still here on earth to see me bring my first book to life. Your words flowed through my fingers, and I hope I am making you proud. I love you to the moon and back.

And last, to all those who have experienced trauma—you are the bravest and strongest among us. May you always remember your light. This book is for you.

Resources

BOOKS

Brogan, Kelly. *A Mind of Your Own: The Truth About Depression and How Women Can Heal Their Bodies to Reclaim Their Lives.* New York: Harper Wave, 2016.

Campbell-McBride, Natasha. *Gut and Psychology Syndrome: Natural Treatment for Autism, Dyspraxia, A.D.D., Dyslexia, A.D.H.D, Depression, and Schizophrenia.* Cambridge, UK: Medinform Publishing, 2004.

Chapman, Alexander, Kim Gratz, and Matthew Tull. *The Dialectical Behavior Therapy Skills Workbook for Anxiety: Breaking Free from Worry, Panic, PTSD & Other Anxiety Symptoms.* Oakland, CA: New Harbinger, 2011.

Emerson, David, and Elizabeth Hopper. *Overcoming Trauma Through Yoga: Reclaiming Your Body.* Berkeley, CA: North Atlantic, 2011.

Herman, Judith. *Trauma and Recovery: The Aftermath of Violence—from Domestic Abuse to Political Terror.* New York: Basic Books, 1992.

Korn, Leslie. *Nutrition Essentials for Mental Health: A Complete Guide to the Food-Mood Connection.* New York: W. W. Norton, 2016.

Levine, Peter A. *Healing Trauma: A Pioneering Program for Restoring the Wisdom of Your Body.* Boulder, CO: Sounds True, 2008.

———. *In an Unspoken Voice: How the Body Releases Trauma and Restores Goodness.* Berkeley, CA: North Atlantic, 2010.

———. *Waking the Tiger: Healing Trauma.* Berkeley, CA: North Atlantic, 1997.

Maté, Gabor. *When the Body Says No: Understanding the Stress-Disease Connection.* New York: Random House, 2011.

Mayer, Emeran. *The Mind-Gut Connection: How the Hidden Conversation Within Our Bodies Impacts Our Mood, Our Choices, and Our Overall Health.* New York: Harper Wave, 2016.

Perlmutter, David. *Grain Brain: The Surprising Truth About Wheat, Carbs, and Sugar—Your Brain's Silent Killers.* New York: Little, Brown, 2013.

Ratey, John, with Eric Hagerman. *Spark: The Revolutionary New Science of Exercise and the Brain.* New York: Little, Brown, 2008.

Ross, Julia. *The Mood Cure: The 4-Step Program to Take Charge of Your Emotions—Today.* New York: Penguin, 2002.

Scott, Trudy. *The Antianxiety Food Solution: How the Foods You Eat Can Help You Calm Your Anxious Mind, Improve Your Mood & End Cravings.* Oakland, CA: New Harbinger, 2011.

Van der Kolk, Bessel. *The Body Keeps the Score: Brain, Mind, and Body in the Healing of Trauma.* New York: Viking, 2014.

Wolynn, Mark. *It Didn't Start with You: How Inherited Family Trauma Shapes Who We Are and How to End the Cycle.* New York: Viking, 2016.

NATIONAL HOTLINES

National Child Abuse Hotline
(800) 422-4453
www.childhelp.org/hotline

National Domestic Violence Hotline
(800) 799-7233 (SAFE) or (800) 787-3224
www.thehotline.org

National Parent Helpline
(855) 427-2736
www.nationalparenthelpline.org

National Suicide Prevention Lifeline
(800) 273-8255
www.suicidepreventionlifeline.org

National Teen Dating Abuse Helpline
(866) 331-9474
www.loveisrespect.org

Trevor Lifeline
(866) 488-7386

24/7 crisis support for LGBTQ youth
www.thetrevorproject.org

Rape, Abuse, and Incest National Hotline
(800) 656-4673 (HOPE)
www.rainn.org

Veterans Crisis Line
(800) 273-8255, press 1 or text to 838255
www.veteranscrisisline.net

YOGA AND MINDFULNESS PROGRAMS
Give Back Yoga Foundation
A national nonprofit organization offering yoga programs for underserved populations, including veterans, incarcerated men and women, cancer survivors, people with eating disorders, and those in recovery for drug and alcohol addictions.
900 Baseline Road 13B
Boulder, CO 80302
www.givebackyoga.org

Integrative Restoration Institute (iRest)
A nonprofit organization offering iRest yoga nidra programs in schools, yoga studios, community centers, hospitals, hospices, VA hospitals, military bases, and homeless shelters across the United States.
900 Fifth Avenue, Suite 204
San Rafael, CA 94901
(415) 456-3909
www.irest.us

Mindful Yoga Therapy
An organization that supports veterans and others with PTSD through mindful yoga practices.
122 Market Square
Newington, CT 06111
(860) 757-3200
www.mindfulyogatherapy.org

Purple Dot Yoga Project
A nonprofit organization supporting and empowering individuals impacted by domestic violence and trauma using yoga as a healing tool.
email: info@purpledotyogaproject.org
www.purpledotyogaproject.org

Warriors at Ease
A nonprofit organization supporting the health and resiliency of military communities across the globe through evidence-based yoga and meditation.
8400 Cedar Street
Silver Spring, MD 20910
(512) 516-5031
email: info@warriorsatease.org
www.warriorsatease.org

TRAUMA EDUCATION, RESEARCH, TREATMENT MODALITIES, AND GENERAL SUPPORT
EMDR Institute
National database to find EMDR (eye movement desensitization and reprocessing) clinicians.
www.emdr.com

National Center for PTSD
Government resource for research and education on trauma and PTSD.
www.ptsd.va.gov

National Center on Domestic Violence, Trauma & Mental Health
Provides training, support, and consultation to advocates, mental health and substance abuse providers, legal professionals, and policymakers.
www.nationalcenterdvtraumamh.org

National Child Traumatic Stress Network
Provides resources, education, and services for children and adolescents exposed to traumatic events.
www.nctsn.org

National Institute of Mental Health
Largest scientific organization in the world dedicated to research focused on the understanding, treatment, and prevention of mental disorders and the promotion of mental health.
www.nimh.nih.gov

Sensorimotor Psychotherapy Institute
Offers somatic psychotherapy education, practice, and research worldwide.
www.sensorimotorpsychotherapy.org

Somatic Experiencing
A body-oriented approach to healing trauma and other stress disorders, founded by Dr. Peter A. Levine.
www.traumahealing.com/somatic-experiencing

Tension & Trauma Releasing Exercises (TRE)
A body-based modality to release muscular patterns of stress, tension, and trauma, founded by Dr. David Berceli.
www.traumaprevention.com

The Trauma Center at Justice Resource Institute
A nonprofit organization founded by Dr. Bessel van der Kolk offering resources for special populations, various trauma treatment approaches, research, lectures, and courses.
www.traumacenter.org

Notes

INTRODUCTION

1. J. Douglas Bremner, "Traumatic Stress: Effects on the Brain," *Dialogues in Clinical Neuroscience* 8(4) (December 2006): 445–61, https://www.ncbi.nlm.nih.gov/pmc/articles/PMC3181836/.
2. Adverse Childhood Experiences Resources, ACE Study Infographic, https://www.cdc.gov/violenceprevention/acestudy/resources.html.
3. Bessel van der Kolk, *The Body Keeps the Score* (New York: Viking Penguin, 2014), 203–4.

A PROPER INTRODUCTION

1. Bessel van der Kolk et al., "Yoga as an Adjunctive Therapy for PTSD," *Journal of Clinical Psychiatry* 75(6) (June 2014): 559–65.
2. Madhav Goyal et al., "Meditation Programs for Psychological Stress and Well-Being," *JAMA Internal Medicine* 174(3) (2014): 357–68.
3. Emeran Mayer, *The Mind-Gut Connection* (New York: Harper Wave, 2016), 21.
4. Brené Brown, *I Thought It Was Just Me: Women Reclaiming Power and Courage in a Culture of Shame* (New York: Avery, 2007).

CHAPTER 1: TRAUMA IS MORE COMMON THAN YOU THINK

1. Van der Kolk, *The Body Keeps the Score*, 31.
2. Roger Saint-Laurent et al., "Somatic Experiencing: How Trauma Can Be Overcome," *Psychology Today*, March 26, 2015, https://www.psychologytoday.com/blog/the-intelligent-divorce/201503/somatic-experiencing.
3. U.S. Department of Veterans Affairs, "What Is PTSD?," https://www.ptsd.va.gov/public/PTSD-overview/basics/what-is-ptsd.asp.
4. National Center for Injury Prevention and Control of the Centers for Disease Control and Prevention, "National Intimate Partner and Sexual Violence Survey: 2010 Summary Report," https://www.cdc.gov/violenceprevention/pdf/nisvs_report2010-a.pdf.
5. U.S. Department of Veterans Affairs, "How Common Is PTSD?," https://www.ptsd.va.gov/public/ptsd-overview/basics/how-common-is-ptsd.asp.
6. Van der Kolk, *The Body Keeps the Score*, 21.

CHAPTER 2: HOW TRAUMA WORKS

1. Viktor E. Frankl, *Man's Search for Meaning* (Boston, MA: Beacon Press, 2006), 112.
2. Peter A. Levine, *Healing Trauma: A Pioneering Program for Restoring the Wisdom of Your Body* (Boulder, CO: Sounds True, 2008), 9.
3. About the CDC-Kaiser ACE Study: https://www.cdc.gov/violenceprevention/acestudy/about.html.

CHAPTER 3: THE TRAUMA CYCLE

1. Judith Herman, *Trauma and Recovery: The Aftermath of Violence—From Domestic Abuse to Political Terror* (New York: Basic Books, 2015), 7–8.
2. Christine Wolf Harlow, "Prior Abuse Reported by Inmates and Probationers," Bureau of Justice Statistics, April 1999, NCJ 172879.
3. E. Romano and R. V. De Luca, "Exploring the Relationship Between Childhood Sexual Abuse and Adult Sexual Perpetration," *Journal of Family Violence* 12(1) (March 1997): 85–98.
4. Harlow, "Prior Abuse Reported by Inmates and Probationers."
5. Christine Grella and Nena Messina, "Childhood Trauma and Women's Health Outcomes in a California Prison Population," *American Journal of Public Health* 96(10) (October 2006): 1842–48.
6. Brené Brown, *The Gifts of Imperfection: Let Go of Who You Think You're Supposed to Be and Embrace Who You Are* (Center City, MN: Hazelden, 2010).
7. Bessel van der Kolk, "The Compulsion to Repeat the Trauma: Re-enactment, Revictimization, and Masochism," *Psychiatric Clinics of North America* 12(2) (June 1989): 389–411.

CHAPTER 4: TRAUMA AND YOUR BRAIN

1. Jordan Grafman and Michael Koenigs, "Post-traumatic Stress Disorder: The Role of Medial Prefrontal Cortex and Amygdala," *Neuroscientist* 15(5) (October 2009): 540–48.
2. Peter A. Levine, *In an Unspoken Voice: How the Body Releases Trauma and Restores Goodness* (Berkeley, CA: North Atlantic Books, 2010), 58.

CHAPTER 5: CREATING A HEALING PATH

1. Centers for Disease Control and Prevention, "Mental Health and Mental Disorders (MHMD)," *Healthy People 2020*, ch. 28, https://www.cdc.gov/nchs/data/hpdata2020/HP2020MCR-C28-MHMD.pdf.

2. Carolyn Gregoire, "Why the Science Behind Anti-Depressants May Be Completely 'Backwards,'" *Huffington Post*, February 28, 2015, http://www.huffingtonpost.com/2015/02/28/how-anti-depressants-work_n_6707272.html.

3. Sharon Begley, "Why Antidepressants Are No Better Than Placebos," *Newsweek*, January 28, 2010, http://www.newsweek.com/why-antidepressants-are-no-better-placebos-71111.

4. Tracy Harrison, "Depression & Anxiety, Part 1," School of Applied Functional Medicine, Depression and Anxiety Solutions Clinical Course transcript, 2016, 4.

5. Ana Swanson, "Big Pharmaceutical Companies Are Spending Far More on Marketing Than Research," *Washington Post*, February 11, 2015, https://www.washingtonpost.com/news/wonk/wp/2015/02/11/big-pharmaceutical-companies-are-spending-far-more-on-marketing-than-research/?utm_term=.125a30221be3.

6. E. H. Turner et al., "Selective Publication of Antidepressant Trials and Its Influence on Apparent Efficacy," *New England Journal of Medicine* 358(3) (January 17, 2008): 252–60.

7. Jay Fournier et al., "Antidepressant Drug Effects and Depression Severity: A Patient-Level Meta-analysis," *Journal of the Medical Association* (2010) 303(1): 47–53, http://jamanetwork.com/journals/jama/article-abstract/185157.

8. Begley, "Why Antidepressants Are No Better Than Placebos."

9. Irving Kirsch, "Antidepressants and the Placebo Effect," *Zeitschrift für Psychologie* 222(3) (January 2014): 128–34, https://www.ncbi.nlm.nih.gov/pmc/articles/PMC4172306/.

10. Kelly Brogan, *A Mind of Your Own: The Truth About Depression and How Women Can Heal Their Bodies to Reclaim Their Lives* (New York: Harper Wave, 2016), 3.

11. Ibid., 63.

CHAPTER 6: MOVEMENT IS MEDICINE

1. Rodolfo R. Llinás, *I of the Vortex: From Neurons to Self* (Cambridge, MA: The MIT Press, 2002), 15–17, 35.

2. Gretchen Reynolds, "Which Type of Exercise Is Best for the Brain?," *New York Times*, February 17, 2016, https://well.blogs.nytimes.com/2016/02/17/which-type-of-exercise-is-best-for-the-brain/?mcubz=0.

3. Ibid.

4. Amanda Macmillan, "It's Official: Yoga Helps Depression," *Time*, March 8, 2017, http://time.com/4695558/yoga-breathing-depression/.

5. Charles Engel et al., "Yoga Nidra as an Adjunctive Therapy for Post-Traumatic Stress Disorder: A Feasibility Study," Samueli Institute (2007) http://www.irest.us/sites/default/files/WRAMH_PTSD_YN_Results_0.pdf.; Neal Pollack, "Warriors at Peace," *Yoga Journal*, 230 (August 2010): 74–77; van der Kolk, "Clinical Implications of Neuroscience Research in PTSD," *Annals of New York Academy of Sciences* 1071 (July 26, 2006): 277–293; Denise Kersten Wills, "Healing Life's Traumas with Yoga," *Yoga Journal* 203 (October 23, 2007): 41–44.

6. Van der Kolk, "Clinical Implications of Neuroscience Research in PTSD."

7. D. D. Blake et al., "The Development of a Clinician-Administered PTSD Scale," *Journal of Traumatic Stress* 8 (1) (January 1995): 75–90; van der Kolk, "Clinical Implications of Neuroscience Research in PTSD."

8. Charles Engel et al., "Yoga Nidra as an Adjunctive Therapy for Post-Traumatic Stress Disorder: A Feasibility Study."

CHAPTER 7: THE HEALING POWER OF BREATH

1. David Coulter, *Anatomy of Hatha Yoga: A Manual for Teachers, Students, and Practitioners* (Body & Breath, 2001), 105.

2. Bangalore G. Kalyani et al., "Neurohemodynamic Correlates of 'Om' Chanting: A Pilot Functional Magnetic Resonance Imaging Study," *International Journal of Yoga* 4(1) (2011): 3–6, http://www.ijoy.org.in/article.asp?issn=0973–6131;year=2011;volume=4;issue=1;spage=3;epage=6;aulast=Kalyani.

CHAPTER 9: MOVEMENT SEQUENCES FOR PHYSICAL AND EMOTIONAL HEALING

1. John Ratey, with Eric Hagerman, *Spark: The Revolutionary New Science of Exercise and the Brain* (New York: Little, Brown, 2008), 140.

2. "Facts & Statistics," Anxiety and Depression Association of America, https://adaa.org/about-adaa/press-room/facts-statistics.

3. Jeff Green, "#MeToo Snares More Than 400 High-Profile People," Bloomberg, June 25, 2018, https://www.bloomberg.com/news/articles/2018-06-25/metoo-snares-more-than-400-high-profile-people-as-firings-rise

4. American Psychological Association, "Social Isolation, Loneliness Could Be Greater Threat to Public Health than Obesity," *Science Daily*, August 5, 2017, https://www.sciencedaily.com/releases/2017/08/170805165319.htm.

5. Michelle Janelsins et al., "Yoga for the Treatment of Insomnia Among Cancer Patients: Evidence, Mechanisms of Action, and Clinical Recommendations," *Oncology and Hematology Review* 10(2) (2014): 164–68, https://www.ncbi.nlm.nih.gov/pmc/articles/PMC4386006/.

6. Michael J. Breus, "Yoga Can Help with Insomnia," *Psychology Today*, October 4, 2012, https://www.psychologytoday.com/blog/sleep-newzzz/201210/yoga-can-help-insomnia.

7. Thomas Beggs and Susan Holtzman, "Yoga for Chronic Low Back Pain: A Meta-analysis of Randomized Controlled Trials," *Pain Research and Management* 18(5) (September–October 2013): 18(5): 267–72, https://www.ncbi.nlm.nih.gov/pmc/articles/PMC3805350/.

8. Christopher Bergland, "How Does Yoga Relieve Chronic Pain? Yoga Has the Opposite Effect on Your Brain as Chronic Pain," *Psychology Today*, May 27, 2015, https://www.psychologytoday.com/blog/the-athletes-way/201505/how-does-yoga-relieve-chronic-pain.

9. C. Villemure et al., "Insular Cortex Mediates Increased Pain Tolerance in Yoga Practitioners," *Cerebral Cortex*, May 21, 2013, https://www.ncbi.nlm.nih.gov/pubmed/23696275.

10. T. Alraek et al., "Traditional Chinese Medicine for Chronic Fatigue Syndrome: A Systematic Review of Randomized Clinical Trials," *Complementary Therapies in Medicine* 22(4) (2014): 826–33, https://www.ncbi.nlm.nih.gov/books/NBK292885/.

11. Don Rauf, "High-Intensity Exercise May Be Bad for the Bowels," *Chicago Tribune*, June 23, 2017, http://www.chicagotribune.com/lifestyles/health/sc-high-intensity-exercise-bowels-health-0628–20170623-story.html.

CHAPTER 10: WIRED TO WANDER

1. National Institutes of Health, "Fact Sheet—Pain Management," https://report.nih.gov/nihfactsheets/ViewFactSheet.aspx?csid=57

2. Nancy Shappell, *A Voice in the Tide: How I Spoke My Truth in the Undertow of Denial and Self-Blame* (Amazon Digital Services LLC, 2015).

3. Fadel Zeidan et al., "Brain Mechanisms Supporting the Modulation of Pain by Mindfulness Meditation," *Journal of Neuroscience* 31(14) (April 2011): 5540–48.

4. Amanda Macmillan, "Yoga and Meditation Can Change Your Genes, Study Says," *Time*, June 16, 2017, http://time.com/4822302/yoga-meditation-genes-stress/.

5. Jancee Dunn, "Save Yourself from Stress," *Time*, August 25, 2017, 19.

6. Gabor Maté, *When the Body Says No: Exploring the Stress-Disease Connection* (New York: Wiley, 2003), 3.

7. Van der Kolk, *The Body Keeps the Score*, 212.

8. Qing Li, "Effect of Forest Bathing Trips on Human Immune Function," *Environmental Health and Preventative Medicine* 15(1) (2010): 9–17, https://www.ncbi.nlm.nih.gov/pmc/articles/.PMC2793341/.

9. Lisa Quast, "Want to Be More Productive? Stop Multitasking," *Forbes*, February 6, 2017.

10. Mary Elizabeth Williams, "Why Every Mind Needs Mindfulness," *Time*, August 25, 2017.

11. Klaus Manhart, "The Limits of Multitasking," *Scientific American Mind* 14(5) (December 2004–January 2005): 62–67.

12. Deloitte, "Global mobile consumer survey: US edition", https://www2.deloitte.com/us/en/pages/technology-media-and-telecommunications/articles/global-mobile-consumer-survey-us-edition.html.

13. Patti Neighmon, "For the Children's Sake, Put Down That Smartphone," *Morning Edition*, April 21, 2014, https://www.npr.org/sections/health-shots/2014/04/21/30/4196338/for-the-childrens-sake-put-down-that-smartphone.

CHAPTER 12: MEDITATIONS AND MINDFULNESS PRACTICES FOR HEALING

1. Brown, *The Gifts of Imperfection*.

2. Pamela Pence, Lori Katz, Cristi Huffman, and Geta Cojucar, "Delivering Integrative Restoration-Yoga Nidra Meditation (iRest®) to Women with Sexual Trauma at a Veteran's Medical Center: A Pilot Study," *International Journal of Yoga Therapy* 24(1) (2014): 53-62.

3. Danny Penman, "Can Mindfulness Meditation Really Reduce Pain and Suffering?," *Psychology Today*, January 9, 2015.

CHAPTER 13: ALL HEALTH BEGINS IN THE GUT

1. Mayer, *The Mind-Gut Connection*, 10–11.

2. Ibid., 44.

3. Ibid., 130–31.

4. Ibid., 45–46.

5. Jennifer S. Labus et al., "Differences in Gut Microbial Composition Correlate with Regional Brain Volumes in Irritable Bowel Syndrome," *Microbiome*, May 1, 2017, https://microbiomejournal.biomedcentral.com/articles/10.1186/s40168–017–0260-z.

6. Christopher Bergland, "Is Gut Microbiome a New Biomarker for PTSD Susceptibility?," *Psychology Today*, October 27, 2017, https://www.psychologytoday.com/blog/the-athletes-way/201710/is-gut-microbiome-new-biomarker-ptsd-susceptibility.

7. Stellenbosch University. "Role of Gut Microbiome in Posttraumatic Stress Disorder: More Than a Gut Feeling." *ScienceDaily*, October 25, 2017, https://www.sciencedaily.com/releases/2017/10/171025103140.htm.

8. Natasha Campbell-McBride, *Gut and Psychology Syndrome: Natural Treatment for Autism, A.D.H.D., Dyslexia, Dyspraxia, Depression, and Schizophrenia* (Cambridge, UK: Medinform Publishing, 2004), 35.

9. Christiane Bode and J. Christian, "Alcohol's Role in Gastronintestinal Tract Disorders," *Alcohol Health and Research World* 21(1) (1997): 76–83, https://pubs.niaaa.nih.gov/publications/arh21–1/76.pdf.

CHAPTER 14: FOOD HEROES AND ZEROS

1. Matt Payton, "Sugar Addiction 'Should Be Treated as a Form of Drug Abuse,'" *The Independent*, April 12, 2016, http://www.independent.co.uk/news/science/sugar-has-similar-effect-on-brain-as-cocaine-a6980336.html.

2. Brogan, *A Mind of Your Own*, 107.

3. Andrew Weil, "An Allergy Impasse?," March 15, 2007, https://www.drweil.com/health-wellness/body-mind-spirit/allergy-asthma/an-allergy-impasse/.

4. Brogan, *A Mind of Your Own*, 90–91.

5. David Perlmutter, *Grain Brain: The Surprising Truth About Wheat, Carbs, and Sugar—Your Brain's Silent Killers* (New York: Little, Brown, 2013), 49.

6. Ibid., 53.

7. Brogan, *A Mind of Your Own*, 90.

8. Trudy Scott, *The Antianxiety Food Solution: How the Foods You Eat Can Help You Calm Your Anxious Mind, Improve Your Mood & End Cravings* (Oakland, CA: New Harbinger, 2011), 74.

9. D. R. Lara, "Caffeine, Mental Health, and Psychiatric Disorders," *Journal of Alzheimer's Disease* 20 (Suppl. 1) (2010): S239–48.

10. G. L. Clementz and J. W. Dailey, "Psychotropic Effects of Caffeine," *American Family Physician* 37(5) (1988): 167–72, quoted in Trudy Scott, *The Antianxiety Food Solution: How the Foods You Eat Can Help You Calm Your Anxious Mind, Improve Your Mood & End Cravings* (Oakland, CA: New Harbinger Publications, 2011),

11. J. E. Pizzorno and M. T. Murray, *Textbook of Natural Medicine* (London: Harcourt, 2000).

12. D. S. Charney, G. R. Heninger, and P. I. Jatlow, "Increased Anxiogenic Effects of Caffeine in Panic Disorders," *Archives of General Psychiatry* 42(3) (1985): 233–43.

13. Scott, *The Antianxiety Food Solution*, 60.

14. Mark Hyman, "Ten Reasons to Quit Your Coffee!" June 13, 2012, http://drhyman.com/blog/2012/06/13/ten-reasons-to-quit-your-coffee/.

15. Pizzorno and Murray, *Textbook of Natural Medicine*.

16. A. A. Badaway, "Alcohol and Violence and the Possible Role of Serotonin," *Criminal Behaviour and Mental Health* 12(1) (2003): 31–44.

17. Scott, *The Antianxiety Food Solution*, 63–64.

18. Scott, *The Antianxiety Food Solution*, 65.

19. Perlmutter, *Grain Brain*, 72.

20. Perlmutter, *Grain Brain*, 90.

21. V. Pitozzi et al., "Effects of Dietary Extra-Virgin Olive Oil on Behavior and Brain Biochemical Parameters in Ageing Rats," *British Journal of Nutrition* 103(11) (2010): 1674–83.

22. Pizzorno and Murray, *Textbook of Natural Medicine*.

23. P. M. Kris-Etherton et al., "Polyunsaturated Fatty Acids in the Food Chain in the United States," *American Journal of Clinical Nutrition* 71(1) (January 2000): S179–88.

24. The Center for Genetics, Nutrition, and Health, "The Importance of the Ratio of Omega-6/Omega-3 Essential Fatty Acids," *Bloomed Pharmacother* 56(8) (October 2002): 365–79, https://www.ncbi.nlm.nih.gov/pubmed/12442909.

25. Perlmutter, *Grain Brain*, 187.

26. Ibid., 186.

27. Leslie Korn, *Nutrition Essentials for Mental Health: A Complete Guide to the Food-Mood Connection* (New York: W. W. Norton, 2016), 187.

28. Andrew Weil, "Top 3 Reasons to Use Turmeric" https://www.drweil.com/diet-nutrition/nutrition/3-reasons-to-eat-turmeric/.

29. Shahin Akhondzadeh et al., "Comparison of Crocus sativus L. and Imipramine in the Treatment of Mild to Moderate Depression: A Pilot Double-Blind Randomized Trial," *BMC Complementary and Alternative Medicine* 4 (September 2, 2004):12, https://bmccomplementalternmed.biomedcentral.com/articles/10.1186/1472–6882–4–12.

30. M Mazidi et al., "A Double-Blind, Randomized and Placebo-Controlled Trial of Saffron (Crocus sativus L.) in the Treatment of Anxiety and Depression," *Journal of Complementary and Integrative Medicine* 13(2) (June 1, 2016): 195–99, https://www.ncbi.nlm.nih.gov/pubmed/27101556.

31. Korn, *Nutrition Essentials for Mental Health*, 51.

32. D. J. Armstrong et al., "Vitamin D Deficiency Is Associated with Anxiety and Depression in Fibromyalgia," *Clinical Rheumatology* 26(4) (April 2007): 551–54, https://www.ncbi.nlm.nih.gov/pubmed/16850115.

Index

NOTE: Page references in *italics* refer to photos of recipes.

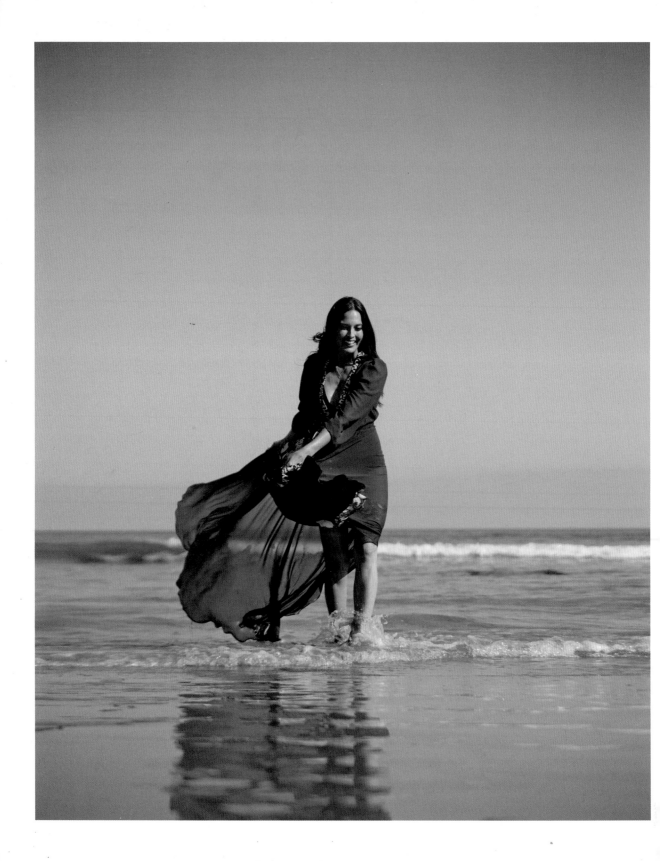